Impact of Bioactive Peptides on Human Health

Impact of Bioactive Peptides on Human Health

Special Issue Editor

Kaustav Majumder

MDPI • Basel • Beijing • Wuhan • Barcelona • Belgrade

Special Issue Editor
Kaustav Majumder
University of Nebraska-Lincoln
USA

Editorial Office
MDPI
St. Alban-Anlage 66
4052 Basel, Switzerland

This is a reprint of articles from the Special Issue published online in the open access journal *Nutrients* (ISSN 2072-6643) in 2018 (available at: https://www.mdpi.com/journal/nutrients/special_issues/Peptides_Health)

For citation purposes, cite each article independently as indicated on the article page online and as indicated below:

LastName, A.A.; LastName, B.B.; LastName, C.C. Article Title. *Journal Name* **Year**, *Article Number*, Page Range.

ISBN 978-3-03897-620-2 (Pbk)
ISBN 978-3-03897-621-9 (PDF)

Contents

About the Special Issue Editor . . . . **vii**

Preface to "Impact of Bioactive Peptides on Human Health" . . . . **ix**

Lilia M. Beltrán-Barrientos, Adrián Hernández-Mendoza, Aarón F. González-Córdova, Humberto Astiazarán-García, Julián Esparza-Romero and Belinda Vallejo-Córdoba
Mechanistic Pathways Underlying the Antihypertensive Effect of Fermented Milk with *Lactococcus lactis* NRRL B-50571 in Spontaneously Hypertensive Rats
Reprinted from: *Nutrients* **2018**, *10*, 262, doi:10.3390/nu10030262 . . . . **1**

Qingyu Ma, Qiuming Liu, Ling Yuan and Yongliang Zhuang
Protective Effects of LSGYGP from Fish Skin Gelatin Hydrolysates on UVB-Induced MEFs by Regulation of Oxidative Stress and Matrix Metalloproteinase Activity
Reprinted from: *Nutrients* **2018**, *10*, 420, doi:10.3390/nu10040420 . . . . **16**

Paulina Keska and Joanna Stadnik
Stability of Antiradical Activity of Protein Extracts and Hydrolysates from Dry-Cured Pork Loins with Probiotic Strains of LAB
Reprinted from: *Nutrients* **2018**, *10*, 521, doi:10.3390/nu10040521 . . . . **28**

Stepheny C. de Campos Zani, Jianping Wu and Catherine B. Chan
Egg and Soy-Derived Peptides and Hydrolysates: A Review of Their Physiological Actions against Diabetes and Obesity
Reprinted from: *Nutrients* **2018**, *10*, 549, doi:10.3390/nu10050549 . . . . **43**

Oscar Guzmán-Gómez, Rosa Virginia García-Rodríguez, Lucía Quevedo-Corona, Ricardo Pérez-Pastén-Borja, Nora Lilia Rivero-Ramírez, Emmanuel Ríos-Castro, Salud Pérez-Gutiérrez, Julia Pérez-Ramos and Germán Alberto Chamorro-Cevallos
Amelioration of Ethanol-Induced Gastric Ulcers in Rats Pretreated with Phycobiliproteins of *Arthrospira (Spirulina) Maxima*
Reprinted from: *Nutrients* **2018**, *10*, 763, doi:10.3390/nu10060763 . . . . **58**

MartaŻebrowska-Gamdzyk, Mateusz Maciejczyk, Anna Zalewska, Katarzyna Guzińska-Ustymowicz, Anna Tokajuk and Halina Car
Whey Protein Concentrate WPC-80 Intensifies Glycoconjugate Catabolism and Induces Oxidative Stress in the Liver of Rats
Reprinted from: *Nutrients* **2018**, *10*, 1178, doi:10.3390/nu10091178 . . . . **73**

Leticia Mora, Marta Gallego and Fidel Toldrá
ACEI-Inhibitory Peptides Naturally Generated in Meat and Meat Products and Their Health Relevance
Reprinted from: *Nutrients* **2018**, *10*, 1259, doi:10.3390/nu10091259 . . . . **91**

Anna Mas-Capdevila, Zara Pons, Amaya Aleixandre, Francisca I. Bravo and Begoña Muguerza
Dose-Related Antihypertensive Properties and the Corresponding Mechanisms of a Chicken Foot Hydrolysate in Hypertensive Rats
Reprinted from: *Nutrients* **2018**, *10*, 1295, doi:10.3390/nu10091295 . . . . **103**

Emily Mason, Lamia L'Hocine, Allaoua Achouri and Salwa Karboune
Hairless Canaryseed: A Novel Cereal with Health Promoting Potential
Reprinted from: *Nutrients* **2018**, *10*, 1327, doi:10.3390/nu10091327 . . . . **115**

Yasutaka Shigemura, Yu Iwasaki, Mana Tateno, Asahi Suzuki, Mihoko Kurokawa, Yoshio Sato and Kenji Sato
A Pilot Study for the Detection of Cyclic Prolyl-Hydroxyproline (Pro-Hyp) in Human Blood after Ingestion of Collagen Hydrolysate
Reprinted from: *Nutrients* **2018**, *10*, 1356, doi:10.3390/nu10101356 . . . . **131**

Yu-Hsin Lin, Guan-Wen Chen, Chin Hsi Yeh, Helena Song and Jenn-Shou Tsai
Purification and Identification of Angiotensin I-Converting Enzyme Inhibitory Peptides and the Antihypertensive Effect of *Chlorella sorokiniana* Protein Hydrolysates
Reprinted from: *Nutrients* **2018**, *10*, 1397, doi:10.3390/nu10101397 . . . . **143**

Kazumi Ninomiya, Shigenobu Ina, Aya Hamada, Yusuke Yamaguchi, Makoto Akao, Fumie Shinmachi, Hitoshi Kumagai and Hitomi Kumagai
Suppressive Effect of the α-Amylase Inhibitor Albumin from Buckwheat (*Fagopyrum esculentum* Moench) on Postprandial Hyperglycaemia
Reprinted from: *Nutrients* **2018**, *10*, 1503, doi:10.3390/nu10101503 . . . . **157**

Subhadeep Chakrabarti, Snigdha Guha and Kaustav Majumder
Food-Derived Bioactive Peptides in Human Health: Challenges and Opportunities
Reprinted from: *Nutrients* **2018**, *10*, 1738, doi:10.3390/nu10111738 . . . . **169**

Maria João Pena, Alex Pinto, Anne Daly, Anita MacDonald, Luís Azevedo, Júlio César Rocha and Nuno Borges
The Use of Glycomacropeptide in Patients with Phenylketonuria: A Systematic Review and Meta-Analysis
Reprinted from: *Nutrients* **2018**, *10*, 1794, doi:10.3390/nu10111794 . . . . **186**

About the Special Issue Editor

Kaustav Majumder is an Assistant Professor at the Department of Food Science, University of Nebraska, Lincoln, USA. He has a Bachelor's degree in biotechnology from the West Bengal University of Technology, in India and holds an MSc and Ph.D. in Food Science and Technology from the University of Alberta, Canada with a research focus on bioactive food proteins and peptides. After completing his degrees, he was a postdoctoral fellow at the University of Guelph, Canada in the Department of Food Science. His research program at the University of Nebraska explores the beneficial health effects of food-derived bioactive proteins and peptides and evaluates their therapeutic potential for the treatment, prevention, and management of hypertension, type-2 diabetes, and associated metabolic disorders. His research delineates the molecular mechanisms of food-derived bioactive compounds to reduce the pathogenesis of hypertension and related metabolic disorders.

Preface to "Impact of Bioactive Peptides on Human Health"

Research from the last two decades has shown that dietary bioactive peptides can exhibit various biological activities that are beneficial to health, above and beyond their known nutritional value. These small fragments of peptides, generally 2–20 amino-acids long, can be produced either naturally (plant seed development, muscle ripening), through food processing (microbial fermentation and enzymatic hydrolysis), or during gastrointestinal digestion. Dietary bioactive peptides have vast potential for application as nutraceutical and functional foods (NFFs) for the treatment of chronic diseases. Over the past two decades, several bioactive peptides from different food components have been identified as having various beneficial effects against chronic disease conditions, such as hypertension and type-2 diabetes. So far, the majority of the studies have identified peptides with anti-microbial activity, antioxidant activity, anti-hypertensive activity, and anti-inflammatory activity. Peptides from both animal (egg, milk, fish, meat) and plant (soybean, pea, bean) protein sources have been explored and have shown different biological activities. Additionally, peptides with biological activities have also been identified from different protein-rich agricultural by-products.

Although the research on bioactive peptides has been gaining momentum, the translation of findings into commercial or practical use has been delayed. The most prominent reasons for this delay are as follows:

1) Isolated bioactive peptides are often studied in in-vitro chemical and cellular assays. The biological activities found are then directly applied in in-vivo studies without considering the absorption, distribution, metabolism, and excretion (ADME) properties of the peptides. As a result, these peptides fail to exhibit similar efficacy in the in-vivo studies.

2) The measurement of the bioaccessibility and bioavailability of bioactive peptides in the human blood can be challenging, as some bioactive peptides have a very short half-life and thus, their plasma concentration can be low. The gastrointestinal stability and absorption of bioactive peptide sequences are not yet clearly understood. Therefore, preliminary studies on pharmacokinetics are required before human interventional studies can be conducted.

3) The molecular mechanisms of action of many bioactive peptides are still unknown as they participate in complex metabolic pathways in the human body. This area of research is particularly important to elucidate the specific pathways involved so that targeted specific activity can be developed.

4) Although a large number of in-vitro chemical and cellular studies and in-vivo animal studies have been conducted, there is a considerable gap of knowledge in regard to clinical studies and human trials.

The current manuscript collection, a total of 14 articles, presents a compilation of recent advances and research developments, providing new insights into food-derived bioactive peptide research. Along with information about diverse bioactivities in the prevention of various metabolic diseases, the manuscripts have valuable information about their modes of action, bioavailability, and other associated challenges that could be helpful for future research development.

Kaustav Majumder
Special Issue Editor

nutrients MDPI

Article

Mechanistic Pathways Underlying the Antihypertensive Effect of Fermented Milk with *Lactococcus lactis* NRRL B-50571 in Spontaneously Hypertensive Rats

Lilia M. Beltrán-Barrientos, Adrián Hernández-Mendoza, Aarón F. González-Córdova, Humberto Astiazarán-García, Julián Esparza-Romero and Belinda Vallejo-Córdoba *

Centro de Investigación en Alimentación y Desarrollo, A.C. (CIAD), Carretera a La Victoria Km. 0.6, Apartado 1735, Hermosillo, Sonora 83304, Mexico; lilia.beltranb@gmail.com (L.M.B.-B.); ahernandez@ciad.mx (A.H.-M.); aaronglz@ciad.mx (A.F.G.-C.); hastiazaran@ciad.mx (H.A.-G.); julian@ciad.mx (J.E.-R.)

* Correspondence: vallejo@ciad.mx; Tel.: +52-662-289-2400

Received: 27 January 2018; Accepted: 23 February 2018; Published: 26 February 2018

Abstract: It has been reported that fermented milk (FM) with *Lactococcus lactis* NRRL B-50571 had an antihypertensive effect in spontaneously hypertensive rats (SHR) and prehypertensive subjects. Therefore, the objective of the present study was to evaluate the possible mechanisms involved (angiotensin converting enzyme inhibition (ACEI), enhancement of nitric oxide production, antioxidant activity and opioid effect), in the antihypertensive effect of FM with SHR. First, twenty one SHR were randomized into three groups to either receive in a single-oral dose of purified water (negative control), FM, or naloxone (opioid receptor antagonist) + FM. In a parallel study, twenty seven SHR were randomized into three groups to either receive ad libitum purified water (negative control), Captopril or FM. After six weeks of treatment ACEI activity, enhancement of nitric oxide production, and antioxidant activity were evaluated in plasma. Results indicated that opioid receptors were not involved in the hypotensive effect of FM. However, ACEI activity (94 U/L), the oxidative stress index (malondialdehyde/catalase + glutathione peroxidase) 0.9, and nitric oxide in plasma (4.4 ± 1.3 U/L), were significantly different from the negative control, and not significantly different from the Captopril group. Thus, these results suggested that these mechanisms are involved in the hypotensive effect of FM.

Keywords: fermented milk; *Lactococcus lactis*; angiotensin converting enzyme inhibition; nitric oxide; antioxidant activity; opioid effect

---

1. Introduction

Hypertension is an important risk factor for cardiovascular diseases, a leading risk factor for death and disability. It has been estimated that hypertension affects more than 40% of people over 25 [1]. The high cost and adverse effects associated with pharmacological therapy have encouraged the scientists to search for new alternatives [2]. Therefore, there has been a rising interest in fermented dairy foods that, besides being nutritional, may promote health or reduce diseases, such as hypertension [3,4]. The beneficial effects of dairy products are attributed to several bioactive components, such as calcium, medium-chain fatty acids, lactose, conjugated linoleic acid and bioactive peptides [5]. Bioactive peptides from milk are liberated from the native protein through proteolysis during gastrointestinal digestion or food processing, such as fermentation with lactic acid bacteria (LAB) [6]. In fact, multifunctional properties of milk-derived peptides are increasingly recognized [7].

The antihypertensive effect of fermented milk products has been attributed to bioactive peptides [8] and/or gamma-amminobutyric acid (GABA) [9] produced during milk fermentation. In fact, the antihypertensive effect of bioactive peptides is often attributed to angiotensin-I converting enzyme inhibition (ACEI), an enzyme that plays a crucial role in blood regulation through the renin angiotensin system (RAS) [10]. Nevertheless, it has been reported that in some cases there is no correlation between in vitro and in vivo ACEI activity, due to peptides undergoing further degradation during gastrointestinal digestion, which may cause less bioavailability to reach target organs and cause the beneficial effect [8]. However, peptides with antioxidant [11], nitric oxide pathway [12], and opioid receptor binding activities [13] might also exhibit antihypertensive activity. Hence, antihypertensive bioactive peptides in fermented milks, may be acting via multiple mechanisms [8].

It has been previously reported that a fermented skim milk product with *Lactococcus* (*L.*) *lactis* NRRL B-50571 had ACEI activity in vitro; and this effect was strain-dependent [14,15]. Furthermore, fermented milk with *L. lactis* NRRL B-50571 reduced systolic blood pressure (SBP) and diastolic blood pressure (DBP), heart rate and had a hypolypidemic effect on spontaneously hypertensive rats (SHR) [16,17]. Additionally, in a pilot randomized double blind controlled clinical trial with prehypertensive subjects a blood pressure lowering effect of fermented milk with *L. lactis* NRRL-B50571 was observed [18]. Afterwards, we assessed that the antihypertensive effect of fermented milk with *L. lactis* was not due to the GABA present when it was administered to SHR [19]. Hence, the antihypertensive effect may be attributed to bioactive peptides present in this fermented milk; yet, it is not clear which mechanism is involved in the hypotensive effect. Therefore, the aim of the present study was to determine in SHR if the antihypertensive effect of fermented milk with *L. lactis* NRRL B-50571 was through the nitric oxide pathway, the opioid receptor binding, or the ACEI and antioxidant activities.

2. Materials and Methods

2.1. Strains and Growth Conditions

L. lactis strain NRRL B-50571 was propagated as previously reported by Rodríguez-Figueroa et al. [14] in 10 mL of sterile lactose (10%, *w*/*v*) M17 broth (DIFCO, Sparks, MD) and incubated at 30 °C for 24 h. Fresh precultures were obtained by repeating the same procedure twice to allow growth until reaching 10^6 to 10^7 cfu/mL. To obtain a working culture, a fresh culture was inoculated (3%) in sterile (110 °C, 10 min) nonfat dry milk reconstituted (10%, *w*/*w*) and incubated at 30 °C for 12 h.

2.2. Sample Preparation

Fermented milk with *L. Lactis* NRRL B-50571 (FM) was prepared as previously reported [18]. Reconstituted (10%, *w*/*v*) commercial skim milk was pasteurized (80 °C for 30 min), inoculated with 3% working culture and fermented at 30 °C for 48 h. To inactivate LAB, fermentation was stopped by applying heat treatment (75 °C, 15 min), followed by quick cooling; subsequently fermented milk was frozen (−20 °C), for further analysis.

To obtain the lyophilized water-soluble extracts from *L. lactis* fermented milk with NRRL B-50571 (WSE-FM) for the evaluation of the opioid effect, WSE-FM were obtained by centrifugation (ThermoScientific, Chelmsford, MA, USA) at 5000 rpm for 40 min at 4 °C; then lyophilized with a freeze-dryer (Labconco, Kansas City, MO, USA), and kept at 4 °C until use for further analysis. Total protein content (Method 960.52 AOAC, 1998) of the lyophilized extracts was evaluated.

2.3. In Vivo Experimental Protocols

A total of twenty-nine male SHR (4 weeks old; 44.7 ± 5.15 g body weight (BW)) were obtained from Charles River Laboratories International, Inc. (Wilmington, MA, USA). Rats were housed in individual cages at 21 ± 2 °C, 12 h light–dark cycles and 52 ± 6% relative humidity, with an ad libitum intake of a standard diet (Purina, Cd. México, México) and purified water. Blood pressure was monitored every week until all rats developed hypertension according to Okamoto and Aoki [20]. SBP and DBP were taken 3 times using the non-invasive blood pressure system using a photoelectric sensor, amplifier, manual inflation cuff and software (Model 229; IITC Life Science Inc., (Woodland Hills, CA, USA). Once all rats were hypertensive, the possible antihypertensive mechanisms (opioid, ACEI, antioxidant, and nitric oxide pathway) were evaluated. All procedures involving animals were approved by the Bioethics Committee of the Research Center for Food and Development (Spanish acronym, CIAD), Hermosillo, Sonora, Mexico, (CE/009/2015).

2.4. Evaluation of Opioid Effect

When SHR were 16 weeks old (320.8 ± 16 g BW, 187.6 ± 15.6 mmHg SBP and 129.6 ± 16.9 mmHg DBP); twenty-one SHR were randomized into three groups (Table 1) of seven rats ($n = 7$). Treatments were assigned randomly to each group to either receive in a single dose: purified water (negative control); 35 mg protein of WSE-FM/kg animal BW; or 1 mg/kg animal BW of naloxone (μ-opioid antagonist receptor) (PiSa Farmacéutica, Cd. México, México) + 35 mg protein of FM-WSE/kg animal BW. FM-WSE from fermented milk was dissolved in purified water.

In order to prepare the corresponding dose of naloxone and WSE-FM, the SHR were weighed before administration. Conscious SHR received via subcutaneous (s.c.) naloxone, and afterwards a single oral dose of WSE-FM through a gastric cannula between 8:00 and 10:00 hours to eliminate circadian cycles. SBP and DBP were monitored before treatment administration and every 10 min until 60 min post-administration.

2.5. Long-Term Effect of FM on Blood Pressure

Twenty-seven male SHR (19 weeks old, 346.4 ± 17.7 g BW, 201.5 ± 15.4 mmHg SBP and 153.4 ± 24.6 mmHg DBP), were randomized into three groups (Table 2) of nine rats ($n = 9$). SHR from the first study had a three-week washout period, before group allocation; during this time, blood pressure was monitored to assess any residual effect. Treatments were assigned randomly to each group to either receive: purified water (negative control); Captopril (a proven hypotensive drug, 40 mg/kg of BW, Sigma-Aldrich Co., St. Louis, MO, USA); or FM. All SHR had free access (ad libitum) to each treatment during the 6 weeks as part of the protocol. SBP and DBP were measured 3 times, once a week between 8:00 and 10:00 hours to eliminate circadian cycles. After six weeks of treatment, rats were sacrificed and blood samples were collected to immediately obtain plasma, and freezed −80 °C for further analysis.

2.6. ACEI Activity in Plasma

Plasma was used for measuring the ACEI activity according to the method of Cushman and Cheung [21]. Hippuryl-L-histidyl-L-leucine (a substrate for ACE) (Sigma-Aldrich Co., St. Louis, MO, USA) was dissolved in 0.1 mol/L sodium borate buffer (pH 8.3) containing 0.3 mol/L NaCl. The reaction was initiated by the addition of 100 μL of the serum and vascular tissue enzyme extract, then incubated for 30 min at 37 °C and stopped by the addition of 250 μL of 1 mol/L HCl. The hippuric acid liberated by ACE was extracted with 1.5 mL ethyl acetate, dissolved by addition of 1.0 mL of Milli-Q water, after removal of ethyl acetate by heating for 20 min at 75 °C, and measured at 228 nm. One unit (U) of activity was defined as the amount of enzyme, which released 1.0 mmol of hippuric acid/min under the above conditions. The specific activity of ACE in serum is expressed as U/L.

2.7. Nitric Oxide Pathway

Nitric oxide pathway was estimated through nitric oxide (NO) production. Plasma NO concentration was determined by the Griess reaction with a colormetric assay kit (Cell Biolabs, Inc., San Diego, CA, USA). This assay is based on the conversion of nitrate to nitrite by nitrate reductase, followed by quantification of nitrate after the Griess reaction. NO concentration in plasma was expressed as μmol/L.

2.8. Antioxidant Activity

Antioxidant activity from peptides was assessed indirectly by determining oxidative stress index/ratio. This index indicates the balance between lipoperoxidation (as malondialdehyde, MDA) and total antioxidant enzyme activity (catalase, CAT, and glutathione peroxidase, GPx) [22].

2.8.1. Superoxide Dismutase Activity (SOD)

The determination of SOD activity in plasma was determined as described by Superoxide Dismutase assay kit (Cayman Chemical Company, Ann Arbor, MI, USA). In this assay, it determines the ability to inhibit the reduction of tetrazolium salt induced by xanthine-xanthine oxidase. One unit of SOD is defined as the amount of enzyme needed to exhibit 50% dismutation of the superoxide radical; and was expressed as U/mL.

2.8.2. Catalase Activity Determination (CAT)

CAT activity in plasma determination was based on the decomposition of hydrogen peroxide (30 µM) at 240 nm [23]. CAT activity was defined as the amount of enzyme that removed 1 µmol H_2O_2 in 1 min. CAT activity was expressed as µmol H_2O_2/min/L.

2.8.3. Glutathione Peroxidase (GPx) Activity

GPx activity in plasma was evaluated as described as the manufacturer for Glutathione peroxidase assay kit (Cayman Chemical Company, Ann Arbor, MI, USA). The GPx activity was determined 340 nm and is expressed as nmol/min/mL.

2.8.4. Determination of Lipid Peroxidation

The degree of lipid peroxidation in plasma was determined as described by Todorova et al. [24], with some modifications. This method uses thiobarbituric acid (TBA), which measures malondialdehyde (MDA) reactive products. 200 µL of plasma were mixed with 200 µL of PBS, and 200 µL trichloroacetic acid (25%). Afterwards, mixtures were centrifuged (2000 g, 20 min) and supernatants were mixed with 150 µL of TBA (1%), followed by heated at 95 °C for 1 h. After cooling absorbance was determined at 532 nm. The MDA concentration was calculated by using an extinction coefficient of 155 (1/mM·cm). MDA was expressed as µmol/L.

2.9. Statistical Analysis

Baseline systolic and diastolic blood pressures were defined as the mean of the values measured in the first run-in period. The blood pressure outcomes were presented as the mean value with standard deviations (SD) for all SHR in each group. For the evaluation of opioid effect the blood pressure (min 50 and 60 post-treatment) between groups were analyzed with one-way ANOVA. Differences among means were assessed by Scheffe multiple comparison test and considered significant when $p < 0.05$. For the long-term effect of FM on blood pressure, the outcomes for each week between groups were analyzed with one-way ANOVA. Differences among means were assessed by Scheffe multiple comparison test and considered significant when $p < 0.05$. The outcomes for ACEI activity, superoxide dismutase, GPx activity, MDA, and oxidative stress index, were analyzed with Kruskal–Wallis test since they did not presented a normal distribution; data are presented as medians and were considered significant when $p < 0.05$. The outcomes for nitric oxide and CAT activity were analyzed with one-way ANOVA. Differences among means were assessed by Scheffe multiple comparison test and considered significant when $p < 0.05$. Data are presented as means ± SEM.

3. Results and Discussion

The use of *Lactococcus lactis* NRRL B-50571 as a starter for fermented milk with antihypertensive effect has been reported in SHR [16,17] and prehypertensive subjects [18], and this hypotensive effect has been attributed to ACEI. Moreover, 21 identified peptides in this fermented milk possessed ACEI activity [15]. However, in several studies it has been reported that there is a lack of correlation between the in vitro and in vivo ACEI activity. This may be due to peptide degradation throughout gastrointestinal digestion, and this may implicate difficulty to reach the target organs in a sufficient amount to exert ACEI effect. However, it should not be disregarded that other mechanisms may be involved in the antihypertensive effect mediated through the interaction with receptor located at the gut [25]. Hence, to the best of our knowledge this is the first study that evaluates the possible mechanisms where peptides may be involved in the hypotensive effect; such as opioid, ACEI, antioxidant and NO pathway (by NO production).

3.1. *Opioid Effect*

Twenty one SHR with blood pressure higher than 186/126 mmHg for systolic and diastolic blood pressures were eligible for randomization (Table 1). As expected, there were no significant differences ($p > 0.05$) between groups on clinical characteristics (systolic blood pressure, diastolic blood pressure, heart rate and weight).

Table 1. Clinical characteristics of SHR.

Groups	Negative Control (Purified Water)	WSE-FM NRRL B-50571	Naloxone + WSE-FM NRRL B-50571	*p* Value
Weight	319 ± 20.1	321.9 ± 16	322.6 ± 10.24	0.97
SBP (mmHg)	188.1 ± 21.8	186.3 ± 20	189 ± 8.8	0.99
DBP (mmHg)	126.2 ± 24.3	127 ± 13.2	131.6 ± 10.7	0.83
Heart rate (beats/min)	488.8 ± 35.1	465.2 ± 27.7	453.7 ± 28.9	0.13

SHR: spontaneously hypertensive rats; SBP: systolic blood pressure; DBP: diastolic blood pressure; WSE: water soluble extract; FM: fermented milk.

Figures 1 and 2 depicts the changes of SBP and DBP every 10 min for 60 min after a single oral dose of purified water (negative control); WSE-FM; or naloxone + WSE-FM. After 50 and 60 min post-treatments, reductions on SBP from WSE-FM group and naloxone + WSE-FM group were 13.8 ± 26.1 and 7.7 ± 9.3 mmHg; and 15.2 ± 29.8 and 12.7 ± 17.7 mmHg, respectively; and were significantly different ($p < 0.05$) from the negative control. Though, DBP were not significantly different ($p > 0.05$) between all groups, DBP from groups receiving WSE-FM or naloxone + WSE-FM, tended to be slightly lower.

It has been previously reported that milk derived peptides possess opioid-like effect, and that this effect may exert a hypotensive effect through binding a specific μ opioid receptor [13]. In fact, the common structural feature for opioid milk peptides is the presence of tyrosine at the N-terminal end, and the presence of another aromatic residue [26]. Meanwhile, it was previously reported that three peptides with tyrosine at the N-terminal (YPSYGL, YPSYG and YIPIQYVLS) where present in the fermented milk with *L. lactis* NRRL B-50571 [15], therefore, we evaluated if the antihypertensive effect may be due to milk peptides binding to opioid receptors.

In the present study μ-opioid receptors were blocked with antagonist opioid receptor (naloxone), and blood pressure reduction was not significantly different ($p > 0.05$) in WSE-FM group and naloxone + WSE-FM group. Hence, in this study the blood pressure lowering effect may not be attributed to peptides binding to opioid receptors.

On the other hand, it was reported that the mechanism of the blood pressure lowering effect of a tetrapeptide from milk whey, after a single subcutaneous administration to SHR, was by opioid receptors, since the response was antagonized with naloxone [13]. Thus, it should not be disregarded that if SHR were administered subcutaneously with specific peptides present in the fermented milk with *L. lactis* NRRL B-50571) [15], the antihypertensive effect could be via binding opioid receptors.

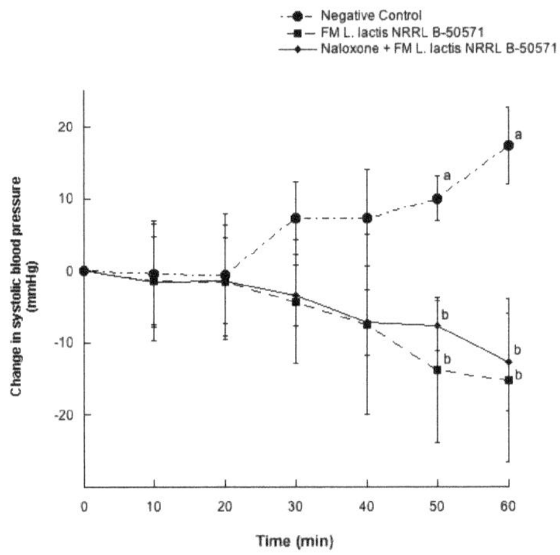

Figure 1. Change in systolic blood pressure in spontaneously hypertensive rats with different treatments. Negative control: purified water; FM *L. lactis* NRRL B-50571: lyophilized water-soluble extract (35 mg protein/kg body weight) of fermented milk with *Lactococcus lactis* NRRL B-50571; Naloxone: (1 mg/kg body weight) Antagonist μ opioid receptor + FM *L. lactis* NRRL B-50571: lyophilized water-soluble extract (35 mg protein/kg body weight) of fermented milk with *Lactococcus lactis* NRRL B-50571. Data are presented as means ± SEM. Data points sharing the same letter within a week was not significantly different ($p > 0.05$).

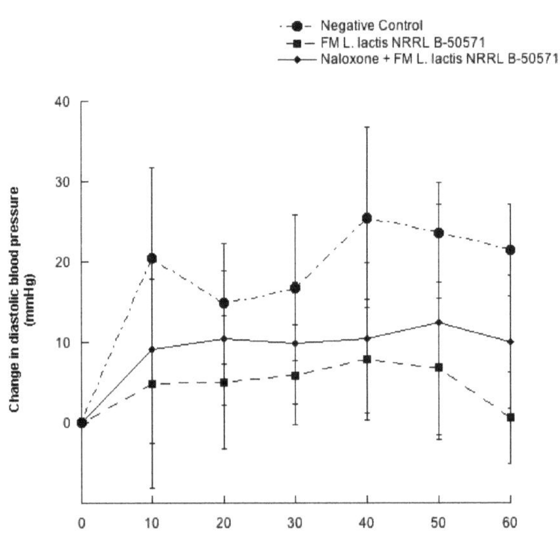

Figure 2. Change in diastolic blood pressure in spontaneously hypertensive rats with different treatments. Negative control: purified water; FM *L. lactis* NRRL B-50571: lyophilized water-soluble extract (35 mg protein/kg body weight) of fermented milk with *L. lactis* NRRL B-50571; Naloxone: (1 mg/kg body weight) Antagonist μ opioid receptor + FM *L. lactis* NRRL B-50571: lyophilized water-soluble extract (35 mg protein/kg body weight) of fermented milk with *L. lactis* NRRL B-50571. Data are presented as means ± SEM.

3.2. Long-Term Effect of FM on Blood Pressure

In a parallel study, twenty seven SHR with blood pressure higher than 200/150 mmHg for systolic and diastolic blood pressures were selected for randomization (Table 2). As expected, there were no significant differences ($p > 0.05$) between groups on clinical characteristics (systolic blood pressure, diastolic blood pressure, heart rate and weight). In this study, we evaluated the other possible mechanisms involved in the antihypertensive effect of fermented milk with *L. lactis*, after six weeks of administration. Changes in SBP and DBP for every week are represented in Figures 3 and 4. Both SBP and DBP values from the Captopril group and FM group were significantly different from the negative control group ($p > 0.05$), but they were not significantly different ($p < 0.05$) between them. Maximal SBP decreases from the FM group was of 49.9 ± 14.2 mmHg, after 6 weeks of treatment, while the Captopril group SBP decreased 45.2 ± 23.6 mmHg on the same week of intervention. After six weeks of intervention, SHR were sacrificed to obtain plasma and evaluate ACEI activity, NO production and antioxidant effect.

Table 2. Clinical characteristics of SHR.

Groups	Negative Control (Purified Water)	Captopril	FM NRRL B-50571	*p* Value
Weight	341.5 ± 18.5	357.2 ± 12.3	340.5 ± 17.9	0.70
SBP (mmHg)	200.8 ± 16.1	201.8 ± 18.3	201.8 ± 13.1	0.98
DBP (mmHg)	152 ± 23.3	158 ± 30.2	150.1 ± 21.8	0.78
Heart rate (beats/min)	461.7 ± 33.5	442.6 ± 40.1	433.7 ± 38	0.28

SHR: spontaneously hypertensive rats; SBP: systolic blood pressure; DBP: diastolic blood pressure; FM: fermented milk.

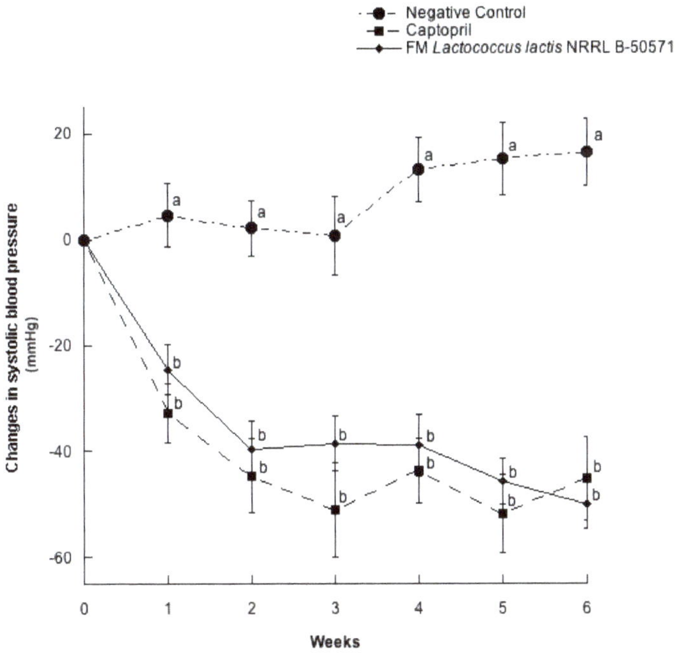

Figure 3. Change in systolic blood pressure in spontaneously hypertensive rats with different treatments. Negative control: purified water; Captopril: 40 mg/kg body weight; FM *L. lactis* NRRL B-50571 (ad libitum): fermented milk with *L. lactis* NRRL B-50571. Data are presented as means ± SEM. Data points sharing the same letter within a week was not significantly different ($p > 0.05$).

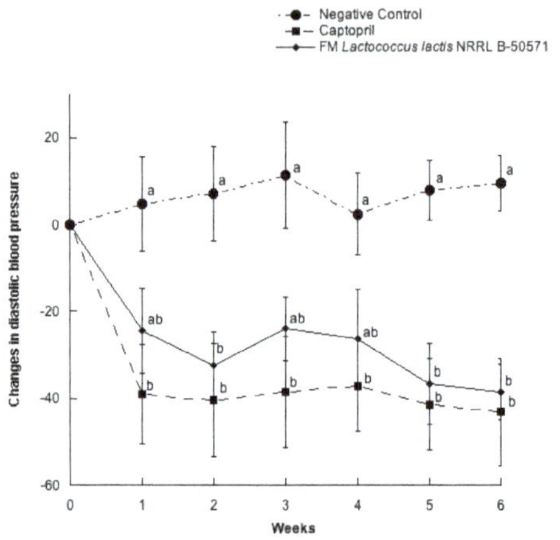

Figure 4. Change in diastolic blood pressure in spontaneously hypertensive rats with different treatments. Negative control: purified water; Captopril: 40 mg/kg body weight; FM *L. lactis* NRRL B-50571 (ad libitum): fermented milk with *L. lactis* NRRL B-50571. Data are presented as means ± SEM. Data points sharing the same letter within a week was not significantly different ($p > 0.05$).

3.3. ACEI Activity

One method to determine *in vivo* ACEI activity indirectly from peptides is through the determination of circulating ACEI activity in plasma [27]. Figure 5 represents the ACEI activity in plasma of SHR after six weeks post-treatment. Plasma ACEI activity was reduced in SHR treated with Captopril (a potent ACE inhibitor) and FM groups, and was not significantly different between them ($p > 0.05$). Moreover, ACEI activity in plasma from the negative control group was 5.5 times higher than the FM group, and was significantly different ($p < 0.05$) from the groups treated with FM or Captopril. Thus, the effect may be attributed to the in vivo ACE inhibition from bioactive peptides in FM, because circulating ACE activity was reduced.

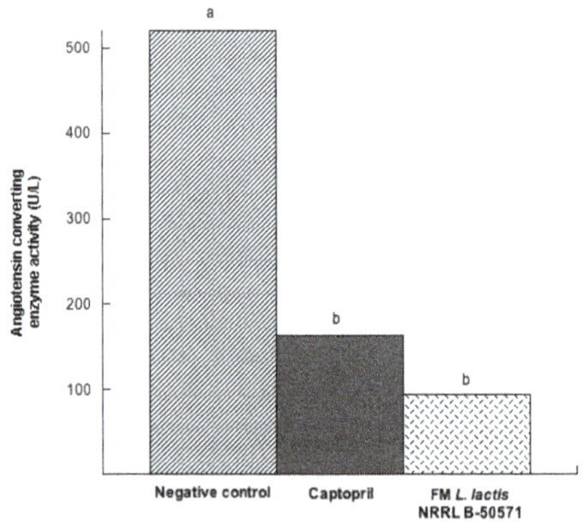

Figure 5. Angiotensin converting enzyme activity (U/L) in plasma from spontaneously hypertensive rats after long-term treatments. Negative control: purified water; Captopril: 40 mg/kg body weight; FM *L. lactis* NRRL B-50571 (ad libitum): fermented milk with *L. lactis* NRRL B-50571. Data are presented as median; and was analyzed by non-parametric test (Kruskal–Wallis $p < 0.05$). Data sharing the same letter was not significantly different ($p > 0.05$).

A similar finding of ACEI activity in vivo after long-term effect of lactoferrin hydrolysates in SHR was evaluated [28]. In another study where there was a single intake of lactoferrin-derived peptides, there were also reductions in circulating ACE activity (40%) after 1 h post-administration; furthermore, these effects were similar to the SHR group, which received Captopril [29], henceforth angiotensin converting enzyme is an enzyme that plays a crucial role in blood regulation through the renin angiotensin system (RAS), thus its inhibition exerts antihypertensive effects [30]. In the present study, since reductions of the ACEI activity in circulating plasma were similar in the FM group and Captopril group; henceforth we may assume that this mechanistic pathway may be involved in the hypotensive effect of FM with *L. lactis* NRRL B-50571.

3.4. NO Pathway

In our present study, NO concentration in plasma was determined (Figure 6). After long-term effect of each treatment, plasma NO concentrations were significantly ($p < 0.05$) higher in the FM group and Captopril group than in the negative control group. Actually, plasma NO was 1.6 times higher in the FM group than in the negative control group; and was significantly different ($p < 0.05$). Recent studies have reported that some antihypertensive peptides may improve NO bioavailability through antioxidant effects, but certain peptides may also enhance NO production, improve endothelial function and improve blood pressure [31]. NO is an important bioregulatory molecule, which improves endothelial function, improves vasodilatation and controls blood pressure; therefore it is considered to be the main vasodilator. SHR may develop endothelial dysfunction by reducing bioavailability of NO. Therefore, increased bioavailability of NO may also improve vasodilation and reduce blood pressure [32,33]. Our findings are similar with those by Kim et al. [33]; they reported that fermented milk had an antihypertensive effect in SHR, had less ACEI activity in plasma, and more concentration of NO, compared to their control group. Hence, NO production may also be considered a mechanism involved in the hypotensive effect of FM with *L. lactis* NRRL B-50571.

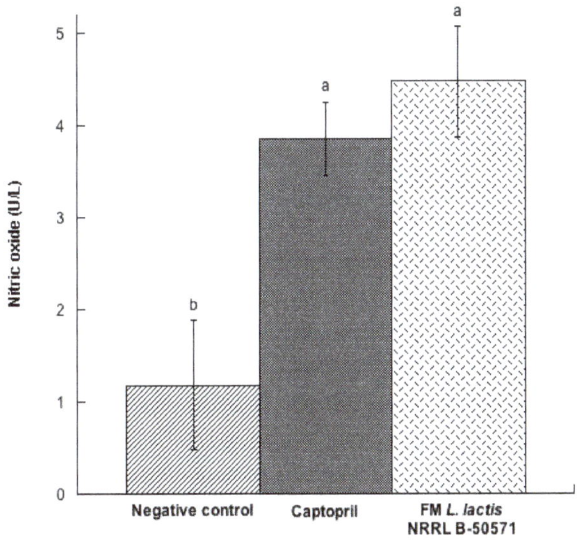

Figure 6. Nitric oxide (U/L) in plasma from spontaneously hypertensive rats after long-term treatments. Negative control: purified water; Captopril: 40 mg/kg body weight; FM *L. lactis* NRRL B-50571 (ad libitum): fermented milk with *Lactococcus lactis* NRRL B-50571. Data are presented as means ± SEM. Data sharing the same letter are not significantly different ($p > 0.05$).

3.5. Antioxidant Effect

To date, there is growing evidence that oxidative stress is one of the main responsible factors for the initiation or evolution of hypertension and its complications. Increased oxidative stress is also considered to be an important causative factor of the vascular endothelial dysfunction, causing decrement of NO production [34]. Therefore, there has been a rising interest on the pursuit for bioactive peptides with antioxidant activity, which may provide additional benefit to the endogenous antioxidant defense system [35]. Moreover, lipid peroxidation plays a major role in oxidative stress. Hence, bioactive components that may reduce lipoperoxidation may help decrease oxidative stress [34]. It has been reported that food bioactive peptides have strong antioxidant effect without significant side effects [36], and that milk derived peptides are the most studied [25]. In fact, it has been reported that whey protein has beneficial effects through enhancement of antioxidant enzymes and down regulation of oxidative markers such as lipoperoxidation [37].

In the present study, we evaluated the concentration of three antioxidant enzymes in plasma post-treatments. Results indicated that SOD (Figure 7) and CAT (Figure 8) were not significantly different ($p > 0.05$) in either group; nevertheless, values were higher in the Captopril group and the FM group than in the negative control group. Moreover, GPx activity (Figure 9) in the Captopril group was significantly higher ($p < 0.05$) than in the FM group and negative control group; however, GPx activity value from the FM group was slightly higher than in the negative control group. Additionally we evaluated lipoperoxidation in plasma through TBA, by detecting MDA products (Figure 10). In this study, although we did not detect differences between all groups ($p > 0.05$), MDA values from the FM group and Captopril group were lower than in the negative control.

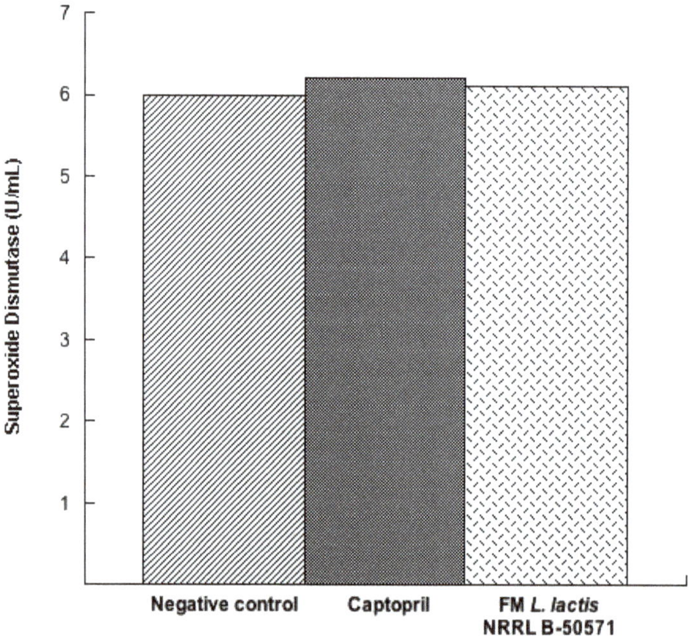

Figure 7. Superoxide dismutase (U/mL) in plasma from spontaneously hypertensive rats after long-term treatments. Negative control: purified water; Captopril: 40 mg/kg body weight; FM *L. lactis* NRRL B-50571 (ad libitum): fermented milk with *Lactococcus lactis* NRRL B-50571. Data are presented as median; and were analyzed by non-parametric test (Kruskal–Wallis $p < 0.05$).

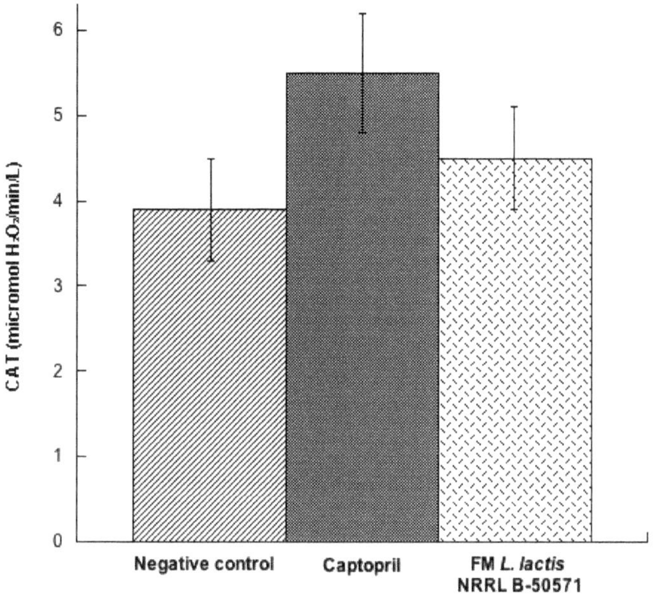

Figure 8. Catalase activity (CAT) (micromol H_2O_2/min/L) in plasma from spontaneously hypertensive rats after long-term treatments. Negative control: purified water; Captopril: 40 mg/kg body weight; FM *L. lactis* NRRL B-50571 (ad libitum): fermented milk with *L. lactis* NRRL B-50571. Data are presented as means ± SEM, and were analyzed by one-way ANOVA.

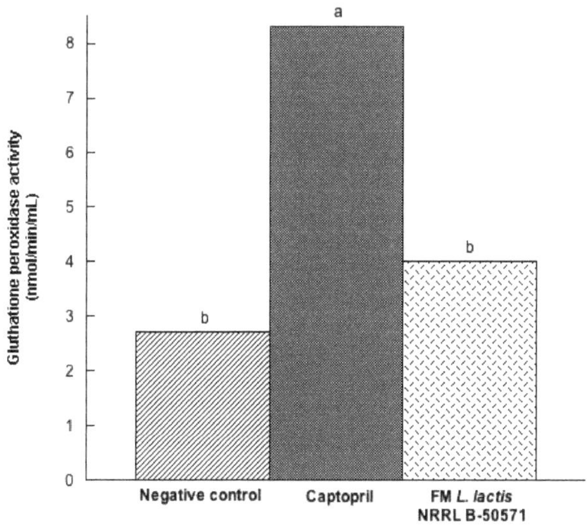

Figure 9. Glutathione peroxidase activity (nmol/min/mL) in plasma from spontaneously hypertensive rats after long-term treatments. Negative control: purified water; Captopril: 40 mg/kg body weight; FM *L. lactis* NRRL B-50571 (*ad libitum*): fermented milk with *Lactococcus lactis* NRRL B-50571. Data are presented as median; and was analyzed by non-parametric test (Kruskal–Wallis $p < 0.05$). Data sharing the same letter are not significantly different ($p > 0.05$).

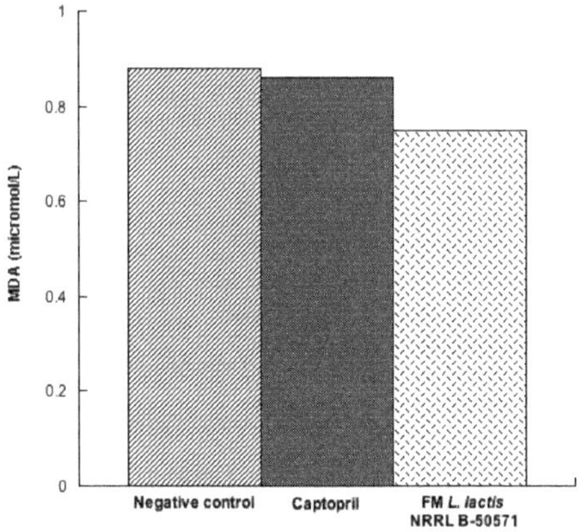

Figure 10. Lipid peroxidation represented as malondialdehyde (MDA) content in plasma from spontaneously hypertensive rats after long-term treatments. Negative control: purified water; Captopril: 40 mg/kg body weight; FM *L. lactis* NRRL B-50571 (ad libitum): fermented milk with *L. lactis* NRRL B-50571. Data are presented as median; and were analyzed by non-parametric test (Kruskal–Wallis $p < 0.05$).

Nonetheless, after the evaluation of the oxidative stress index (Figure 11), which indicates the balance between lipoperoxidation (as malondialdehyde, MDA) and total antioxidant enzyme activity (CAT and GPx), results demonstrated that the Captopril group and the FM group were not significantly different ($p > 0.05$), yet they were significantly different ($p < 0.05$) from the negative control group. Since FM decreased oxidative stress in SHR, antioxidant activity may also be considered as an underlying mechanism pathway on the antihypertensive effect of FM. Thus, daily consumption of fermented milk with *L. lactis* NRRL B-50571 may help lower high blood pressure, as well as MDA levels and oxidative stress index, ACEI activity, and an enhancement of NO production.

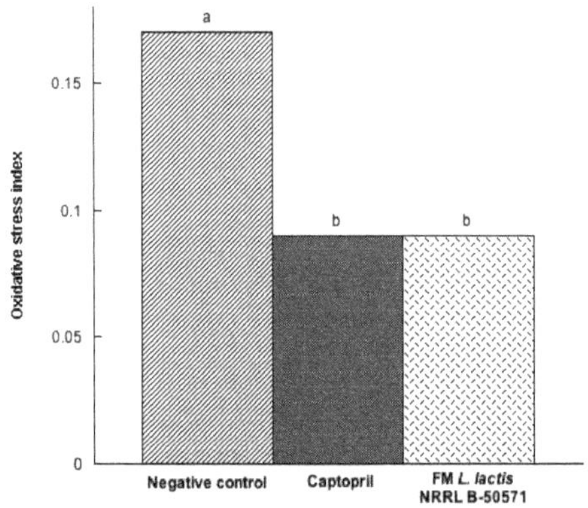

Figure 11. Oxidative stress index represented as the balance between lipid peroxidation (MDA) and antioxidant enzymes (Catalase and Glutathione peroxidase), from spontaneously hypertensive rats after long-term treatments. Negative control: purified water; Captopril: 40 mg/kg body weight; FM *L. lactis* NRRL B-50571 (ad libitum): fermented milk with *L. lactis* NRRL B-50571. Data are presented as median; and was analyzed by non-parametric test (Kruskal–Wallis $p < 0.05$). Data sharing the same letter was not significantly different ($p > 0.05$).

Similarly, it was reported that the antihypertensive effect of whey protein concentrate hydrolysates in SHR was through ACEI activity, oxidative damage reduction, and enhancement of NO production [38].

4. Conclusions

The antihypertensive effect of fermented milk with *Lactococcus lactis* NRRL B-50571 in SHR and prehypertensive subjects was previously reported. Nonetheless, this is the first study that elucidates the basic mechanistic pathways underlying the hypotensive effect of fermented milk with *Lactococcus lactis* NRRL B-50571. Results indicated that fermented milk with *Lactococcus lactis* NRRL B-50571 seem to act as angiotensin converting enzyme inhibitor, nitric oxide production enhancer and as an antioxidant; which overall helped reduce blood pressure in SHR.

Acknowledgments: The authors would like to thank Alejandro Santos-Espinosa, Anahí Gaxiola-Villa and Lourdes Santiago-López for their technical assistance.

Author Contributions: The author's responsibilities were as follows: Belinda Vallejo-Córdoba, Aarón F. González-Córdova, Adrián Hernández-Mendoza and Lilia María Beltrán-Barrientos designed the study. Lilia María Beltrán-Barrientos conducted the study and wrote the manuscript. Belinda Vallejo-Córdoba revised the manuscript and had primary responsibility for the final content of the manuscript. Aarón F. González-Córdova, Adrián Hernández-Mendoza, Humberto Astiazarán-García and Julián Esparza-Romero supplied valuable knowledge and scientific consultation throughout the study; and all authors read and approved the final manuscript.

Conflicts of Interest: The authors hereby declare no conflict of interests. This study was supported by the Mexican Council of Science and Technology (CONACYT; México City, Mexico) research project 240338 CONACYT. CONACYT had no role in the design of the study; in the collection, analyses, or interpretation of data; in the writing of the manuscript, or in the decision to publish the results.

References

1. O'Shea, P.M.; Griffin, T.P.; Fitzgibbon, M. Hypertension: The role of biochemistry in the diagnosis and management. *Clin. Chim. Acta* **2017**, *465*, 131–143. [CrossRef] [PubMed]
2. Miller, G.D.; Jarvis, J.K.; McBean, L.D. Dairy foods and hypertension. In *Handbook of Dairy Foods and Nutrition*, 3rd ed.; CRC Press: Boca Raton, FL, USA, 2007; pp. 99–139.
3. Flambard, B.; Johansen, E. Developing a functional dairy product: From research on *Lactobacillus helveticus* to industrial application of Cardi-04TM in novel antihypertensive drink yogurts. In *Functional Dairy Products*; Saarela, M., Ed.; CRC Press LLC: Boca Raton, FL, USA, 2007; pp. 506–520.
4. Beltrán-Barrientos, L.M.; Hernández-Mendoza, A.; Torres-Llanez, M.J.; González-Córdova, A.F.; Vallejo-Córdoba, B. Invited review: Fermented milk as antihypertensive functional food. *J. Dairy Sci.* **2016**, *99*, 4099–4110. [CrossRef] [PubMed]
5. Ebringer, L.; Ferencik, M.; Krajcovic, J. Beneficial health effects of milk and fermented dairy products. *Folia Microbiol. (Praha)* **2008**, *53*, 378–394. [CrossRef] [PubMed]
6. González-Córdova, A.F.; Torres-Llanez, M.J.; Rodríguez-Figueroa, J.C.; Espinoza-De-Los-Monteros, J.J.; García, H.S.; Vallejo-Cordoba, B. Actividad inhibidora de la enzima convertidora de angiotensina en leches fermentadas con cepas de *Lactobacillus*. *CYTA J. Food* **2011**, *9*, 146–151. [CrossRef]
7. Mohanty, D.P.; Mohapatra, S.; Misra, S.; Sahu, P.S. Milk derived bioactive peptides and their impact on human health—A review. *Saudi J. Biol. Sci.* **2016**, *23*, 577–583. [CrossRef] [PubMed]
8. Udenigwe, C.; Mohan, A. Mechanisms of food protein-derived antihypertensive peptides other than ACE inhibition. *J. Funct. Foods* **2014**, *8*, 45–52. [CrossRef]
9. Hayakawa, K.; Kimura, M.; Kamata, K. Mechanism underlying gamma-aminobutyric acid-induced antihypertensive effect in spontaneously hypertensive rats. *Eur. J. Pharmacol.* **2002**, *438*, 107–113. [CrossRef]
10. Perazella, M.A.; Setaro, J.F. Renin-angiotensin-aldosterone system: Fundamental aspects and clinical implications in renal and cardiovascular disorders. *J. Nucl. Cardiol.* **2003**, *10*, 184–196. [CrossRef] [PubMed]
11. Del Mar Contreras, M.; Carron, R.; Montero, M.J.; Ramos, M.; Recio, I. Novel casein-derived peptides with antihypertensive activity. *Int. Dairy J.* **2009**, *19*, 566–573. [CrossRef]

12. Yamaguchi, N.; Kawaguchi, K.; Yamamoto, N. Study of the mechanism of antihypertensive peptides VPP and IPP in spontaneously hypertensive rats by DNA microarray analysis. *Eur. J. Pharmacol.* **2009**, *620*, 71–77. [CrossRef] [PubMed]
13. Nurminen, M.L.; Sipola, M.; Kaarto, H.; Pihlanto-Leppala, A.; Piilola, K.; Korpela, R.; Tossavainen, O.; Korhonen, H.; Vapaatalo, H. α-Lactorphin lowers blood pressure measured radiotelemetry in normotensive and spontaneously hypertensive rats. *Life Sci.* **2000**, *66*, 1535–1543. [CrossRef]
14. Rodríguez-Figueroa, J.C.; Reyes-Díaz, R.; González-Córdova, A.F.; Troncoso-Rojas, R.; Vargas-Arispuro, I.; Vallejo-Cordoba, B. Angiotensin-converting enzyme inhibitory activity of milk fermented by wild and industrial *Lactococcus lactis* strains. *J. Dairy Sci.* **2010**, *93*, 5032–5038. [CrossRef] [PubMed]
15. Rodríguez-Figueroa, J.C.; González-Córdova, A.F.; Torres-Llanez, M.J.; García, H.S.; Vallejo-Cordoba, B. Novel angiotensin I-converting enzyme inhibitory peptides produced in fermented milk by specific wild *Lactococcus lactis* strains. *J. Dairy Sci.* **2012**, *95*, 5536–5543. [CrossRef] [PubMed]
16. Rodríguez-Figueroa, J.C.; González-Córdova, A.F.; Astiazarán-Gacía, H.; Vallejo-Córdoba, B. Hypotensive and heart rate lowering effects in rats receiving milk fermented by specific *Lactococcus lactis* strains. *Br. J. Nutr.* **2013**, *109*, 827–833. [CrossRef] [PubMed]
17. Rodríguez-Figueroa, J.C.; González-Córdova, A.F.; Astiazarán-Gacía, H.; Vallejo-Cordoba, B. Antihypertensive and hypolipidemic effect of milk fermented by specific *Lactococcus lactis* strains. *J. Dairy Sci.* **2013**, *96*, 4094–4099. [CrossRef] [PubMed]
18. Beltrán-Barrientos, L.M.; González-Córdova, A.F.; Hernández-Mendoza, A.; Torres-Inguanzo, E.H.; Astiazarán-García, H.; Esparza-Romero, J.; Vallejo-Córdoba, B. Randomized double-blind controlled clinical trial of the blood pressure lowering effect of fermented milk with *Lactococcus lactis*: A pilot study. *J. Dairy Sci.* **2018**. [CrossRef] [PubMed]
19. Beltrán-Barrientos, L.M.; Estrada-Montoya, C.; Reyes-Díaz, R.; Hernández-Mendoza, A.; González-Córdova, A.F.; Vallejo-Córdoba, B. Assessment of the potential role of gamma-aminobutyric acid on the antihypertensive effect of fermented milk with *Lactococcus lactis* NRRL B-50571. *J. Funct. Foods* **2018**, in press.
20. Okamoto, K.; Aoki, K. Development of a strain of spontaneously hypertensive rats. *Jpn. Circ. J.* **1963**, *27*, 282–293. [CrossRef] [PubMed]
21. Cushman, D.W.; Cheng, H.S. Spectrophotometric assay and properties of the angiotensin converting enzyme of rabbit lung. *Biochem. Pharmacol.* **1971**, *20*, 1637–1648. [CrossRef]
22. Ruas, C.B.G. Oxidative stress biomarkers of exposure in the blood of cichlid species from a metal-contaminated river. *Ecotox. Environ. Safe* **2008**, *71*, 86–93. [CrossRef] [PubMed]
23. Hwang, J.W.; Kim, E.K.; Lee, S.J.; Kim, Y.S.; Choi, D.K.; Park, T.K.; Moon, S.H.; Jeon, B.T.; Park, P.J. Antocyanin effectively scavenges free radicals and protects retinal cells from H_2O_2-triggered G2/M arrest. *Eur. Food Res. Technol.* **2012**, *234*, 431–439. [CrossRef]
24. Todorova, I.; Simeonova, G.; Kyuchukova, D.; Dinev, D.; Gadjeva, V. Reference values of oxidative stress parameters (MDA, SOD, CAT) in dogs and cats. *Comp. Clin. Pathol.* **2005**, *13*, 190–194. [CrossRef]
25. Hernández-Ledesma, B.; García-Nebot, M.J.; Fernández-Tomé, S.; Amigo, L.; Recio, I. Dairy protein hydrolysates: Peptides for health benefits. *Int. Dairy J.* **2014**, *38*, 82–100. [CrossRef]
26. Meisel, H.; FitzGerald, R.J. Opioid peptides encrypted in intact milk protein sequences. *Br. J. Nutr.* **2000**, *84*, 27–31. [CrossRef]
27. Manzanares, P.; Salom, J.B.; García-Tejedor, A.; Fernández-Musoles, R.; Ruiz-Jiménez, P.; Gimeno-Alcañiz, J.V. Unraveling the mechanisms of action of lactoferrin-derived antihypertensive peptides: ACE inhibition and beyond. *Food Funct.* **2015**, *6*, 2440–2452. [CrossRef] [PubMed]
28. Fernández-Musoles, R.; Manzanares, P.; Burguete, M.C.; Alborch, E.; Salom, J.B. In vivo angiotensin I-converting enzyme inhibition by long-term intake of antihypertensive lactoferrin hydrolysate in spontaneously hypertensive rats. *Food Res. Int.* **2013**, *54*, 627–632. [CrossRef]
29. Ruiz-Giménez, P.; Ibáñez, A.; Salom, J.B.; Marcos, J.F.; López-Díez, J.J.; Vallés, S.; Torregrosa, G.; Alborch, E.; Manzanares, P. Antihypertensive properties of lactoferricin B-derived peptides. *J. Agric. Food Chem.* **2010**, *58*, 6721–6727. [CrossRef] [PubMed]
30. Majumder, K.; Wu, J. Molecular targets of antihypertensive peptides: understanding the mechanisms of action based on the pathophysiology of hypertension. *Int. J. Mol. Sci.* **2015**, *16*, 256–283. [CrossRef] [PubMed]
31. Chakrabarti, S.; Wu, J. Bioactive peptides on endothelial function. *Food Sci. Hum. Wellness* **2016**, *5*, 1–7. [CrossRef]

32. Ceriello, A. Possible role of oxidative stress in the pathogenesis of hypertension. *Diabetes Care* **2008**, *31*, 181–184. [CrossRef] [PubMed]
33. Kim, S.M.; Park, S.; Choue, R. Effects of fermented milk peptides supplement on blood pressure and vascular function in spontaneously hypertensive rats. *Food Sci. Biotechnol.* **2010**, *19*, 1409–1413. [CrossRef]
34. Yuan, W.; Wang, J.; Zhou, F. In vivo hypotensive and physiological effects of a silk fibroin hydrolysate on spontaneously hypertensive rats. *Biosci. Biotechnol. Biochem.* **2012**, *76*, 1987–1989. [CrossRef] [PubMed]
35. Erdmann, K.; Cheung, B.W.Y.; Schroder, H. The possible roles of food-derived bioactive peptides in reducing the risk of cardiovascular disease. *J. Nutr. Biochem.* **2008**, *19*, 643–654. [CrossRef] [PubMed]
36. Sarmadi, B.H.; Ismail, A. Antioxidative peptides from food proteins: A review. *Peptides* **2010**, *31*, 1949–1956. [CrossRef] [PubMed]
37. Hsieh, C.C.; Hernández-Ledesma, B.; Fernández-Tolomé, S.; Weinborn, V.; Barile, D.; de Moura, J.M.L. Milk proteins, peptides, and oligosaccharides: Effects against the 21st century disorders. *BioMed. Res. Int.* **2015**. [CrossRef] [PubMed]
38. Park, E.; Seo, B.Y.; Yoon, Y.C.; Lee, S.M. Beneficial effects of hydrolysates of whey proteins in spontaneously hypertensive rats. *J. Food Nutr. Res.* **2017**, *5*, 794–800. [CrossRef]

nutrients

MDPI

Article

Protective Effects of LSGYGP from Fish Skin Gelatin Hydrolysates on UVB-Induced MEFs by Regulation of Oxidative Stress and Matrix Metalloproteinase Activity

Qingyu Ma, Qiuming Liu, Ling Yuan and Yongliang Zhuang *

Yunnan Institute of Food Safety, Kunming University of Science and Technology, No. 727 South Jingming Road, Kunming 650500, Yunnan, China; mqy0323@hotmail.com (Q.M.); kgqml2012@163.com (Q.L.); ly15145551312@163.com (L.Y.)

* Correspondence: ylzhuang@kmust.edu.cn; Tel./Fax: +86-871-6592-0216

Received: 2 February 2018; Accepted: 26 March 2018; Published: 28 March 2018

Abstract: A previous study has shown that tilapia fish skin gelatin hydrolysates inhibited photoaging in vivo, and that, Leu-Ser-Gly-Tyr-Gly-Pro (LSGYGP) identified in the hydrolysate had a high hydroxyl radical scavenging activity. In this study, activities of LSGYGP were further evaluated using ultraviolet B (UVB)-induced mouse embryonic fibroblasts (MEFs). UVB irradiation significantly increased the intercellular reactive oxygen species (ROS) production and matrix metalloproteinases (MMPs) activities and decreased the content of collagen in MEFs. LSGYGP reduced the intercellular ROS generation in UVB-induced MEFs. Meanwhile, the decrease of superoxide dismutase (SOD) activity and the increase of malondiaidehyde (MDA) content were inhibited by LSGYGP. LSGYGP reduced MMP-1 and MMP-9 activities in a dose-dependent manner. Molecular docking simulation indicated that LSGYGP inhibited MMPs activities by docking the active sites of MMP-1 and MMP-9. Furthermore, LSGYGP also affected the intercellular phosphorylation of UVB-induced the mitogen-activated protein kinase pathway. LSGYGP could protect collagen synthesis in MEFs under UVB irradiation by inhibiting oxidative stress and regulating MMPs activities.

Keywords: LSGYGP; UVB radiation; oxidant stress; matrix metalloproteinases; MAPK pathway

1. Introduction

Ultraviolet (UV) irradiation, including ultraviolet A (UVA) (315–400 nm) and ultraviolet B (UVB) (290–320 nm), can generate reactive oxygen species (ROS)/nitrogen species. Excessive oxidative stress can cause photoaging and even apoptotic or necrotic skin cell death [1]. Compared with UVA, UVB irradiation produces greater biological effects. UVB may pass through the epidermis, penetrate the upper part of the dermis, and induce the generation of excessive ROS [2]. The matrix metalloproteinases (MMPs) are a family of zinc-dependent endopeptidases and can degrade all components of extracellular matrix protein and connective tissues [3]. UV irradiation increases MMPs expression and protein kinases phosphorylation by mitogen-activated protein kinases (MAPK) pathway, which causes intercellular collagen destruction. Three distinct MAPK signal transduction pathways, including extracellular signal-regulated kinases (ERKs), c-Jun N-terminal kinases (JNKs), and p38, have important effects on signaling pathways that regulate MMPs expression [4].

ROS scavengers inhibit the intercellular UVB-induced damage by attenuating MMPs activity. The decline of ROS plays a role in photoaging activities and is possibly via the suppression of MMPs production [5,6]. In recent years, most studies focus on peptides derived from marine animal sources, including jumbo squid skin [7], pacific hake [8], spiny head croaker [9], sea cucumber [10], which possess good radical scavenging activities. Furthermore, previous studies showed that some peptides have good inhibitory photoaging activities. Zhuang et al. [11] showed that jellyfish collagen peptides could protect collagen fibers of photoaged mice skin. Chen et al. [12] indicated that hydrolysates from Pacific cod skin could block the up-regulation of MMPs expression in photoaging mice. Some studies showed that peptides from different sources have inhibitory MMPs activities in cells [13–16]. Chen et al. [13] reported that Chlorella-derived peptide had MMP-1 inhibitory activity in human skin fibroblast irradiated with UVB. Nguyen et al. [14] found that AELPSLPG had the MMPs inhibitory effects on the human fibrosarcoma. Ryu et al. [15] discovered that the peptide LEDPFDKDDWDNWK from sea horse inhibited the MMP expression in osteoblastic MG-63 cell. Lu et al. [16] reported that the hydrolysates from cod skin gelatin inhibited MMP-1 activity in UVB-induced mice fibroblasts, and two peptides (GEIGPSGGRGKPGKDGDAGPK and GFSGLDGAKGD) were identified.

A number of compounds can decrease MMPs activities by docking the active sites of MMPs [17]. A structure-activity relationship study is required to determine the interaction between peptides and MMP catalytic sites. It could be a powerful technology to use the structure-activity relationship for development of MMPs inhibitor using molecular docking simulation.

In our previous study, the effect of tilapia skin gelatin hydrolysates (TGHs) on UV-induced mice skin damages was determined. The results showed that TGHs regulated the UV-induced abnormal changes of antioxidant indicators in photoaging mice. TGHs could protect mice skin collagen fibers from UV irradiation damages. The action mechanisms of TGHs mainly involved antioxidant abilities and repaired to endogenous collagen synthesis. Fractionation of TGH led to the identification of peptide LSGYGP which displayed a high hydroxyl radical scavenging activity [18]. In this study, we aim to study the protective effects of LSGYGP on intercellular collagen formation, ROS generation and MMP levels in UVB-induced mouse embryonic fibroblasts (MEFs). The interaction between MMP active sites and LSGYGP was analyzed by molecular docking simulation. Furthermore, the regulation of LSGYGP on the intercellular phosphorylation of the MAPK signal pathway was studied.

2. Materials and Methods

2.1. Materials and Regents

LSGYGP was provided by Shanghai Synpeptide Co., Ltd. (Shanghai, China). Fetal bovine serum (FBS), dulbecco's modified Eagle's medium (DMEM), phosphate buffered saline (PBS), and trypsin (0.25%) were purchased from Gibco (New York, NY, USA). 3-(4,5 dimethylthiazol-2-yl)-2,5-diphenyltetrazolium bromide (MTT) was provided from Sigma Chemical Co. (St. Louis, MO, USA). 2′,7′-dichlorodihydrofluorescein diacetate ROS assay kit was purchased from Beyotime Biotechnology Co., Ltd. (Shanghai, China). Superoxide dismutase (SOD) and malondialdehyde (MDA) commercial kits were provided from Nanjing Jiancheng Institute of Biotechnology (Nanjing, China). The ELISA kits of Collagen I, MMP-1, MMP-9, p-JNK, p-ERK, and p-p38 were purchased from R&D (Systems Inc., Minneapolis, MN, USA).

2.2. Cell Culture

MEFs were isolated from the dermis of ICR fetal mice according to the previous method [16,19] and cultured in 5% CO_2 at 37 °C in DMEM with FBS (10%, *v*/*v*), penicillin (100 U/mL), and streptomycin (100 mg/L). The generations 5–7 of MEFs were selected for further assays.

2.3. UVB Irradiation and Cell Viability Assay

MEFs (2×10^4 cells/well) were plated in 96-well plates containing DMEM with FBS (10%, *v*/*v*) and incubated in 5% CO_2 at 37 °C for 24 h. MEFs were further incubated in culture medium with LSGYGP (20, 40 and 80 μM) for 24 h, and then the cells were placed in a thin layer of PBS. MEFs-treated were exposed to UVB using two lamps (Beijing Zhongyiboteng-tech Co., Ltd., Beijing, China) that emitted UVB peaking at 313 nm, which delivered uniform irradiation at a distance of 30 cm. MEFs were irradiated by UVB with a dose of 30 mJ/cm^2, which was determined with a UV-313 radiometer

(Photoelectric Instrument Factory of Beijing Normal University, China). The PBS was replaced by the culture medium with LSGYGP and incubated at 37 °C for an additional 12 h. Finally, MEFs and culture supernatants were obtained for further study. The normal control (NC) group was cultured at the same condition without UVB irradiation and LSGYGP, and the model control (MC) group was exposed to UVB irradiation without LSGYGP.

Cell viability was evaluated with MTT assay [20]. The collected cells were treated with 150 μL MTT reagents (0.5 mg/mL) for 4 h at 37 °C. Subsequently, the MTT reagent was removed, and the amount of MTT formazan was solubilised with 150 μL of dimethyl sulfoxide (DMSO). The absorbance of each well was measured using ELISA (Spectra Max M5; Molecular Devices, Winooski, VT, USA) at 570 nm.

2.4. Determination of Generated Intracellular ROS

The levels of intracellular ROS were determined with fluorescence assay using a DCFH-DA ROS assay kit [21]. MEFs (2 × 10^4 cells/well) were plated in 12-well plates, and UVB irradiation was the same with that in Section 2.3. The collected cells were resuspended in freshly prepared serum-free medium that contained 10 μM DCFH-DA at 37 °C for 20 min in the dark. MEFs were then harvested and washed with PBS. The oxidative formation of DCFH-DA via intracellular ROS was immediately examined at λex of 485 nm and λem of 535 nm using a flow cytometer (Guava easyCyte 6-2L; EMD Millipore, Hayward, CA, USA). The result was expressed by relative content compared with that of the NC group.

2.5. Analysis of Intracellular SOD and MDA

MEFs (2 × 10^4 cells/well) were plated in 12-well plates, and the UVB irradiation was the same with that in Section 2.3. The collected cells resuspended in PBS and lysates were prepared under ultrasonic and centrifuged. The supernatants were quantified using BCA protein assay. Intracellular SOD activity and MDA content was measured by the respective kits, and they were expressed by U/mg protein (prot) and nM/mg prot.

2.6. ELISA Assays of Collagen I, MMP-1, and MMP-9

MEFs (2 × 10^4 cells/well) were plated in 6-well plates, and the UVB irradiation was same with that in Section 2.3. The culture supernatants were collected and the collagen I content and the MMP-1 and MMP-9 activities were determined by ELISA, which were performed according to the manufacturer's protocol of the respective kits.

2.7. Molecular Docking Analysis

The three-dimensional structures of MMP-1 (966c.pdb) and MMP-9 (1gkc.pdb) were obtained from the Protein Data Bank. Water molecules were removed, and the cofactors zinc and chloride atoms were retained in the MMPs model [22]. The structure of LSGYGP was built by using SYBYL2.1.1 software (Tripos Associates, St. Louis, MO, USA). Hydrogen atoms were added to crystal structures 966c and 1gkc in SYBYL. The docking of LSGYGP onto the active sites of MMP-1 and MMP-9 was performed by molecular visualization. T-score, C-score, hydrogen bond, and distance were calculated by SYBYL [22].

2.8. ELISA Analysis of JNK, ERK, and p38

MEFs (2 × 10^4 cells/well) were plated in 6-well plates, and the UVB irradiation was the same with that in Section 2.3. The collected cells were lysed by rapid freezing and thawing, and the contents of p-ERK, p-JNK, and p-p38 were tested by respective kits, which were operated according to the manufacturer's protocol.

2.9. Statistical Analysis

The outcomes for cell viability, collagen production, intercellualar SOD activity and MDA content, ROS production, MMPs activity and phosphorylation of MAPK were presented as the mean value with standard deviation. The significant differences between different groups were analyzed with multiple comparison test using SPSS (version 17.0, IBM Inc., Chicago, IL, USA). The statistical differences were considered significant at $p < 0.05$ and the significant differences were expressed using different lowercase letters. The molecular docking visualization, T-score, C-score, hydrogen bond and distance were evaluated by SYBYL 2.1.1 software (Tripos, Associaties, Inc., St. Louis, MO, USA).

3. Results

3.1. Cell Viability

As shown in Figure 1, the effect of LSGYGP on the viability of MEFs was determined. UVB irradiation significantly decreased the viability of MEFs compared with that of the NC group ($p < 0.05$). LSGYGP had high protective effect on cell viability against UV irradiation, and the effect of LSGYGP was in a dose-dependent manner. LSGYGP with a dose of 40 µM had significantly different with MC group ($p < 0.05$).

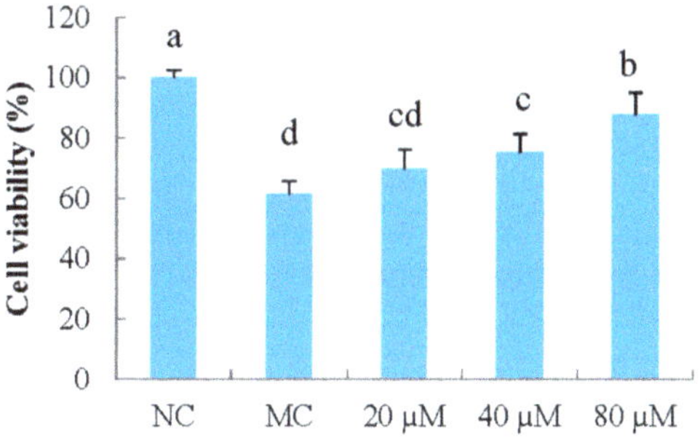

Figure 1. The effect of LSGYGP with different concentrations (20, 40, 80 µM) on cell viability in mouse embryonic fibrolasts (MEFs) ultraviolet B (UVB)-induced. Bar values with different letters were significant difference ($p < 0.05$). NC: nomal control; MC: model control.

3.2. Collagen I

Figure 2 shows different concentrations of LSGYGP inhibiting decrease in collagen content in MEFs UVB-induced. Compared with that of NC group, the collagen content of MC group significantly decreased by 56.2% ($p < 0.05$). LSGYGP potently increased the collagen production in MEFs, and the effect was in a dose-dependent manner. Intracellular collagen contents were significantly increased more than twice at LSGYGP with the concentration of 80 µM compared with that of MC group.

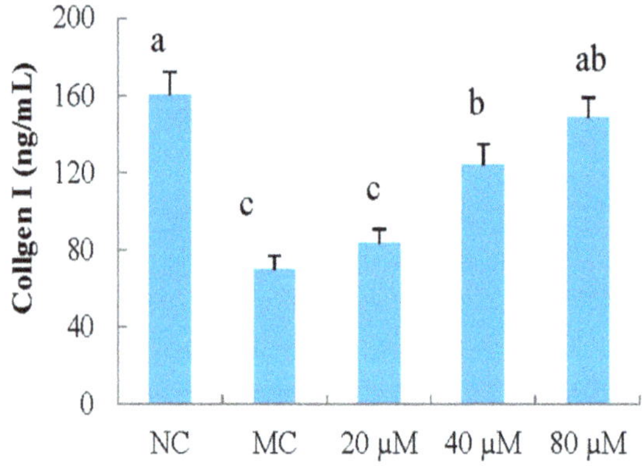

Figure 2. The effect of LSGYGP on collagen production in mouse embryonic fibrolasts (MEFs) ultraviolet B (UVB)-induced. Bar values with different letters were significant difference ($p < 0.05$).

3.3. Antioxidant Indicators

As shown in Figure 3A, the activities of SOD enzymes were decreased by UVB irradiation, and the activities of MC group decreased by 56.0% compared with that of NC group. LSGYGP protected intercellular SOD activities against the UVB damages in a dose-dependent manner. LSGYGP with a dose of 40 μM was significantly higher than that in MC group ($p < 0.05$).

The results (Figure 3B) showed that UVB irradiation caused the MDA content in MC group to increase by 136.4%, compared with that of NC group ($p < 0.05$). MDA increase was significantly inhibited by LSGYGP ($p < 0.05$), and the inhibitory ability of LSGYGP was in a dose-dependent manner. Compared with NC group, it had no significant difference with LSGYGP at a dose of 80 μM ($p > 0.05$).

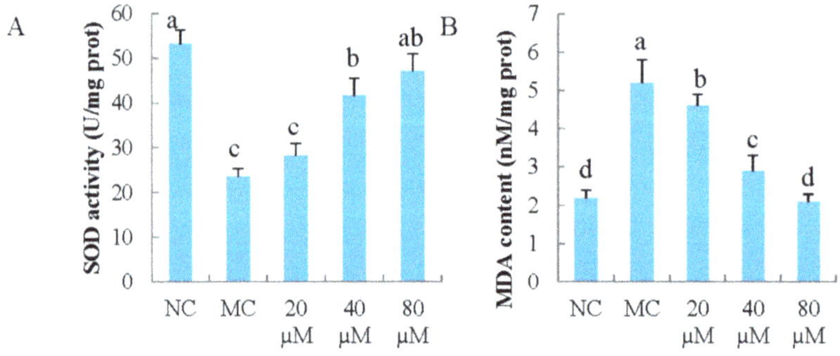

Figure 3. The effect of LSGYGP on intercellular superoxide dismutase (SOD) activity (**A**) and malondiaidehyde (MDA) content (**B**) in mouse embryonic fibrolasts (MEFs) ultraviolet B (UVB)-induced. Bar values with different letters were significant difference ($p < 0.05$).

3.4. ROS Generation

A previous study showed excessive ROS generation from UVB irradiation can induce photoaging [5]. In this study, the effect of LSGYGP on UVB-induced ROS production in MEFs was evaluated. The results showed that UVB irradiation markedly increased ROS production by 32.4%, compared with that in NC group (Figure 4). LSGYGP regulated the intercellular ROS generation under UVB irradiation, and this inhibitory activity was in a dose-dependent manner.

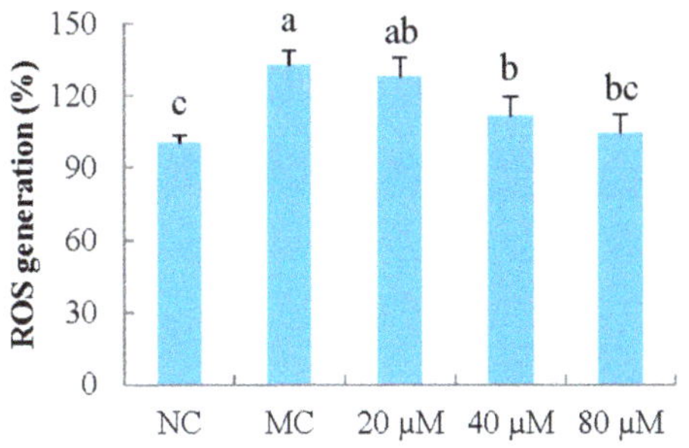

Figure 4. The effect of LSGYGP on intercellular reactive oxygen species (ROS) production in mouse embryonic fibrolasts (MEFs) ultraviolet B (UVB)-induced. Bar values with different letters were significant difference ($p < 0.05$).

3.5. *Intercellular MMP-1 and MMP-9 Activity*

As shown in Figure 5, UVB irradiation dramatically increased the activities of MMP-1 and MMP-9 in MEFs ($p < 0.05$). LSGYGP significantly decreased the up-regulated activities of MMP-1 and MMP-9 ($p < 0.05$) in a dose-dependent manner. Meanwhile, the LSGYGP with 40 μM group significantly inhibited of MMP-1 and MMP-9 activities ($p < 0.05$), compared with that of the MC group.

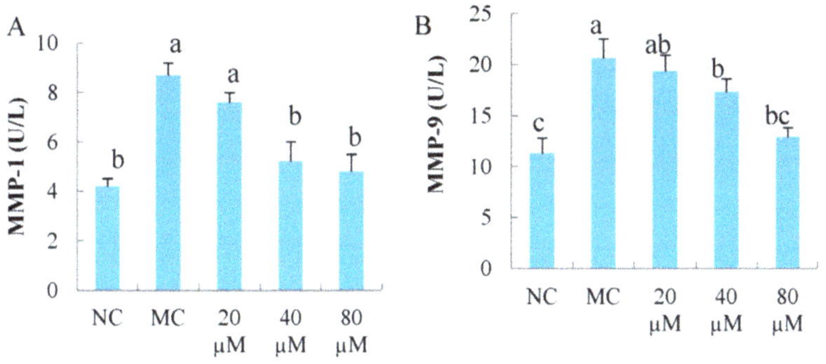

Figure 5. The effect of LSGYGP on intercellular matrix metalloprpteinases (MMP)-1 (**A**) and MMP-9 (**B**) activity in mouse embryonic fibrolasts (MEFs) ultraviolet B (UVB)-induced. Bar values with different letters were significant difference ($p < 0.05$).

3.6. *Molecular Docking*

Figure 6 shows the binding of LSGYGP at the active sites of MMP-1 and MMP-9. LSGYGP entered the narrow $S_1{}'$-subpocket and created strong interactions with the enzymes. The docking simulation of LSGYGP at the MMP-1 and MMP-9 active sites in the presence of Zn(II) showed the best docking pose, and the total scores were 7.30 and 8.53 (Table 1), respectively. Table 1 indicated the all possible direct hydrogen bond interactions. After docking, the peptide LSGYGP had eight hydrogen bonds with MMP-1 residues, including Glu219, Tyr240, Thr241, Tyr237, and Leu235. Seven hydrogen bonds of MMP-9 and LSGYGP were formed with Pro421, Leu188, Ala189, and Glu402, and four hydrogen bonds were formed between LSGYGP and Glu402 of MMP-9. The short 1.98 Å and 2.02 Å hydrogen bonds were found between LSGYGP and Zn(II) of MMP-1 and MMP-9, respectively.

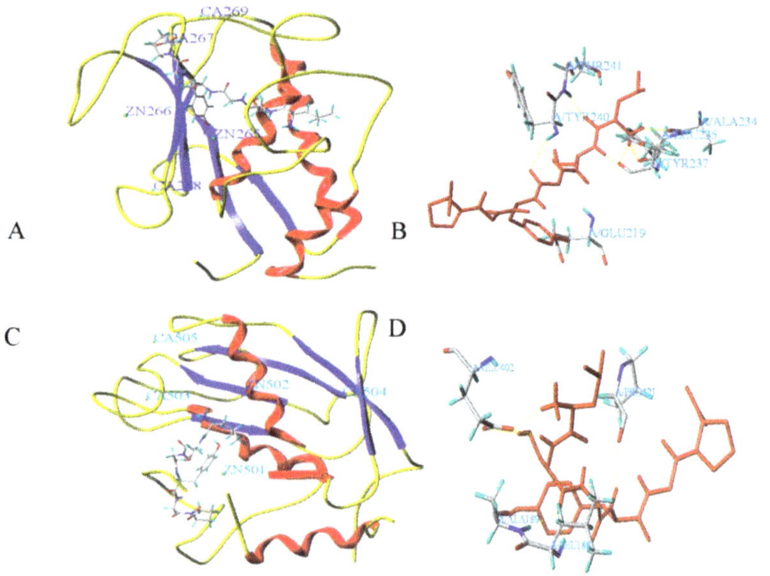

Figure 6. The molecular docking between LSGYGP and matrix metalloprpteinases (MMP). (**A**) and (**B**): docking of LSGYGP and MMP-1; (**C**) and (**D**): docking of LSGYGP and MMP-9.

Table 1. The data of molecular docking between LSGYGP and matrix metalloprpteinases (MMP).

LSGYGP	T-Score	C-Score	Hydrogen Bond Number	Distance (Å)
MMP-1	7.30	5	8	Glu219: 2.06; Tyr240: 2.62; Thr241: 2.02; Tyr237: 2.10/2.05; Leu235: 1.90/1.81/2.58 Zn265: 1.98
MMP-9	8.53	4	7	Pro421: 2.33; Leu188: 1.65; Ala189: 2.27; GLU402: 2.44/2.27/1.93/2.31; Zn1450: 2.02

3.7. The Phosphorylation of ERK, JNK, and p38 in MEFs

In this study, the effect of LSGYGP via the MAPK pathway on the up-regulated expressions of MMPs was investigated. As shown in Figure 7, UVB irradiation caused a significant increase in p-ERK, p-JNK, and p-p38 levels in MEFs ($p < 0.05$). LSGYGP regulated the phosphorylation of ERK, JNK, and p38 in a dose-dependent manner. A significant difference occurred in the phosphorylation of ERK, JNK, and p38 levels between LSGYGP with 80 μM group and MC group ($p < 0.05$). Our results indicated that LSGYGP could inhibit the phosphorylation of ERK, JNK, and p38 in the MAPK signaling pathway.

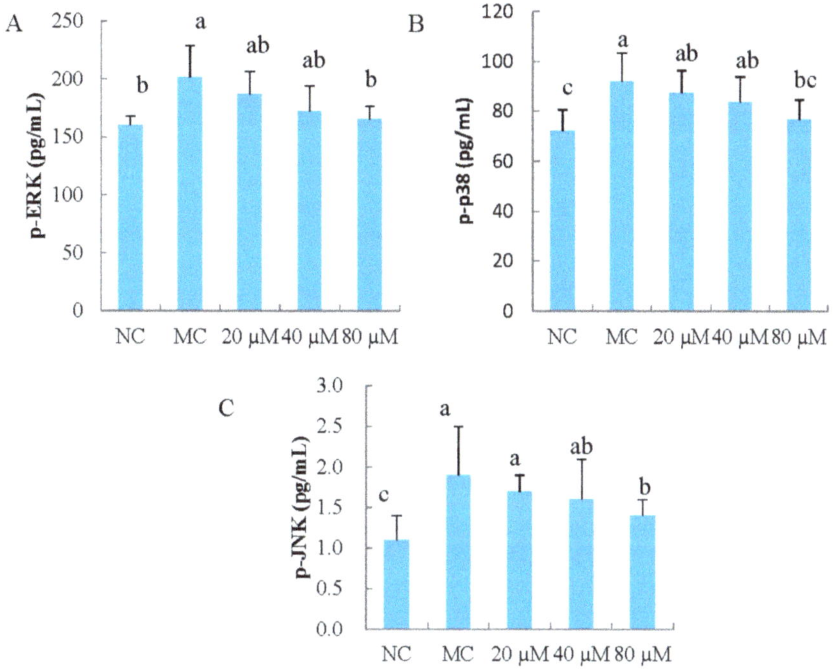

Figure 7. The effect of LSGYGP on the phosphorylation of extracellular signal-regulated kinases (ERK) (**A**), p38 (**B**) and jun N-terminal kinases (JNK) (**C**) of mitogen-activated protein kinases (MAPK) signaling pathway in mouse embryonic fibrolasts (MEFs) ultraviolet B (UVB)-induced. Bar values with different letters were significant difference ($p < 0.05$).

4. Discussion

In photoaging damage, the decrease of collagen formation is a main characteristic feature. UVB-irradiation increases the production of ROS within the cells. ROS plays a significant role in the declension of collagen synthesis [6]. In our previous study, TGHs was shown to inhibit photoaging damage changes in mice UV-induced model, and successive separation of TGHs led to the identification of LSGYGP that displayed a strong hydroxyl radical scavenging activity in vitro [18]. In this study, collagen in MEFs was severely destroyed by UVB irradiation, and the collagen content decreased by 47.9% after 30 mJ/cm^2 of UVB radiation. LSGYGP could significantly inhibit UVB-induced collagen decrease. The previous studies indicated UVB irradiation affected many biological functions involving the synthesis of MMPs [2]. MMPs can destroy collagen synthesis in the skin dermis. Concerning the action mechanisms of decreasing MMPs levels, the blocking of the MMP secretion and bonding of enzyme activity sites may be mainly involved in inhibiting the catalytic reaction of MMPs. Several studies reported peptides with Leu and Pro had high inhibitory MMPs activities [14,23], and LSGYGP was in accordance to this characteristic. To understand the potential mechanisms of the LSGYGP effects on photoaging, we study whether LSGYGP regulates oxidant stress and inhibits MMPs using MEFs UVB-induced model. Furthermore, the effect of LSGYGP of direct docking active sites of MMPs was evaluated.

Intracellular ROS content directly reflects reducing power in cells [6]. Compared with normal MEFs, UVB irradiation significantly increased intracellular ROS content in this study. LSGYGP can inhibit the increase of UVB-induced ROS significantly. In normal physiological conditions, the formation of oxidants is balanced by efficient removal of antioxidative enzymes, including SOD,

CAT, and GSH-Px. SOD is the initial enzyme in the enzymatic defense system in vivo and converts superoxide radicals into hydrogen peroxide [24]. The activities of intracellular SOD were decreased by UVB irradiation-induced ROS. LSGYGP can inhibit the decrease of SOD activities. Meanwhile, intercellular ROS UVB-induced enhances the oxidative stress of skin cell membrane lipids, which causes a large amount of lipid peroxidation product MDA. This process consequently induces skin photoaging [25]. In this study, the MDA UVB-induced was significantly decreased by LSGYGP. Therefore, LSGYGP could decrease intercellular lipid peroxidation damages UVB-induced and alleviate photo-oxidative stress of collagen production through regulating the activities of antioxidant enzymes. LSGYGP could affect the collagen metabolism of photoaging cells by the alleviation of intercellular oxidative stress.

The MMP family can cause the degradation of skin collagen and lead to photoaging. Currently, over 20 types of MMPs were divided into collagenases, matrilysins, gelatinases, stromelysins, and membrane-type MMPs, according to their function [26]. MMP-1 belongs to the collagenase and degrades collagen I, which is a major composition in the skin dermis. The increase of MMP-1 expression can cause skin collagen damage. Collagen is the richest protein in the dermal connective tissue and collagen is broken in pieces by MMP-1 [27]. Collagen fragments are further hydrolyzed via other MMPs, such as MMP-2 (gelatinase A) and MMP-9 (gelatinase B). A variety of naturally occurring agents, which have inhibitory MMPs ability, have been widely used to prevent photoaging [26]. Thus, finding of MMP-1 and MMP-9 inhibitors is considered as a promising strategy to increase the type I procollagen production for skin photoaging therapies. In this study, the cell viability and the activities of MMP-1 and MMP-9 of UVB-induced MEFs were examined. UVB irradiation could significantly attenuate MEFs death and increase the activities of intercellular MMP-1 and MMP-9 of MEFs by UV radiation. LSGYGP could regulate the abnormal changes during UVB irradiation.

Previous studies showed that the production of excessive ROS could affect the levels of MMPs [6]. Thus, the effect of LSGYGP on MMPs was due to its scavenging ROS ability. We are interested in finding out whether the LSGYGP has any direct interaction in the active sites of MMP-1 and MMP-9 proteins, which can suppress MMP-1 and MMP-9 activities. The structures of MMPs are similar, and the main differences occur in the S_1' pocket. The S_1' pocket of MMP-1 is short and narrow, and the S_1' specificity site in MMP-9 is described as tunnel [28,29]. The molecular docking simulation could be used as a tool to evaluate the mechanisms of molecular interactions between MMPs and LSGYGP. Our results showed that LSGYGP could enter the S_1'-subpocket of MMP-1 and MMP-9 and give strong interactions with the enzymes. The docking simulation of LSGYGP at the MMP-1 and MMP-9 active sites with Zn(II) displayed the best docking pose (Figure 6) with high T-score and right C-score. Hydrogen bonds interaction force is important in stabilizing the docking complex and catalytic reactions [28]. After docking, the peptide LSGYGP formed eight and seven hydrogen bonds with MMP-1 and MMP-9 residues, respectively. Previous studies showed that Tyr 240 and Thr 241 were key hydrophobic and polar amino acids of the S_1 pocket of MMP-1 [22], and the essential glutamic acid residue (402) was key to the catalytic center of MMP-9 [22,29]. Our results showed that LSGYGP could form hydrogen bonds with the Tyr 240 and Thr 241 of MMP-1 and the Glu 402 of MMP-9, respectively. The results suggested that LSGYGP effectively interacted with the active sites of MMPs, which enhanced its inhibitory MMPs activities. Zn(II) at the MMPs active sites often plays an important part for MMPs activity [22,28]. The distances of the oxygen atoms of LSGYGP and Zn(II) were determined in this study. The short 1.98 Å and 2.02 Å were found in MMP-1 and MMP-9, suggesting that LSGYGP could effectively interact with the active sites of MMPs and inhibit the enzymatic activity. Furthermore, LSGYGP had a hydrophobic amino acid (Pro) at the carboxy terminal and the aromatic group in Tyr, and the side chains of Pro and the aromatic group of Tyr may accommodate with the S_1' pocket of MMP-1 and MMP-9 and increase inhibitory MMPs potential.

Exposure to UVB irradiation has been shown to stimulate the phosphorylation of protein kinases by the MAPK pathway. The phosphorylation of MAPK pathway directly activates the transcription factor AP-1, which can increase the expression of MMPs. Thus, MAPK pathways play an important role in regulating MMP expression [30]. MAPKs contain three general classes, ERK, JNK, and p38 kinases. The phosphorylation of JNK can activate phospho-c-Jun. Phospho-c-Jun may form AP-1 and further enhance the expressions of MMPs. In addition, the phosphorylation of ERK activates the transcription of c-Fos and c-Jun, which are also known to form AP-1. In this study, we investigated whether the MMPs via the MAPK signaling pathway were influenced by LSGYGP. Our data suggested that LSGYGP regulated the phosphorylation of ERK, p38, and JNK in the MAPK pathway, thereby inhibiting the up-regulation of UVB-induced MMP expression. Therefore, the effect of LSGYGP on the MAPK signaling pathway may be one of the key mechanisms to suppress the up-regulated expression of MMPs caused by UVB irradiation.

5. Conclusions

LSGYGP showed high hydroxyl radical scavenging activities in our previous study. We further study the effects of LSGYGP on intercellular MMP activity and oxidative stress in UVB-induced MEFs. Our results indicated, for the first time, that the photoaging signs inhibitory activities of LSGYGP resulted from suppressing intercellular ROS generation, regulating intercellular reducing power, and decreasing the UVB-mediated expression of MMPs, thereby blocking the MAPK pathways. Furthermore, LSGYGP could bind to the active sites of MMP-1 and MMP-9, decrease their activities, and inhibit collagen degradation. Thus, LSGYGP may be a potential agent in tackling the signs of photoaging.

Acknowledgments: We gratefully thank the National Natural Science Foundation of China (Grant No. 31360381) for the financial support on this research.

Author Contributions: Yongliang Zhuang and Qingyu Ma conceived and designed the experiments; Qiuming Liu performed the cell experiments; Ling Yuan performed the molecular docking; Qingyu Ma and Qiuming Liu collected the data; Yongliang Zhuang and Qingyu Ma provided the reagents, analyzed the data and prepared the manuscript. All authors read and approved the final manuscript.

Conflicts of Interest: The authors declare no conflict of interest.

References

1. Fan, J.; Zhuang, Y.; Li, B. Effects of collagen and collagen hydrolysate from jellyfish umbrella on histological and immunity changes of mice photoaging. *Nutrients* **2013**, *5*, 223–233. [CrossRef] [PubMed]
2. Leirós, G.J.; Kusinsky, A.G.; Balañá, M.E.; Hagelin, K. Triolein reduces MMP-1 upregulation in dermal fibroblasts generated by ROS production in UVB-irradiated keratinocytes. *J. Dermatol. Sci.* **2017**, *85*, 124–130. [CrossRef] [PubMed]
3. Mohamed, M.A.; Jung, M.; Lee, S.M.; Lee, T.H.; Kim, J. Protective effect of Disporum sessile D. Don extract against UVB-induced photoaging via suppressing MMP-1 expression and collagen degradation in human skin cells. *J. Photochem. Photobiol. B* **2014**, *133*, 73–79. [CrossRef] [PubMed]
4. Chiang, H.M.; Lin, T.J.; Chiu, C.Y.; Chang, C.W.; Hsu, K.C.; Fan, P.C.; Wena, K.C. *Coffeaarabica* extract and its constituents prevent photoaging by suppressing MMPs expression and MAP kinase pathway. *Food Chem. Toxicol.* **2011**, *49*, 309–318. [CrossRef] [PubMed]
5. Hong, Y.F.; Lee, H.; Jung, B.J.; Jang, S.; Chung, D.K.; Kim, H. Lipoteichoic acid isolated from *Lactobacillus plantarum* down-regulates UV-induced MMP-1 expression and up-regulates type I procollagen through the inhibition of reactive oxygen species generation. *Mol. Immunol.* **2015**, *67*, 248–255. [CrossRef] [PubMed]
6. Muller, F.L.; Lustgarten, M.S.; Jang, Y.; Richardson, A.; Van Remmen, H. Trends in oxidative aging theories. *Free Radic. Biol. Med.* **2007**, *43*, 477–503. [CrossRef] [PubMed]
7. Mendis, E.; Rajapakse, N.; Byun, H.G.; Kim, S.K. Investigation of jumbo squid (*Dosidicus gigas*) skin gelatin peptides for their in vitro antioxidant effects. *Life Sci.* **2005**, *77*, 2166–2178. [CrossRef] [PubMed]
8. Cheung, I.W.Y.; Cheung, L.K.Y.; Tan, N.Y.; Li-Chan, E.C.Y. The role of molecular size in antioxidant activity of peptide fractions from Pacific hake (*Merlucciu sproductus*) hydrolysates. *Food Chem.* **2012**, *134*, 1297–1306. [CrossRef] [PubMed]

9. Song, R.; Shi, Q.; Gninguue, A.; Wei, R.; Luo, H. Purification and identification of a novel peptide derived from by-products fermentation of spiny head croaker (*Collichthys lucidus*) with antifungal effects on phytopathogens. *Process Biochem.* **2017**, *62*, 184–192. [CrossRef]
10. Zhou, X.; Wang, C.; Jiang, A. Antioxidant peptides isolated from sea cucumber *Stichopus Japonicus*. *Eur. Food Res. Technol.* **2012**, *234*, 441–447. [CrossRef]
11. Zhuang, Y.; Hou, H.; Zhao, X.; Zhang, Z.; Li, B. Effects of collagen and collagen hydrolysate from jellyfish (*Rhopilema esculentum*) on mice skin photoaging induced by UV irradiation. *J. Food Sci.* **2009**, *74*, H183–H188. [CrossRef] [PubMed]
12. Chen, T.; Hou, H.; Fan, Y.; Wang, S.; Chen, Q.; Si, L.; Li, B. Protective effect of gelatin peptides from pacific cod skin against photoaging by inhibiting the expression of MMPs via MAPK signaling pathway. *J. Photochem. Photobiol. B* **2016**, *165*, 34–41. [CrossRef] [PubMed]
13. Chen, C.L.; Liou, S.F.; Chen, S.J.; Shih, M.F. Protective effects of Chlorella-derived peptide on UVB-induced production of MMP-1 and degradation of procollagen genes in human skin fibroblasts. *Regul. Toxicol. Pharm.* **2011**, *60*, 112–119. [CrossRef] [PubMed]
14. Nguyen, V.T.; Qian, Z.J.; Ryu, B.M.; Kim, K.N.; Kim, D.; Kim, Y.M.; Jeon, Y.J.; Park, W.S.; Choi, I.W.; Kim, G.H.; et al. Matrix metalloproteinases (MMPs) inhibitory effects of an octameric oligopeptide isolated from abalone Haliotis discus hannai. *Food Chem.* **2013**, *141*, 503–509. [CrossRef] [PubMed]
15. Ryu, B.M.; Qian, Z.J.; Kim, S.K. Purification of a peptide from seahorse, that inhibits TPA-induced MMP, iNOS and COX-2 expression through MAPK and NF-kappaB activation, and induces human osteoblastic and chondrocytic differentiation. *Chem. Biol. Int.* **2010**, *184*, 413–422. [CrossRef] [PubMed]
16. Lu, J.; Hou, H.; Fan, Y.; Yang, T.; Li, B. Identification of MMP-1 inhibitory peptides from cod skin gelatin hydrolysates and the inhibition mechanism by MAPK signaling pathway. *J. Func. Foods* **2017**, *33*, 251–260. [CrossRef]
17. Parthasarathy, A.; Gopi, V.; Devi, K.M.S.; Balaji, N.; Vellaichamy, E. Aminoguanidine inhibits ventricular fibrosis and remodeling process in isoproterenol-induced hypertrophied rat hearts by suppressing ROS and MMPs. *Life Sci.* **2014**, *118*, 15–26. [CrossRef] [PubMed]
18. Sun, L.; Zhang, Y.; Zhuang, Y. Antiphotoaging effect and purification of an antioxidant peptide from tilapia (*Oreochromis niloticus*) gelatin peptides. *J. Func. Foods* **2013**, *5*, 154–162. [CrossRef]
19. Ren, S.W.; Li, J.; Wang, W.; Guan, H.S. Protective effects of j-ca3000 + CP against ultraviolet-induced damage in HaCaT and MEF cells. *J. Photochem. Photobiol. B.* **2010**, *101*, 22–30. [CrossRef] [PubMed]
20. Huang, S.; Ma, Y.; Sun, D.; Fan, J.; Cai, S. In vitro DNA damage protection and anti-inflammatory effects of Tartary buckwheats (*FagopyrumtataricumL. Gaertn*) fermented by filamentous fungi. *Int. J. Food Sci. Technol.* **2017**, *52*, 2006–2017. [CrossRef]
21. Zhuang, Y.; Ma, Q.; Guo, Y.; Sun, L. Protective effects of rambutan (*Nephelium lappaceum*) peel phenolics on H_2O_2-induced oxidative damages in HepG2 cells and d-galactose-induced aging mice. *Food Chem. Toxicol.* **2017**, *108*, 554–562. [CrossRef] [PubMed]
22. Sun, L.; Liu, Q.; Fan, J.; Li, X.; Zhuang, Y. Purification and Characterization of Peptides Inhibiting MMP-1 Activity with C Terminate of Gly-Leu from Simulated Gastrointestinal Digestion Hydrolysates of Tilapia (*Oreochromis niloticus*) Skin Gelatin. *J. Agric. Food Chem.* **2018**, *66*, 593–601.
23. Roomi, M.W.; Ivanov, V.; Niedzwiecki, A.; Rath, M. Synergistic antitumor effect of ascorbic acid, lysine, proline, and epigallocatechin gallate on human fibrosarcoma cells HT1080. *Ann. Cancer Res. Ther.* **2004**, *12*, 146–156. [CrossRef]
24. Hou, H.; Li, B.; Zhao, X.; Zhuang, Y.; Ren, G.; Yan, M.; Zhang, X.; Chen, L.; Fan, Y. The effect of pacific cod (*Gadusmacrocephalus*) skin gelatin polypeptides on UV radiation induced skin photoaging in ICR mice. *Food Chem.* **2009**, *115*, 945–950. [CrossRef]
25. Ma, Q.; Guo, Y.; Sun, L.; Zhuang, Y. Anti-diabetic effects of phenolic extract from rambutan peels (*Nephelium lappaceum*) in high-fat diet and streptozotocin-induced diabetic mice. *Nutrients* **2017**, *9*, 801. [CrossRef]
26. Fanjul-Fernández, M.; Folgueras, A.R.; Cabrera, S.; López-Otín, C. Matrix metalloproteinases: Evolution, gene regulation and functional analysis in mouse models. *Biochim. Biophys. Acta* **2010**, *1803*, 3–19. [CrossRef] [PubMed]

27. You, G.E.; Jung, B.J.; Kim, H.R.; Kim, H.G.; Kim, T.R.; Chung, D.K. Lactobacillus sakei lipoteichoic acid inhibits MMP-1 induced by UVA in normal dermal fibroblasts of human. *J. Microbiol. Biotechnol.* **2013**, *23*, 1357–1364. [CrossRef] [PubMed]
28. Yuan, H.; Lu, W.; Wang, L.; Shan, L.; Li, H.; Huang, J.; Sun, Q.; Zhang, W. Synthesis of derivatives of methyl rosmarinate and their inhibitory activities against matrix metalloproteinase-1 (MMP-1). *Eur. J. Med. Chem.* **2013**, *62*, 148–157. [CrossRef] [PubMed]
29. Sarkar, J.; Nandy, S.K.; Chowdhury, A.; Chakraborti, T.; Chakraborti, S. Inhibition of MMP-9 by green tea catechins and prediction of their interaction by molecular docking analysis. *Biomed. Pharm.* **2016**, *84*, 340–347. [CrossRef] [PubMed]
30. Chao, W.; Deng, J.; Huang, S.; Li, P.; Liang, Y.; Huang, G. 3, 4-dihydroxybenzalacetone attenuates lipopolysaccharide-induced inflammation in acute lung injury via down-regulation of MMP-2 and MMP-9 activities through suppressing ROS-mediated MAPK and PI3K/AKT signaling pathways. *Int. Immunopharm.* **2017**, *50*, 77–86. [CrossRef] [PubMed]

nutrients

Article

Stability of Antiradical Activity of Protein Extracts and Hydrolysates from Dry-Cured Pork Loins with Probiotic Strains of LAB

Paulina Kęska and Joanna Stadnik *

Department of Animal Raw Materials Technology, Faculty of Food Science and Biotechnology, University of Life Sciences in Lublin, Skromna 8, 20-704 Lublin, Poland; paulina.keska@up.lublin.pl

* Correspondence: joanna.stadnik@up.lublin.pl; Tel.: +48-81-462-3341

Received: 2 March 2018; Accepted: 19 April 2018; Published: 22 April 2018

Abstract: The application of starter cultures to improve quality and safety has become a very common practice in the meat industry. Probiotic strains of lactic acid bacteria (LAB) can also bring health benefits by releasing bioactive peptides. The aim of this work was to evaluate the stability of antiradical activity of protein extracts from LAB-inoculated dry-cured pork loins during long-term aging and evaluate their hydrolysates after simulated gastrointestinal digestion. Analyses of hydrolysates by using liquid chromatography-tandem mass spectrometry (LC-MS/MS) were strengthened with in silico analysis. The highest antiradical activity of the protein extracts was observed after 180 days of aging. The influence of the strain used (LOCK, BAUER, or BB12) on the inactivation ability of ABTS radicals varied during long-term aging. The IC_{50} values indicated the higher antiradical properties of salt-soluble (SSF) compared to water-soluble fraction (WSF) of proteins. The peptides generated by in vitro digestion have MW between 700 and 4232 Da and their length ranged from 5 to 47 amino acids in a sequence where Leu, Pro, Lys, Glu, and His had the largest share. This study demonstrates that the degradation of pork muscle proteins during gastrointestinal digestion may give rise to a wide variety of peptides with antiradical properties.

Keywords: antiradical peptides; dry-cured meat products; in vitro digestion

1. Introduction

During the last several decades, the application of starter cultures has become a common practice in the production of more consistent and stable fermented meat products in order to improve their quality and safety, reduce variability, and enhance sensory characteristics. The starter groups used in meat fermentation are, by order of importance, lactic acid bacteria (LAB) (mainly *Lactobacillus* spp. and *Pediococcus* spp.), nonpathogenic coagulase-negative staphylococci (primarily *Staphylococcus* spp. and *Kocuria* spp.), molds (*Penicillium*), and yeasts (*Debaryomyces*) [1,2]. LAB play a significant role in meat fermentation by creating unfavorable conditions for pathogens and spoilage microorganisms via several mechanisms of action (e.g., competition for nutrients and living place on the product) or the production of substances inhibiting their growth especially lactic acid and/or acetic acid, acetoin, diacetyl, hydrogen peroxide, and bacteriocins. This contributes to product stability and safety [3,4]. The production of lactic acid also has a direct impact on the sensory properties of the product by providing a mild acidic taste and by supporting the drying process, which requires a sufficient decline in pH. Moreover, LAB influence the sensory characteristics of the fermented meats by producing small amounts of acetic acid, ethanol, acetoin, carbon dioxide, pyruvic acid, and their ability to initiate the production of aromatic compounds from proteinaceous precursors. Microorganisms other than LAB involved in meat fermentation mainly bring about and stabilize the desired sensory properties [5].

Use of probiotic starter cultures for the production of fermented meat products has attracted attention in recent years [6]. Probiotic LAB strains, in addition to shaping the technological and sensory characteristics of the product, can also bring health benefits [7]. Recent studies involving the use of LAB strains with probiotic properties, i.e., *Lactobacillus rhamnosus* LOCK900 (LOCK), *Bifidobacterium animalis* spp. *lactis* BB12 (BB12) and a potentially probiotic strain *Lactobacillus acidophilus* Bauer Ł0938 (BAUER) have confirmed the suitability of using them in dry-cured meat product formulations, which underlines their favorable effects on hygienic quality and sensory characteristics of the products [8,9]. Regardless of the health benefits of LAB bacteria strains resulting due to their probiotic character, the proteolytic system of LAB is very efficient in releasing bioactive peptides from food proteins [10,11]. Meat protein-derived bioactive peptides are promising candidates for ingredients of functional meat products [12]. Bioactive peptides are inactive in the parent protein sequence until they are released by enzymatic hydrolysis. This process occurs naturally within the gastrointestinal tract during normal metabolism of dietary proteins. The same process happens during fermentation or aging in meat processing [13,14]. Previous in silico studies have shown that pork meat has great potential for influencing the physiological functions of the body as a source of peptides with biological activities such as antioxidative or angiotensin I-converting enzyme (ACE) inhibitory properties as well as dipeptidyl peptidase IV (DPP-4) inhibitors [15]. Bioactive peptides exhibiting ACE inhibitory activity have been found after in vitro digestion of Spanish dry-cured ham by gastrointestinal proteases [16]. Moreover, the in vivo antihypertensive activity of bioactive peptides of dry-cured ham has been reported in animal models of hypertension [17]. Recent studies suggest that dry-cured ham rich in bioactive peptides may exert a plethora of activities over the cardiovascular system including lipid and glucose metabolism in healthy subjects with pre-hypertension [18].

Our preceding study [19] demonstrated that inoculation with the above mentioned probiotic or potentially probiotic strains of LAB influenced the antioxidant activity of peptides isolated from dry-cured pork loins. Since aging time and gastrointestinal digestion influence the activity of bioactive peptides, the study of the antiradical activity during aging and after in vitro gastrointestinal digestion would be of interest. Consequently, the aim of this study was to evaluate the stability of antiradical activity (by ABTS assay) of protein extracts from LAB-inoculated dry-cured pork loins during long-term aging and evaluate their hydrolysates after simulated gastrointestinal digestion with pepsin and pancreatin. Analyses of hydrolysates with the highest antiradical properties using liquid chromatography-tandem mass spectrometry (LC-MS/MS) were strengthened by in silico analysis.

2. Results and Discussion

The significance levels of the factors included in the experiment and obtained by the ANOVA are presented in Table 1. Treatment (inoculation), aging time, and the interaction between them showed a significant effect on proteolytic changes expressed as primary amino groups (-NH_2) and antiradical activity (ABTS) before and after each step of in vitro gastrointestinal digestion and simulated absorption of dry-cured loins.

Table 1. Significance levels showed by the experimental factors and their interactions for the antiradical activity of dry-cured loins during long-term aging and in vitro gastrointestinal digestion.

Factor	-NH_2 (μM/mL)		Antiradical Activity			
			(%)		IC_{50} (μM/mL)	
	WSF	SSF	WSF	SSF	WSF	SSF
			before digestion			
Treatment (T)	**	**	**	**	**	**
Aging time (S)	**	**	**	**	**	**
TxS	**	**	**	**	**	n.s.

Table 1. *Cont.*

Factor	-NH_2 (μM/mL)		Antiradical Activity			
			(%)		IC_{50} (μM/mL)	
	WSF	SSF	WSF	SSF	WSF	SSF
			after pepsin hydrolysis			
Treatment (T)	**	**	**	**	**	n.s.
Aging time (S)	**	**	**	**	**	**
TxS	**	**	**	**	**	*
			after pepsin/pancreatin hydrolysis			
Treatment (T)	**	**	**	**	**	**
Aging time (S)	**	**	**	**	**	**
TxS	**	**	**	**	**	**
			after simulated absorption			
Treatment (T)	**	**	**	**	**	**
Aging time (S)	**	**	**	**	**	**
TxS	**	**	**	**	**	**

-NH_2, the content of primary amino groups; WSF, water-soluble fraction; SSF, salt-soluble fraction; * $p < 0.05$; ** $p < 0.01$; n.s.: not significant.

2.1. *Stability of Antiradical Activity during Long-Term Aging*

The highest antiradical activity against ABTS (%) was noted with the protein fractions extracted from dry-cured loins after 180 days of aging (see Table 2). However, the influence of either the strain used (LOCK, BAUER, or BB12) or the aging time on the inactivation ability of radicals generated from ABTS was ambiguous. Generally, the increase of antiradical activity of protein extracts up to 180 days of aging (expressed as percentage scavenging activity) was observed and followed by a systematic decrease during further aging stages. As far as WSF is concerned, at the first sampling point (after 28 days of aging), the highest antiradical activity ($p < 0.05$) was noted for the LOCK sample (69.94%).

Table 2. Antiradical activity of protein extracts obtained from undigested dry-cured pork loins (mean ± standard deviation).

Sample	Aging Time (Days)	WSF			SSF		
		-NH_2 (μM/mL)	Radical Scavenging (%)	IC_{50} (μM/mL)	-NH_2 (μM/mL)	Radical Scavenging (%)	IC_{50} (μM/mL)
C	28	8.08 ^{a,A} ± 0.04	65.63 ^{a,A} ± 2.14	0.28 ^{a,A} ± 0.01	6.22 ^{a,A} ± 0.83	65.30 ^{a,A} ± 1.87	0.26 ^{a,A} ± 0.03
	90	8.54 ^{a,A} ± 0.17	72.78 ^{b,A} ± 1.08	0.30 ^{a,A} ± 0.01	9.04 ^{b,A,B} ± 0.66	65.60 ^{a,A} ± 2.20	0.20 ^{b,A} ± 0.02
	180	16.10 ^{b,A} ± 1.20	79.14 ^{c,A,D} ± 1.35	0.29 ^{a,A} ± 0.01	7.72 ^{a,b,A} ± 0.82	75.70 ^{b,A} ± 1.44	0.14 ^{c,A} ± 0.01
	270	18.68 ^{c,A} ± 0.86	64.23 ^{a,A,B} ± 1.81	1.02 ^{b,A} ± 0.01	7.27 ^{a,b,A} ± 0.84	59.24 ^{c,A} ± 1.22	0.30 ^{d,A} ± 0.01
	360	29.96 ^{d,A} ± 1.22	59.15 ^{d,A} ± 0.66	2.40 ^{c,A} ± 0.11	11.21 ^{c,A} ± 0.82	51.29 ^{d,A} ± 1.11	0.35 ^{e,A} ± 0.01
LOCK	28	9.02 ^{a,A} ± 0.41	69.94 ^{a,B} ± 2.40	0.23 ^{a,B} ± 0.01	5.57 ^{a,A,B} ± 0.53	62.60 ^{a,B} ± 3.22	0.18 ^{a,B} ± 0.02
	90	9.68 ^{a,B} ± 0.45	75.55 ^{b,A,B} ± 2.26	0.24 ^{a,B} ± 0.01	7.42 ^{a,b,A} ± 1.12	66.96 ^{b,A,B} ± 1.38	0.14 ^{b,B} ± 0.01
	180	17.61 ^{b,A} ± 2.36	78.82 ^{b,A} ± 2.93	0.33 ^{a,B} ± 0.01	7.10 ^{a,b,A} ± 0.76	76.42 ^{c,A} ± 3.31	0.11 ^{c,B} ± 0.01
	270	21.31 ^{c,B} ± 0.05	66.27 ^{c,A} ± 2.28	1.42 ^{b,B} ± 0.08	7.34 ^{a,b,A} ± 0.01	56.54 ^{d,B} ± 1.41	0.35 ^{d,B} ± 0.01
	360	23.44 ^{d,B} ± 0.94	62.48 ^{d,B} ± 1.61	1.68 ^{c,B} ± 0.13	10.78 ^{b,B} ± 0.63	48.82 ^{e,B} ± 0.96	0.28 ^{e,B} ± 0.01
BAUER	28	10.28 ^{a,B} ± 0.95	65.53 ^{a,A} ± 2.38	0.28 ^{a,A} ± 0.02	6.46 ^{a,A} ± 0.18	56.35 ^{a,C} ± 2.53	0.28 ^{a,A} ± 0.03
	90	9.37 ^{a,A,B} ± 0.20	77.53 ^{b,B} ± 2.42	0.27 ^{a,C} ± 0.01	8.90 ^{b,A,C} ± 0.80	66.17 ^{b,A,B} ± 0.39	0.24 ^{a,C} ± 0.01
	180	20.62 ^{b,A} ± 1.83	83.89 ^{c,C} ± 1.86	0.27 ^{a,C} ± 0.01	11.22 ^{c,B} ± 0.29	63.55 ^{c,B} ± 2.31	0.18 ^{b,C} ± 0.05
	270	22.76 ^{b,C} ± 1.21	62.89 ^{d,B} ± 1.13	1.46 ^{b,B,C} ± 0.16	10.78 ^{c,B} ± 0.36	68.68 ^{d,C} ± 1.62	0.35 ^{c,B} ± 0.03
	360	30.91 ^{c,A} ± 0.71	61.52 ^{d,A,B} ± 1.11	1.66 ^{b,B} ± 0.16	12.58 ^{c,A} ± 1.22	43.31 ^{e,C} ± 1.18	0.34 ^{c,B} ± 0.01
BB12	28	10.68 ^{a,B} ± 0.15	64.99 ^{a,A} ± 2.33	0.29 ^{a,A} ± 0.01	4.95 ^{a,B} ± 0.45	60.04 ^{a,D} ± 1.63	0.20 ^{a,B} ± 0.01
	90	10.89 ^{a,C} ± 0.56	76.12 ^{b,B} ± 3.53	0.29 ^{a,A} ± 0.01	10.31 ^{b,B,C} ± 2.62	67.83 ^{b,B} ± 2.70	0.18 ^{a,D} ± 0.01
	180	17.63 ^{b,A} ± 1.30	81.17 ^{c,D} ± 1.10	0.22 ^{a,D} ± 0.01	9.47 ^{b,c,B} ± 0.56	72.31 ^{c,C} ± 1.41	0.13 ^{b,A} ± 0.01
	270	26.26 ^{c,D} ± 0.02	74.12 ^{b,C} ± 1.41	1.79 ^{b,C} ± 0.16	7.04 ^{c,A} ± 0.61	62.50 ^{d,D} ± 1.52	0.26 ^{c,A} ± 0.17
	360	29.07 ^{c,A} ± 2.32	61.42 ^{d,A,B} ± 0.70	1.66 ^{b,B} ± 0.16	10.22 ^{b,A,B} ± 0.62	51.70 ^{e,A,B} ± 2.41	0.25 ^{c,A} ± 0.01

-NH_2, the content of primary amino groups; WSF, water-soluble fraction; SSF, salt-soluble fraction; C, control sample; LOCK, sample inoculated with *Lactobacillus rhamnosus* LOCK900; BAUER, sample inoculated with *Lactobacillus acidophilus* Bauer Ł0938; BB12, sample inoculated with *Bifidobacterium animalis* ssp. *lactis* BB-12; $^{a–e}$ Within the same treatment, means followed by a common letter do not differ significantly ($p < 0.05$); $^{A–D}$ Within the same aging time, means followed by a common letter do not differ significantly ($p < 0.05$).

However, in the subsequent steps (90, 180, and 270 days), the *Lactobacillus rhamnosus* LOCK900 strain was less effective in generating antiradical components with no statistically significant differences between LOCK and C sample. The highest antiradical effects were achieved for loins with BAUER after 90 and 180 days of aging (77.53% and 83.89%, respectively) and BB12 in 270 days (74.12%). The varied effect of probiotic LAB strains on generating antiradical molecules during long-term aging was also observed for SSF. Lower ($p < 0.05$) antiradical values were observed for batches with LAB compared with the variant that underwent spontaneous fermentation (C) at day 28. After this time, the behavior of this parameter in inoculated samples was ambiguous during the rest of the aging period. The biggest differences in antiradical activity (%) were noted between the sample subjected to spontaneous fermentation (C) and BB12 after 28, 90, 180, and 270 days. The LOCK batches had statistically significantly lower antiradical properties (%) compared to C ($p < 0.05$) at 28, 270, and 360 days. BAUER batches had significantly lower values ($p < 0.05$) of radical scavenging activity after 28, 180, and 360 days of aging as compared to C batches.

Antiradical properties were also defined as the concentration of the sample required to inhibit 50% of the radical-scavenging effect (IC_{50}). Generally, the IC_{50} values clearly indicated the higher antiradical properties of protein-released components during long-term aging from SSF compared to WSF (see Table 2). With respect to the WSF, the antiradical activity of the hydrolysis products was stable between 28 and 180 day of aging ($p > 0.05$) and then decreased in all samples. SSF fractions were characterized by greater fluctuations of this parameter especially between 28 and 180 days of aging ($p < 0.05$).

Quantitative analysis was also used for investigating the correlation between antiradical activities and the content of protein degradation products in both fractions of muscle proteins. The correlation between the antiradical activity (expressed as percent inhibition and $1/IC_{50}$ (not IC_{50}) showing parallelism with antiradical activity) and the primary amino groups content (μM/mL) was therefore determined [20].

As shown in Table 3, there was no positive correlation between the content of protein degradation products and the antiradical activity, which corresponds with other studies [21–23]. However, the strong negative correlation between the antiradical activity of the WSF fraction (expressed as $1/IC_{50}$) and the content of components with potential antiradical properties indicated the loss of bioactive properties during aging, which corresponds with the results presented in Table 1.

Therefore, the progressive degradation of proteins by endogenous meat enzymes and exogenous microbial proteases during 360 days of aging results in the disappearance of biological activity of protein-related compounds at a later stage. This may be a result of an overly extensive hydrolysis of the peptide chains [23].

Table 3. The Pearson's correlation coefficients between ABTS $1/IC_{50}$ values and the content of protein degradation products.

Fraction	Antiradical Activity	$-NH_2$ (μM/mL)
WSF	%	−0.399
	$1/IC_{50}$	−0.833
SSF	%	−0.273
	$1/IC_{50}$	−0.247

$-NH_2$, the content of primary amino groups; WSF, water-soluble fraction; SSF, salt-soluble fraction.

2.2. *Stability of Antiradical Activity during In Vitro Digestion*

Determining the in vitro bioactivity to promote the beneficial effects of bioactive compounds should be carried out in the context of their immunity to digestive enzymes and to estimate their nutritional importance. In this context, hydrolysis of protein extracts obtained from dry-cured pork loin using gastrointestinal enzymes was accomplished using a two-step hydrolysis reaction. The first step was hydrolysis by pepsin (pH 2 at 37 °C for 2 hours) while the second step was the successive hydrolysis by pancreatin (pH 7 at 37 °C for 3 hours). The sequential digestion with pepsin and pancreatin provides a suitable model for evaluating peptides released in the intestinal tract. The effect of gastric in vitro (pepsin) and consecutive intestinal in vitro (pancreatin) digestion on protein extracts of dry-cured loins was discussed. The results are summarized in Tables 4 and 5.

Table 4. Antiradical activity of protein hydrolysates after gastric digestion (mean ± standard deviation).

Sample	Aging Time (Days)	WSF			SSF		
		$-NH_2$ (μM/mL)	Radical Scavenging (%)	IC_{50} (μM/mL)	$-NH_2$ (μM/mL)	Radical Scavenging (%)	IC_{50} (μM/mL)
C	28	15.26 ^{a,A,B} ± 1.28	61.22 ^{a,A} ± 1.15	0.66 ± 0.06 ^{a,A}	14.74 ^{a,A,C} ± 0.72	57.98 ^{a,A,C} ± 1.50	0.87 ^{a,A} ± 0.05
	90	16.20 ^{a,A} ± 0.49	81.77 ^{b,A} ± 1.77	0.92 ± 0.03 ^{b,A}	8.09 ^{b,A} ± 0.54	69.33 ^{b,A} ± 0.76	0.50 ^{b,A} ± 0.01
	180	22.27 ^{b,A} ± 1.16	76.33 ^{c,A} ± 1.68	0.20 ± 0.01 ^{c,A,B}	11.44 ^{c,A} ± 0.60	59.47 ^{a,A} ± 0.91	0.13 ^{c,A} ± 0.01
	270	24.32 ^{b,A} ± 1.36	60.27 ^{a,A} ± 0.97	2.02 ± 0.03 ^{d,A}	9.61 ^{d,A} ± 0.47	47.67 ^{c,A} ± 1.73	0.76 ^{d,A,C} ± 0.04
	360	28.72 ^{c,A,B} ± 1.97	57.32 ^{d,A} ± 1.01	2.39 ± 0.04 ^{e,A}	15.26 ^{a,A} ± 0.50	47.52 ^{c,A} ± 0.97	1.11 ^{e,A} ± 0.07
LOCK	28	16.77 ^{a,A} ± 0.28	61.08 ^{a,A} ± 0.72	0.85 ± 0.05 ^{a,B}	14.10 ^{a,c,A} ± 0.02	58.60 ^{a,A} ± 0.80	0.85 ^{a,A} ± 0.06
	90	17.18 ^{a,A} ± 1.38	83.06 ^{b,A} ± 1.43	0.91 ± 0.06 ^{a,B}	7.39 ^{b,A} ± 0.76	69.42 ^{b,A} ± 0.98	0.42 ^{b,B} ± 0.03
	180	23.65 ^{b,A} ± 0.85	70.77 ^{c,B} ± 2.04	0.19 ± 0.01 ^{b,B}	11.81 ^{a,b,c,A,B} ± 0.78	62.26 ^{c,B} ± 1.34	0.09 ^{c,B} ± 0.05
	270	25.14 ^{b,c,A,B} ± 0.41	59.99 ^{a,A} ± 0.91	1.45 ± 0.06 ^{c,B}	7.97 ^{b,B} ± 0.18	52.73 ^{d,B} ± 0.91	0.85 ^{a,A,B} ± 0.03
	360	25.89 ^{c,A} ± 0.72	52.164 ^{d,B} ± 1.78	1.94 ± 0.18 ^{d,B}	15.64 ^{a,A} ± 3.09	54.12 ^{d,B} ± 2.67	1.08 ^{a,A} ± 0.26
BAUER	28	14.71 ^{a,B} ± 0.63	59.74 ^{a,A} ± 1.36	0.79 ± 0.05 ^{a,B}	12.32 ^{a,B} ± 1.01	54.32 ^{a,B} ± 1.20	0.86 ^{a,A} ± 0.01
	90	19.59 ^{b,B} ± 0.81	83.05 ^{b,A} ± 0.97	0.95 ± 0.03 ^{a,C}	7.40 ^{b,A} ± 1.21	70.61 ^{b,B} ± 0.97	0.35 ^{b,C} ± 0.02
	180	27.94 ^{c,B} ± 0.44	76.68 ^{c,A} ± 1.52	0.21 ± 0.01 ^{b,A}	13.01 ^{a,B} ± 0.27	55.92 ^{c,C} ± 1.19	0.13 ^{c,A} ± 0.014
	270	29.63 ^{d,C} ± 0.32	54.80 ^{d,B} ± 0.86	2.22 ± 0.11 ^{c,C}	10.80 ^{a,b,C} ± 0.41	50.94 ^{d,C} ± 0.80	0.70 ^{d,C} ± 0.04
	360	32.47 ^{e,B} ± 0.76	47.75 ^{e,C} ± 1.83	3.12 ± 0.07 ^{d,C}	19.72 ^{c,A} ± 2.70	47.48 ^{e,A} ± 1.10	1.12 ^{e,A} ± 0.11
BB12	28	15.61 ^{a,A,B} ± 0.85	65.38 ^{a,B} ± 1.63	0.82 ± 0.01 ^{a,B}	15.83 ^{a,C} ± 0.99	56.27 ^{a,C} ± 1.84	0.90 ^{a,A} ± 0.04
	90	21.31 ^{b,C} ± 0.18	86.51 ^{b,B} ± 0.63	0.83 ± 0.03 ^{a,C}	8.74 ^{b,A} ± 1.24	75.18 ^{b,C} ± 0.98	0.44 ^{b,B} ± 0.03
	180	23.10 ^{b,c,A} ± 1.11	73.87 ^{c,C} ± 0.72	0.21 ± 0.01 ^{b,A}	11.95 ^{c,d,A,B} ± 0.62	60.09 ^{c,A} ± 0.68	0.12 ^{c,A,B} ± 0.02
	270	26.18 ^{c,B} ± 1.35	57.57 ^{d,C} ± 0.79	1.99 ± 0.07 ^{c,A}	7.65 ^{b,B} ± 0.02	49.23 ^{d,D} ± 0.60	0.94 ^{a,B} ± 0.08
	360	29.95 ^{d,A,B} ± 2.39	46.56 ^{e,C} ± 1.22	2.87 ± 0.11 ^{d,C}	14.16 ^{d,A} ± 0.48	60.31 ^{c,C} ± 0.70	0.99 ^{a,A} ± 0.04

$-NH_2$, the content of primary amino groups; WSF, water-soluble fraction; SSF, salt-soluble fraction; C, control sample; LOCK, sample inoculated with *Lactobacillus rhamnosus* LOCK900; BAUER, sample inoculated with *Lactobacillus acidophilus* Bauer Ł0938; BB12, sample inoculated with *Bifidobacterium animalis* ssp. *lactis* BB-12; $^{a-e}$ Within the same treatment, means followed by a common letter do not differ significantly ($p < 0.05$);$^{A-D}$ Within the same aging time, means followed by a common letter do not differ significantly ($p < 0.05$).

Table 5. Antiradical activity of protein hydrolysates after gastric-intestinal digestion (mean ± standard deviation).

Sample	Aging Time (Days)	WSF			SSF		
		$-NH_2$ (μM/mL)	Radical Scavenging (%)	IC_{50} (μM/mL)	$-NH_2$ (μM/mL)	Radical Scavenging (%)	IC_{50} (μM/mL)
C	28	21.08 ^{a,A,B} ± 1.24	86.43 ^{a,A} ± 1.00	0.16 ^{a,A} ± 0.01	10.61 ^{a,A} ± 2.39	82.31 ^{a,A} ± 0.64	0.17 ^{a,A} ± 0.01
	90	18.63 ^{a,A} ± 0.42	93.49 ^{b,A} ± 1.73	0.35 ^{b,A} ± 0.02	15.36 ^{b,A,B} ± 1.88	85.71 ^{b,A} ± 0.50	0.28 ^{b,A} ± 0.01
	180	28.88 ^{b,A} ± 1.32	96.01 ^{c,A} ± 0.68	0.17 ^{a,A,B} ± 0.02	12.88 ^{c,A} ± 0.25	87.06 ^{c,A} ± 0.90	0.13 ^{c,A} ± 0.02
	270	18.68 ^{a,A} ± 0.86	94.93 ^{c,A} ± 0.62	0.22 ^{a,A} ± 0.01	7.30 ^{d,A} ± 0.84	95.86 ^{d,A} ± 0.37	0.14 ^{a,c,A} ± 0.01
	360	31.39 ^{b,A,B} ± 2.41	91.73 ^{d,A} ± 0.76	0.51 ^{c,A} ± 0.06	15.87 ^{b,A} ± 2.28	94.84 ^{d,A} ± 1.96	0.14 ^{a,c,A,B} ± 0.01
LOCK	28	20.88 ^{a,A,B} ± 1.30	88.63 ^{a,B} ± 0.72	0.19 ^{a,B} ± 0.02	10.46 ^{a,A} ± 1.49	72.81 ^{a,B} ± 1.91	0.15 ^{a,B} ± 0.01
	90	21.24 ^{a,B} ± 1.27	96.67 ^{b,B} ± 0.69	0.32 ^{b,A} ± 0.01	16.56 ^{b,A} ± 1.45	89.34 ^{b,B} ± 0.74	0.23 ^{b,B} ± 0.01
	180	25.68 ^{b,B} ± 2.01	96.33 ^{b,d,A} ± 0.55	0.19 ^{a,A} ± 0.01	18.81 ^{b,B} ± 2.26	90.05 ^{b,B} ± 1.32	0.11 ^{c,A} ± 0.01
	270	21.31 ^{a,B} ± 0.05	97.83 ^{c,B} ± 0.50	0.21 ^{a,A} ± 0.01	7.34 ^{c,A} ± 0.01	91.01 ^{b,c,B} ± 0.68	0.14 ^{a,c,A} ± 0.01
	360	27.94 ^{b,A} ± 1.10	95.58 ^{d,B} ± 0.66	0.43 ^{c,B} ± 0.01	16.40 ^{b,A} ± 0.50	91.82 ^{c,B} ± 1.19	0.12 ^{c,A} ± 0.01
BAUER	28	19.00 ^{a,B} ± 1.17	85.94 ^{a,A} ± 0.98	0.14 ^{a,A,C} ± 0.01	10.63 ^{a,A} ± 1.17	72.45 ^{a,B} ± 1.03	0.14 ^{a,C} ± 0.01
	90	18.59 ^{a,A} ± 0.14	94.41 ^{b,A} ± 0.38	0.41 ^{b,B} ± 0.02	12.40 ^{a,B} ± 2.07	90.95 ^{b,c,C} ± 0.62	0.20 ^{b,C} ± 0.01
	180	37.16 ^{b,C} ± 2.04	98.06 ^{c,B} ± 0.23	0.13 ^{a,B} ± 0.01	18.12 ^{b,B} ± 2.16	90.14 ^{b,B} ± 1.56	0.12 ^{a,c,A} ± 0.05
	270	22.76 ^{c,C} ± 1.21	95.59 ^{d,A} ± 1.09	0.35 ^{c,C} ± 0.01	10.78 ^{a,B} ± 0.36	92.15 ^{cC} ± 0.54	0.13 ^{a,c,A} ± 0.01
	360	33.28 ^{d,B} ± 1.15	95.71 ^{d,B} ± 1.20	0.47 ^{d,A,B} ± 0.01	19.94 ^{b,B} ± 2.35	88.60 ^{d,C} ± 1.54	0.12 ^{c,A,C} ± 0.01
BB12	28	21.61 ^{a,A} ± 1.35	89.52 ^{a,B} ± 1.44	0.13 ^{a,C} ± 0.02	10.78 ^{a,A} ± 0.45	78.93 ^{a,C} ± 1.28	0.19 ^{a,D} ± 0.01
	90	19.35 ^{a,A} ± 0.09	98.56 ^{bC} ± 0.23	0.32 ^{b,A} ± 0.01	14.87 ^{b,A,B} ± 2.18	92.62 ^{b,c,D} ± 0.85	0.22 ^{b,B,C} ± 0.01
	180	31.80 ^{b,A} ± 0.74	96.95 ^{c,C} ± 0.56	0.13 ^{a,B} ± 0.01	17.71 ^{c,B} ± 0.79	91.86 ^{b,C} ± 0.50	0.11 ^{c,A} ± 0.02
	270	26.26 ^{c,D} ± 0.02	98.08 ^{b,c,B} ± 0.33	0.51 ^{c,B} ± 0.02	7.04 ^{d,A} ± 0.61	93.33 ^{c,D} ± 0.52	0.11 ^{c,B} ± 0.01
	360	28.40 ^{c,A} ± 2.89	94.69 ^{d,B} ± 1.29	0.42 ^{d,B} ± 0.01	18.69 ^{c,C} ± 0.45	93.55 ^{c,A,B} ± 1.54	0.15 ^{d,B} ± 0.01

$-NH_2$, the content of primary amino groups; WSF, water-soluble fraction; SSF, salt-soluble fraction; C, control sample; LOCK, sample inoculated with *Lactobacillus rhamnosus* LOCK900; BAUER, sample inoculated with *Lactobacillus acidophilus* Bauer Ł0938; BB12, sample inoculated with *Bifidobacterium animalis* ssp. *lactis* BB-12; $^{a-d}$ Within the same treatment, means followed by a common letter do not differ significantly ($p < 0.05$); $^{A-D}$ Within the same aging time, means followed by a common letter do not differ significantly ($p < 0.05$).

As noted earlier, the antiradical activity defined as percent inhibition and IC_{50} values were uncorrelated. However, the higher antiradical activity (%) was determined for the WSF fraction, which was probably indirectly related to a higher content of primary amino groups. The IC_{50} values unambiguously indicate SSF as a source of antiradical components and this tendency was maintained during in vitro gastrointestinal digestion (see Tables 4 and 5) and simulated adsorption (see Table 6).

The decrease in the antiradical activity of the dry-cured loin protein hydrolysates determined by the ABTS test (expressed as % and IC_{50}) was observed after gastric digestion (see Table 4) and compared to the undigested samples, which was followed by an increase of biological activity after pancreatin treatment (see Table 5). This observation corresponds with other authors' findings [24–27]. The highest biological activity was achieved after 90 days of aging due to the hydrolytic degradation of proteins under the action of pepsin. During this period, an average of 83.60% was reported for WSF with significantly higher ($p < 0.05$) values of biological activity obtained for BB12 batches (86.51%). With regard to SSF, the antiradical activity after 90 days of aging was at an average level of 69.34% for C and LOCK ($p > 0.05$), while BAUER and BB12 batches was statistically significantly ($p < 0.05$) higher (70.61% and 75.18%, respectively). Pancreatin digested samples (see Table 5) showed values ranging from 85.94 for BAUER (28 days) to 98.56 for BB12 (90 days) for WSF and 72.45 for BAUER (28 days) to 95.86% for C (270 days) in the case of SSF. This suggests that fewer peptides with antiradical properties are associated with pepsin digestion than pancreatin. This may be due to the nature of the enzymes used. While pepsin can break down proteins and large peptides into smaller fragments by shielding the cleavage sites for further enzymes, pancreatin can primarily hydrolyze some of the peptides in smaller peptides and possibly amino acids. Pancreatin contains many enzymes including trypsin and additional proteases that give rise to hydrolysis activity, which leads to deeper breakdown of peptide chains. These results can be explained by the formation of a greater proportion of peptides and amino acids with hydrophilic properties during pancreatic digestion. Moreover, Zhu et al. [28] reported that pepsin cleaves peptides into smaller fragments, which exposes the internal groups to the environment. While trypsin hydrolyzed peptides into smaller chains, it also produced more free amino acids due to its greater hydrolytic activity. Therefore, these amino acids have greater affinity with water. This is because the increase of hydrophobic properties of GI digestion after pepsin treatment makes them less likely to react with the water-soluble ABTS radical. However, the increase of the hydrophilic property of GI digestion after pancreatin treatment favors their trapping of the ABTS radical [24].

After in vitro gastrointestinal digestion and simulated absorption, the antiradical properties of the hydrolysates increased compared to undigested proteins (see Table 6).

Table 6. Antiradical activity of protein hydrolysates after simulated adsorption (mean ± standard deviation).

Sample	Aging Time (Days)	WSF			SSF		
		$-NH_2$ (μM/mL)	Radical Scavenging (%)	IC_{50} (μM/mL)	$-NH_2$ (μM/mL)	Radical Scavenging (%)	IC_{50} (μM/mL)
C	28	$2.79^{a,A} \pm 0.03$	$89.62^{a,A} \pm 0.65$	$0.08^{a,A} \pm 0.01$	$1.72^{a,A,C} \pm 0.24$	$86.19^{a,A} \pm 1.12$	$0.03^{a,A} \pm 0.01$
	90	$2.26^{b,A} \pm 0.21$	$78.46^{b,A} \pm 1.08$	$0.07^{a,A} \pm 0.01$	$1.35^{b,A} \pm 0.19$	$81.32^{b,A,B} \pm 2.90$	$0.03^{a,A} \pm 0.01$
	180	$4.29^{c,A} \pm 0.08$	$80.17^{c,A} \pm 0.86$	$0.03^{b,A} \pm 0.01$	$2.66^{a,A} \pm 0.34$	$90.49^{c,A} \pm 1.37$	$0.02^{a,A} \pm 0.01$
	270	$3.74^{d,A} \pm 0.18$	$83.68^{d,A} \pm 0.88$	$0.15^{c,A,B} \pm 0.02$	$1.38^{b,A} \pm 0.07$	$85.89^{a,A} \pm 1.11$	$0.03^{a,A} \pm 0.01$
	360	$4.39^{c,A} \pm 0.31$	$73.31^{e,A} \pm 0.75$	$0.24^{d,A} \pm 0.01$	$1.68^{b,A} \pm 0.06$	$66.46^{d,A} \pm 1.49$	$0.10^{b,A} \pm 0.02$
LOCK	28	$2.55^{a,B} \pm 0.08$	$91.47^{a,B} \pm 0.81$	$0.08^{a,A} \pm 0.01$	$1.52^{a,d,A,B} \pm 0.18$	$86.98^{a,A} \pm 1.24$	$0.03^{a,b,A} \pm 0.01$
	90	$2.85^{bB} \pm 0.24$	$84.13^{bB} \pm 1.93$	$0.06^{b,A} \pm 0.01$	$1.21^{b,A,B} \pm 0.07$	$79.95^{b,A} \pm 1.56$	$0.03^{a,A} \pm 0.01$
	180	$4.04^{c,d,B} \pm 0.05$	$76.47^{c,B} \pm 0.83$	$0.02^{c,B} \pm 0.01$	$2.10^{c,B} \pm 0.04$	$86.80^{a,B} \pm 0.61$	$0.01^{b,A} \pm 0.01$
	270	$4.25^{c,B} \pm 0.01$	$84.08^{b,A} \pm 0.95$	$0.13^{d,B} \pm 0.01$	$1.34^{a,b,A} \pm 0.18$	$87.26^{a,B} \pm 0.77$	$0.03^{a,B} \pm 0.01$
	360	$3.96^{d,A,B} \pm 0.05$	$70.92^{d,B} \pm 0.72$	$0.23^{e,A} \pm 0.01$	$1.66^{d,A} \pm 0.08$	$70.12^{c,B} \pm 0.87$	$0.10^{c,A} \pm 0.01$
BAUER	28	$2.32^{a,C} \pm 0.08$	$88.61^{a,A} \pm 1.88$	$0.08^{a,A} \pm 0.01$	$1.96^{a,C} \pm 0.31$	$89.63^{a,B} \pm 0.81$	$0.02^{a,B} \pm 0.01$
	90	$3.15^{b,B} \pm 0.34$	$85.65^{b,B} \pm 1.28$	$0.09^{a,B} \pm 0.01$	$1.06^{b,B} \pm 0.01$	$83.63^{b,B} \pm 1.07$	$0.03^{a,A} \pm 0.01$
	180	$4.41^{c,A} \pm 0.17$	$88.96^{a,C} \pm 0.44$	$0.02^{b,B} \pm 0.01$	$1.58^{c,C} \pm 0.06$	$87.26^{cB} \pm 0.67$	$0.02^{a,B} \pm 0.01$
	270	$4.55^{c,C} \pm 0.24$	$68.39^{c,B} \pm 1.01$	$0.15^{c,A} \pm 0.01$	$2.06^{a,B} \pm 0.07$	$83.22^{b,C} \pm 0.76$	$0.03^{a,C} \pm 0.01$
	360	$4.36^{c,A} \pm 0.12$	$74.98^{d,C} \pm 1.35$	$0.17^{d,B} \pm 0.02$	$2.03^{a,A} \pm 0.18$	$72.40^{d,C} \pm 0.91$	$0.11^{b,A} \pm 0.01$

Table 6. *Cont.*

Sample	Aging Time (Days)	WSF			SSF		
		$-NH_2$ (μM/mL)	Radical Scavenging (%)	IC_{50} (μM/mL)	$-NH_2$ (μM/mL)	Radical Scavenging (%)	IC_{50} (μM/mL)
BB12	28	2.46 ^{a,B} ± 0.08	91.74 ^{a,B} ± 1.26	0.07 ^{a,A} ± 0.01	1.23 ^{a,B} ± 0.13	85.92 ^{a,A} ± 0.36	0.03 ^{a,A} ± 0.01
	90	3.03 ^{b,B} ± 0.34	88.30 ^{b,C} ± 1.72	0.090 ^{b,B} ± 0.01	1.24 ^{a,A,B} ± 0.08	71.63 ^{b,C} ± 1.66	0.029 ^{a,A} ± 0.01
	180	3.78 ^{c,C} ± 0.01	80.54 ^{c,A} ± 0.97	0.02 ^{c,B} ± 0.01	1.87 ^{b,B,C} ± 0.39	89.58 ^{c,A} ± 0.96	0.017 ^{b,A} ± 0.01
	270	5.25 ^{d,D} ± 0.01	86.38 ^{d,C} ± 0.66	0.17 ^{d,A} ± 0.01	1.28 ^{a,A} ± 0.05	78.72 ^{d,D} ± 1.09	0.03 ^{a,A,C} ± 0.01
	360	3.46 ^{c,B} ± 0.21	81.05 ^{c,D} ± 1.84	0.14 ^{e,C} ± 0.01	1.76 ^{a,b,A} ± 0.47	68.86 ^{e,B} ± 0.62	0.14 ^{c,B} ± 0.01

$-NH_2$, the content of primary amino groups; WSF, water-soluble fraction; SSF, salt-soluble fraction; C, control sample; LOCK, sample inoculated with *Lactobacillus rhamnosus* LOCK900; BAUER, sample inoculated with *Lactobacillus acidophilus* Bauer Ł0938; BB12, sample inoculated with *Bifidobacterium animalis* ssp. *lactis* BB-12; $^{a–d}$ Within the same treatment, means followed by a common letter do not differ significantly ($p < 0.05$); $^{A–D}$ Within the same aging time, means followed by a common letter do not differ significantly ($p < 0.05$).

As expected, the best antiradical properties were achieved after in vitro gastrointestinal digestion and simulated adsorption of WSF extracted after 28 days of aging. These results are not consistent with the radical scavenging activity expressed by the IC_{50} for which the increase in antiradical properties attain the lowest biological activity (highest antiradical activity) on day 180, which was followed by a systematic decline until the end of the aging period was noted. This tendency was described earlier (see Table 2). In this period (180 days of aging), the statistically significantly higher biological activity as an antiradical within the WSF ($p < 0.05$) was shown for the BAUER and BB12 (IC_{50} = 0.02 μM/mL both; Table 6). With regard to SSF, the best antiradical properties (determined by % and IC_{50}) were recorded after simulated absorption of the digested product after 180 days of aging with the best properties reported ($p < 0.05$) for the spontaneous fermentation (C) and BB12 batches. However, the differences between them were not statistically significant ($p > 0.05$).

2.3. *Stability of Antiradical Activity during In Vitro Digestion*

Dry-cured meats constitute a specific group of products in which the proteolytic processes take place from raw material to finished product, which can take up to 24 months. Proteolytic degradation of proteins takes place through exogenous enzymes of meat as well as by exogenous enzymes derived from microorganisms primarily responsible for fermentation processes that occur on raw meat. The proteolytic activity attributed to bacteria is characteristic of a particular strain. Therefore, different peptide and amino acid profiles are predicted depending on the LAB strains used during production. These aspects are crucial for detecting the specific functions of potentially bioactive peptides especially when digested with enzymes of the human gastrointestinal tract. The digestive tract affects the release of peptides from parent proteins and modifies or degrades peptides that may exhibit antiradical properties. In fact, the specificity of the enzyme affects the amount, size, and composition of the peptides, which influences the biological activity of the digested samples [25,29] and the degree of their absorption through the intestinal membrane.

Therefore, LC-MS/MS analysis was used to evaluate peptides (28, 90, and 180 days) and compare the peptide profile of the samples after in vitro digestion and absorption in the simulated gastrointestinal tract. Peptide sequences were identified and characterized by nano-LC-MS, which confirms the identification by exact mass determination with LTQ-Orbitrap. The cleavage of peptide bonds by digestive proteases leads to the release of peptides that have different lengths and free amino acids. The most typical well-known bioactive peptides are 200–1700 Da with fragment lengths from 2 to 14 amino acids so that they are able to easily pass through the gut lane and are capable of secreting nutritional value and bioactive functions [30].

The peptides found in the digested samples have MW between 700 and 4232 Da and the length of the peptide fragments determined in the study ranged from 5 to 47 amino acids in a sequence, which is in agreement with other peptide profile studies obtained by digestion [31,32]. This probably indicates that they may have biological effects. The influence of individual strains on the peptide profile of the analyzed samples after the digestion and absorption process was summarized in the

Venn diagram (see Figure 1) [33]. Venn diagrams indicated an increase in the number of peptides identified as common for the WSF of batches inoculated with LAB (from 84 to 134 sequences obtained after in vitro digestion and adsorption. At the same time in relation to the SSF, a decrease from 279 to 55 common sequences has been noted. After 180 days of aging, 402 common peptide sequences were identified for the WSF of C and BB12 samples while only 135 identified peptides were common for the C and BAUER batches. By analogy, taking into account the SSF, the C sample had more common peptide sequences with the LOCK (139) and less when compared to the BAUER sample (83).

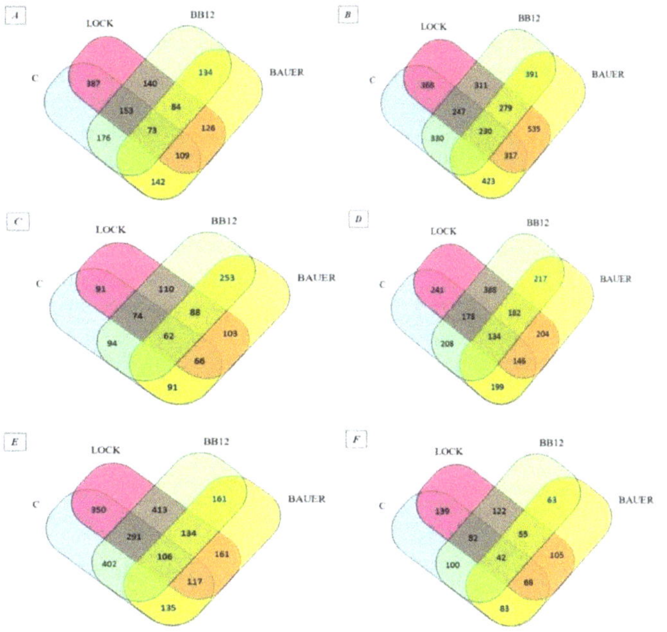

Figure 1. Venn diagrams of peptides obtained from dry-cured pork loins after digestion and simulated absorption: (**A**) peptides obtained from WSF after 28 days of aging, (**B**) peptides obtained from SSF after 28 days of aging, (**C**) peptides obtained from WSF after 90 days of aging, (**D**) peptides obtained from SSF after 90 days of aging, (**E**) peptides obtained from WSF after 180 days of aging, (**F**) peptides obtained from SSF after 180 days of aging. LOCK, sample inoculated with *Lactobacillus rhamnosus* LOCK900; BAUER, sample inoculated with *Lactobacillus acidophilus* Bauer Ł0938; BB12, sample inoculated with *Bifidobacterium animalis* ssp. *lactis* BB-12.

Due to the large number of peptides and, taking into account the highest antiradical activity of protein-released components extracted from the loins after 180 days of aging, the peptides derived from digestion and simulated absorption were identified by chromatographic methods and in silico analysis. The analyses were repeated twice and identical peptide sequences were selected for further analysis. In total, all peptides up to 480 sequences (38.53%) showed potency as antioxidants in the in silico study. In addition, the selected sequences were evaluated by rating capacity for bioactivity.

The peptide sequences with the highest *A* parameter (i.e., above 0.4) are presented in Table 7. Both sarcoplasmic and myofibrillar proteins have been described as precursors of bioactive peptides on the basis of in vitro assays. The amino acid composition, conformation, and hydrophobicity is correlated with antioxidant activity and likely determines the mechanism (transfer of hydrogen (HAT) or single electron (SET)) and the effectiveness of antioxidants [34,35]. It has been found that the peptides possibly containing substances and donating electrons are likely to react with the free radicals to terminate a radical reaction. Cys and Met residues, which contain nucleophilic sulphur side chains as well as Trp, Tyr, and Phe, have aromatic side chains and readily donate hydrogen atoms [28]. The antioxidant activity of peptides with one or more residues of His, Pro, Cys, Tyr, Trp, Phe, or Met and the presence of hydrophobic amino acids might be enhanced [36]. Peptides containing the amino acid residues Val, Leu, Ile, Ala, Phe, Lys, or Cys at the N-terminal and Trp, Tyr, His, or Pro in the sequence had been reported to show antioxidant activity [36,37]. This is caused by acidic or basic amino acid residues (Asp, Glu, His, Arg, or Lys) or hydrophilic amino acids (Ser, Thr) in this position. Moreover, as reported by Power et al. [35], it is suggested that a second amino acid adhering to the C-terminal is a major factor influencing antioxidant activity. If this amino acid has a high hydrogen bond and steric and low hydrophobicity, it will increase its anti-oxidative potential.

Within the peptide sequences identified in the present study (see Table 7), Leu (19.01%), Pro (15.85%), Lys (11.62%), Glu (7.39%), and His (7.04%) had the largest share in their amino acid composition, which corresponds to other authors [17,21]. Their presence is likely to determine the antiradical ability of the peptides due to their ability to quench unpaired electrons or radicals by supporting protons. Other authors also reported that the presence of these nonpolar amino acids such as Leu and Pro has been correlated to the antioxidant activity [21,38]. This contributes to the radical scavenging activity of peptides due to their special structural characteristics. Chen et al. [39] demonstrated that peptides containing His can act as metal ion chelators, active-oxygen quenchers, and hydroxy radical scavengers. Escudero et al. [17] reported about proline-rich peptide SAGNPN, which showed a high radical scavenging activity. Yet, many synthesized peptides like GGSILI, IAKLE, ALGGA, NVLVG, GLAGA, and NAAKL possessed Leu residues. The presence of Leu possibly contributed to the antioxidant activities of peptides [17,40].

Table 7. Peptide sequences with the highest antiradical properties obtained after digestion and simulated adsorption of dry-cured pork loin after 180 days of aging.

Peptide Sequence	Mass	Parental Protein	Protein ID [1]	Bioactive Fragment Location	*A* Parameter	Hydropathicity (GRAVY)	Charge
I**LKP**LE	711.45	Uncharacterized protein	F1SA53; F1SFX4	(2–4) (2–3) (3–4)	0.5000	0.517	0
L**LKP**IE	711.45	Rab GDP dissociation inhibitor beta	Q6Q7J2	(2–4) (2–3) (3–4)	0.5000	0.517	0
L**LKP**LE	711.45	Kinesin-like protein	F1SDL9	(2–4) (2–3) (3–4)	0.5000	0.400	0
LKPDPVA	738.43	Serum albumin	F1RUN2; P08835	(1–3) (1–2) (2–3)	0.4286	−0.114	0
AG**LKPGEL**	783.45	Phosphoglycerate mutase	B5KJG2	(3–5) (3–4) (7–8)	0.5000	−0.050	0
AS**LKP**EF	790.42	Triosephosphate isomerase	D0G7F6; Q29371	(3–5) (3–4) (4–5)	0.4286	−0.200	0
TL**LKP**NM	815.46	Fructose-bisphosphate aldolase	F1RJ25; F1SSB5	(3–5) (3–4) (4–5)	0.4286	−0.029	1
ILKPLED	826.48	Uncharacterized protein	F1SA53; F1SFX4	(2–4) (2–3) (3–4)	0.4286	−0.057	−1
TL**LKP**NM	831.45	Fructose-bisphosphate aldolase	F1RJ25; F1SSB5	(3–5) (3–4) (4–5)	0.4286	−0.029	1
HLPHDPM	845.39	Citrate synthase	F1SLZ4; I3LBB3; P00889	(1–4) (1–2) (3–5)	0.4286	−1.57	0
KN**LHPEL**	849.47	L-lactate dehydrogenase A chain	P00339	(3–4) (5–7) (6–7)	0.4286	−1.157	0
KDTQ**LHL**	853.47	Myosin-4	Q9TV62; F1SS61	(1–2) (5–7) (5–6) (6–7)	0.5714	−1.029	0.5
QDTK**LHL**	853.47	Uncharacterized protein	F1RN91	(5–7) (5–6) (6–7)	0.4286	−1.029	0.5
HLPHDPM	861.38	Citrate synthase	F1SLZ4; I3LBB3; P00889	(1–4) (1–2) (3–5)	0.4286	−1.057	0
A**LKP**T**KPM**	900.51	Phosphoglycerate mutase	B5KJG2	(2–3) (2–4) (3–4) (6–7)	0.5000	−0.525	2
VD**LKP**D**WG**	928.47	Uncharacterized protein	I3LNG8	(3–5) (3–4) (4–5) (7–8)	0.5000	−0.725	−1
YAG**LKPGEL**	946.51	Phosphoglycerate mutase	B5KJG2	(4–6) (4–5) (5–6) (8–9)	0.4444	−0.189	0
ELPEH**LKP**	961.52	Glutathione S-transferase P	F1RVN0; P80031	(1–2) (6–8) (6–7) (7–8)	0.6250	−1.212	−0.5
AG**LKPGEL**PT	981.55	Phosphoglycerate mutase	B5KJG2	(3–5) (3–4) (4–5) (7–8)	0.4000	−0.270	0
QA**LKP**T**KPM**	1012.57	Phosphoglycerate mutase	B5KJG2	(3–5) (3–4) (4–5) (7–8)	0.4444	−0.856	2
ELDQA**LKP**T	1013.54	Phosphoglycerate mutase	B5KJG2	(1–2) (6–8) (6–7)	0.4444	−0.811	−1
YAG**LKPGEL**P	1043.57	Phosphoglycerate mutase	B5KJG2	(4–6) (4–5) (5–6) (8–9)	0.4000	−0.330	0
E**TW**PP**LKP**S	1053.55	Glutathione S-transferase P	F1RVN0; P80031	(2–3) (6–8) (6–7) (7–8)	0.4444	−1.200	0
LVNS**PHLKPA**	1074.62	Uncharacterized protein	F1S557	(5–7) (6–7) (7–9) (7–8) (8–9)	0.5000	−0.100	1.5
RYAG**LKPGEL**	1102.62	Phosphoglycerate mutase	B5KJG2	(5–7) (5–6) (6–7) (9–10)	0.4000	−0.620	1
ELPEH**LKP**F	1108.60	Glutathione S-transferase P	F1RVN0; P80031	(1–2) (5–6) (6–8) (6–7) (7–8)	0.5556	−0.767	−0.5
LDQA**LKP**T**KP**	1109.65	Phosphoglycerate mutase	B5KJG2	(5–7) (5–6) (6–7) (9–10)	0.4000	−0.930	1
DQA**LKP**T**KPM**	1127.60	Phosphoglycerate mutase	B5KJG2	(4–6) (4–5) (5–6) (8–9)	0.4000	−1.120	1
ME**TW**PP**LKP**S	1184.59	Glutathione S-transferase P	F1RVN0; P80031	(3–4) (7–9) (7–8) (8–9)	0.4000	−0.890	0
ELDQA**LKP**T**KPM**	1385.72	Phosphoglycerate mutase	B5KJG2	(1–2) (6–8) (6–7) (7–8) (10–11)	0.4176	−0.908	0
HLHWGSSDDH	1189.49	Carbonic anhydrase 3	Q5S1S4	(1–3) (1–2) (2–3) (2–4) (4–5)	0.5000	−1.570	−0.5
HLHWGSSD**DHG**SE	1462.59	Carbonic anhydrase 3	Q5S1S4	(1–3) (2–3) (1–2) (2–4) (4–5) (9–11)	0.4615	−1.569	−1.5
HLHWGSSD**DHG**SEH	1599.65	Carbonic anhydrase 3	Q5S1S4	(1–3) (1–2) (2–3) (2–4) (4–5) (9–11)	0.4286	−1.686	−1

[1] ID from Uniprot; bold refers to the short fragments with antiradical properties located in peptide sequences.

3. Materials and Methods

3.1. Preparation of Dry-Cured Loins

The pork primal cuts of Polish White Large fatteners (live weight of approximately 120–130 kg) were used in this study. Loins (*M. longissimus thoracis*) were excised at 24 h *post mortem* from half carcasses chilled at 4 °C at a local abattoir (Lublin, Poland). At 48 h post mortem, all loins underwent curing using a surface massage with a mixture of 20 g of sea salt, 9.7 g of curing salt, and 0.3 g of $NaNO_3$ per kg of loin. After 24-hour curing at 4 °C, the loins were randomly divided into four experimental batches with three loins each. One of the batches was regarded as a control sample (C). The other three experimental batches were inoculated with *Lactobacillus rhamnosus* (formerly *Lactobacillus casei* ŁOCK 0900) LOCK900 (LOCK), *Lactobacillus acidophilus* Bauer Ł0938 (BAUER), and *Bifidobacterium animalis* ssp. *lactis* BB-12 (BB12), respectively to achieve an initial level of 10^6–10^7 CFU/g of meat. The inoculum was prepared at the Department of Food Hygiene and Quality Management (WULSSGGW, Warsaw, Poland) according to the procedure previously described by Wójciak et al. [41]. Subsequently, the loins were hung at 16 ± 1 °C in a disinfected laboratory aging chamber with a relative humidity of between 75% and 80% for 14 days. Then the whole pieces of loins were vacuum-packed in PA/PE (80 μm thick) bags (Wispak, Lublin, Poland) and aged at 4 ± 1 °C for 12 months. Three independent experimental trials were conducted with 12 loins utilized in each trial. After 28, 90, 180, 270, and 360 days of aging, the samples were taken for analysis.

3.2. Muscle Proteins Extraction

Water-soluble fraction (WSF) of meat proteins was extracted according to the method described by Molina and Toldrá [42] with modifications suggested by Fadda et al. [43]. To prepare the salt-soluble fraction (SSF), the pellet resulting from the WSF extraction was re-suspended in 0.6 M NaCl in 0.1 M phosphate buffer (pH 6.2) in a ratio of 1:6 and homogenized for 1 min (T25 Basic ULTRA-TURRAX; IKA, Staufen, Germany). The resulting homogenate was deaerated prior to extraction for 18 h at 4 °C. After the centrifugation step at 10,000× *g*, 4 °C for 10 min, the supernatant was filtered through Whatman Filter Paper No. 1. Protein concentration of both fractions was determined by the Biuret method [44] using Liquick Cor-TOTAL PROTEIN 60 kit (Cormay Group, Łomianki, Poland) and bovine serum albumin (BSA) as the standard.

3.3. Simulated In Vitro Digestion and Absorption

Muscle protein fractions (WSF and SSF) have been subjected to in vitro digestion using pepsin and pancreatin [16]. Prior to the simulated gastric digestion, protein fractions were adjusted to pH 2.0 with 1 M HCl. Pepsin solution in 6 M HCl (pH 2.0) was added to protein fractions at the ratio of enzyme to substrate of 1:100. The digestion was carried out at 37 °C for 2 h in darkness and under continuous stirring. Afterward, the solution was neutralized to pH 7.0 with 1 M NaOH. For simulated intestinal digestion, pancreatin was added at a 1:50 enzyme to substrate ratio. After incubation at 37 °C for 3 h in darkness with continuous stirring, the enzyme was inactivated by heating at 95 °C for 10 min. Obtained hydrolysates were dialyzed with membrane tubes (molecular weight cut-off 7 kDa; Spectra/Por®) against phosphate buffered saline (PBS; pH 7.4; 1:4, v/v). The absorption process was carried out without light for 1 h at 37 °C.

3.4. Primary Amino Groups Content

After each step of in vitro digestion and simulated absorption, the protein degradation products were evaluated by measuring the content of primary amino groups according to the trinitrobenzene sulfonic acid (TNBS) method [45]. The content of primary amino groups (-NH_2) was expressed as μM/mL of L-leucine amino equivalent based on the calibration curve.

3.5. Peptide Identification

Hydrolysates obtained after each step of in vitro digestion and simulated absorption were concentrated in the evaporator and dissolved in 2 mL of 0.01 M HCl prior to chromatographic analysis. The separation of the peptide mixture was done using nanoACQUITY (Waters) liquid chromatography (LC) instruments and Orbitrap Velos Mass Spectrometer (Thermo Electron Corp., San Jose, CA, USA). The peptide mixture was applied to a RP-18 (nanoACQUITY Symmetry C18 Waters 186003545) column using a gradient of acetonitrile (0−35% AcN over 180 min) in the presence of 0.05% formic acid at a flow rate of 250 nL/min. The data was processed by Mascot Distiller and Mascot Search (Matrix science, London, UK) and then compared to the Uniprot database. The search parameters for precursor ions and mass tolerance products were 10 ppm and 0.1. Da. Venn diagrams were applied to analyze the similarity of peptides from each batch.

3.6. Determination of Antiradical Activity

3.6.1. In vitro Antiradical Activity

Free radical-scavenging activity of hydrolysates obtained after each step of in vitro digestion and simulated absorption was determined by the ABTS [2,2′-azinobis-(3-ethylbenzothiazoline-6-sulfonic acid)] method according Re et al. [46]. The scavenging activity of the hydrolysates was expressed as the percentage of free radical-scavenging effect using the formula below.

$$\text{Scavenging [\%]} = [1 - (\text{As}/\text{Ac})] \times 100 \quad (1)$$

where As-absorbance of sample is related to Ac-absorbance of control (ABTS solution). The effective concentration of sample required to scavenge ABTS radical by 50% (IC_{50} value) was obtained by linear regression analysis of the dose-response curve by plotting between percent inhibition and concentration. Nine replicates were performed per sample.

3.6.2. In Silico Antioxidant Activity

The peptide sequences, which were obtained as a result of chromatographic analyses of hydrolysates after in vitro digestion and simulated absorption, were analyzed using the in silico approach. The potential of biological activity was evaluated using tools available in the BIOPEP database i.e., "Profiles of potential biological activity" for distinguishing all peptides with antioxidant properties and "Calculations" to determine the frequency of bioactive fragment occurrence in a protein sequence (A parameter) [47]. The selected peptides were characterized for their amino acids composition, hydrophobicity, and net charge using ProtParm tools [48].

3.7. Statistical Analysis

Statistical analysis and comparisons among means were carried out using the SAS statistical software (SAS Institute Inc., Cary, NC, USA). The results were presented as mean ± standard deviation. The data were analyzed by two-way ANOVA. The Tukey's post hoc test was applied for comparing mean values and differences were considered significant at $p < 0.05$.

4. Conclusions

The antiradical activity of WSF and SSF (undigested protein extracts of dry-cured pork loins) and hydrolysates obtained by in vitro digestion have been confirmed. The results suggest that dry-cured pork loin is abundant in natural antioxidants and has the potential to support innate mechanisms to control oxidation processes and can be used to promote human health and food protection. Importantly, the biological activity of these peptides after in vitro digestion at gastrointestinal levels in humans is resistant to the loss of their antiradical bioactivity. It is, however, necessary to establish a correlation between in vitro and in vivo digestion to assess the bioavailability of potential antioxidant peptides.

Author Contributions: Paulina Kęska and Joanna Stadnik conceived and designed the experiments. Paulina Kęska performed the experiments. Paulina Kęska and Joanna Stadnik analyzed the data. Paulina Kęska and Joanna Stadnik wrote the paper.

Conflicts of Interest: The authors declare no conflict of interest.

References

1. Laranjo, M.; Elias, M.; Fraqueza, M.J. The use of starter cultures in traditional meat products. *J. Food Qual.* **2017**, *2017*, 9546026. [CrossRef]
2. Ojha, K.S.; Kerry, J.P.; Duffy, G.; Beresford, T.; Tiwari, B.K. Technological advances for enhancing quality and safety of fermented meat products. *Trends Food Sci. Technol.* **2015**, *44*, 105–116. [CrossRef]
3. Kęska, P.; Stadnik, J.; Zielińska, D.; Kołożyn-Krajewska, D. Potential of bacteriocins from LAB to improve microbial quality of dry-cured and fermented meat products. *Acta Sci. Pol. Technol. Aliment.* **2017**, *16*, 119–126. [CrossRef] [PubMed]
4. Favaro, L.; Todorov, S.D. Bacteriocinogenic LAB strains for fermented meat preservation: Perspectives, challenges, and limitations. *Probiotics Antimicrob.* **2017**, *9*, 444–458. [CrossRef] [PubMed]
5. Kröckel, L. The role of lactic acid bacteria in safety and flavour development of meat and meat products. In *Lactic Acid Bacteria-R & D for Food, Health and Livestock Purposes*, 1st ed.; Kongo, M., Ed.; InTech: London, UK, 2013; Chapter 5; pp. 129–152, ISBN 978-953-51-0955-6. [CrossRef]
6. De Vuyst, L.; Falony, G.; Leroy, F. Probiotics in fermented sausages. *Meat Sci.* **2008**, *80*, 75–78. [CrossRef] [PubMed]
7. Kołożyn-Krajewska, D.; Dolatowski, Z.J. Probiotic meat products and human nutrition. *Process Biochem.* **2012**, *47*, 1761–1772. [CrossRef]
8. Neffe-Skocińska, K.; Okoń, A.; Kołożyn-Krajewska, D.; Dolatowski, Z. Amino acid profile and sensory characteristics of dry fermented pork loins produced with a mixture of probiotic starter cultures. *J. Sci. Food Agric.* **2017**, *97*, 2953–2960. [CrossRef] [PubMed]
9. Wójciak, K.M.; Libera, J.; Stasiak, D.M.; Kołożyn-Krajewska, D. Technological aspect of *Lactobacillus acidophilus* Bauer, *Bifidobacterium animalis* BB-12 and *Lactobacillus rhamnosus* LOCK900 use in dry-fermented pork neck and sausage. *J. Food Process. Preserv.* **2017**, *41*, e12965. [CrossRef]
10. Brown, L.; Pingitore, E.V.; Mozzi, F.; Saavedra, L.; Villegas, J.M.; Hebert, E.M. Lactic acid bacteria as cell factories for the generation of bioactive peptides. *Protein Pept. Lett.* **2017**, *24*, 146–155. [CrossRef] [PubMed]
11. Pessione, E.; Cirrincione, S. Bioactive molecules released in food by lactic acid bacteria: Encrypted peptides and biogenic amines. *Front. Microbiol.* **2016**, *7*, 876. [CrossRef] [PubMed]
12. Arihara, K. Strategies for designing novel functional meat products. *Meat Sci.* **2006**, *74*, 219–229. [CrossRef] [PubMed]
13. Minkiewicz, P.; Darewicz, M.; Iwaniak, A.; Sokołowska, J.; Starowicz, P.; Bucholska, J.; Hrynkiewicz, M. Common amino acid subsequences in a universal proteome-Relevance for food science. *Int. J. Mol. Sci.* **2015**, *16*, 20748–20773. [CrossRef] [PubMed]
14. Stadnik, J.; Kęska, P. Meat and fermented meat products as a source of bioactive peptides. *Acta Sci. Pol. Technol. Aliment.* **2015**, *14*, 181–190. [CrossRef] [PubMed]
15. Kęska, P.; Stadnik, J. Porcine myofibrillar proteins as potential precursors of bioactive peptides-an in silico study. *Food Funct.* **2016**, *7*, 2878–2885. [CrossRef] [PubMed]
16. Escudero, E.; Mora, L.; Toldrá, F. Stability of ACE inhibitory ham peptides against heat treatment and in vitro digestion. *Food Chem.* **2014**, *161*, 305–311. [CrossRef] [PubMed]
17. Escudero, E.; Mora, L.; Fraser, P.D.; Aristoy, M.C.; Arihara, K.; Toldrá, F. Purification and identification of antihypertensive peptides in Spanish dry-cured ham. *J. Proteom* **2013**, *78*, 499–507. [CrossRef] [PubMed]
18. Montoro-García, S.; Zafrilla-Rentero, M.P.; Celdrán-de Haro, F.M.; Piñero-de Armas, J.J.; Toldrá, F.; Tejada-Portero, L.; Abellán-Alemán, J. Effects of dry-cured ham rich in bioactive peptides on cardiovascular health: A randomized controlled trial. *J. Funct. Foods* **2017**, *38*, 160–167. [CrossRef]
19. Kęska, P.; Stadnik, J. Characteristic of antioxidant activity of dry-cured pork loins inoculated with probiotic strains of LAB. *CyTA J. Food* **2017**, *15*, 374–381. [CrossRef]
20. Li, X.; Wu, X; Huang, L. Correlation between antioxidant activities and phenolic contents of radix *Angelicae sinensis* (Danggui). *Molecules* **2009**, *14*, 5349–5361. [CrossRef] [PubMed]

21. Chen, H.M.; Muramoto, K.; Yamauchi, F. Structural analysis of antioxidative peptides from *Soybean Beta-Conglycinin*. *J. Agr. Food Chem.* **1995**, *43*, 574–578. [CrossRef]
22. Klompong, V.; Benjakul, S.; Kantachote, D.; Shahidi, F. Antioxidative activity and functional properties of protein hydrolysate of yellow stripe trevally (*Selaroides leptolepis*) as influenced by the degree of hydrolysis and enzyme type. *Food Chem.* **2007**, *102*, 1317–1327. [CrossRef]
23. You, L.; Zhao, M.; Cui, C.; Zhao, H.; Yang, B. Effect of degree of hydrolysis on the antioxidant activity of loach (*Misgurnus anguillicaudatus*) protein hydrolysates. *Innov. Food Sci. Emerg.* **2009**, *10*, 235–240. [CrossRef]
24. You, L.; Zhao, M.; Regenstein, J.M.; Ren, J. Changes in the antioxidant activity of loach (*Misgurnus anguillicaudatus*) protein hydrolysates during a simulated gastrointestinal digestion. *Food Chem.* **2010**, *120*, 810–816. [CrossRef]
25. Samaranayaka, A.G.; Li-Chan, E. Food-derived peptidic antioxidants: A review of their production, assessment, and potential applications. *J. Funct. Foods* **2011**, *3*, 229–254. [CrossRef]
26. Nalinanon, S.; Benjakul, S.; Kishimura, H.; Shahidi, F. Functionalities and antioxidant properties of protein hydrolysates from the muscle of ornate threadfin bream treated with pepsin from skipjack tuna. *Food Chem.* **2011**, *124*, 1354–1362. [CrossRef]
27. Chang, O.K.; Ha, G.E.; Jeong, S.G.; Seol, K.H.; Oh, M.H.; Kim, D.W.; Ham, J.S. Antioxidant activity of porcine skin gelatin hydrolyzed by pepsin and pancreatin. *Korean J. Food Sci. An.* **2013**, *33*, 493–500. [CrossRef]
28. Zhu, C.Z.; Zhang, W.G.; Kang, Z.L.; Zhou, G.H.; Xu, X.L. Stability of an antioxidant peptide extracted from Jinhua ham. *Meat Sci.* **2014**, *96*, 783–789. [CrossRef] [PubMed]
29. Sarmadi, B.H.; Ismail, A. Antioxidative peptides from food proteins: A review. *Peptides* **2010**, *31*, 1949–1956. [CrossRef] [PubMed]
30. Paolella, S.; Falavigna, C.; Faccini, A.; Virgili, R.; Sforza, S.; Dall'Asta, C.; Galaverna, G. Effect of dry-cured ham maturation time on simulated gastrointestinal digestion: Characterization of the released peptide fraction. *Food Res. Int.* **2015**, *67*, 136–144. [CrossRef]
31. Bauchart, C.; Morzel, M.; Chambon, C.; Mirand, P.P.; Reynès, C.; Buffière, C.; Rémond, D. Peptides reproducibly released by in vivo digestion of beef meat and trout flesh in pigs. *Br. J. Nutr.* **2007**, *98*, 1187–1195. [CrossRef] [PubMed]
32. Escudero, E.; Sentandreu, M.A.; Toldra, F. Characterization of peptides released by in vitro digestion of pork meat. *J. Agr. Food Chem.* **2010**, *58*, 5160–5165. [CrossRef] [PubMed]
33. Li, L.; Liu, Y.; Zhou, G.; Xu, X.; Li, C. Proteome profiles of digested products of commercial meat sources. *Front. Nutr.* **2017**, *4*, 8. [CrossRef] [PubMed]
34. Chen, Y.; Kwon, S.W.; Kim, S.C.; Zhao, Y. Integrated approach for manual evaluation of peptides identified by searching protein sequence databases with tandem mass spectra. *J. Proteome Res.* **2005**, *4*, 998–1005. [CrossRef] [PubMed]
35. Power, O.; Jakeman, P.; FitzGerald, R.J. Antioxidative peptides: Enzymatic production, in vitro and in vivo antioxidant activity and potential applications of milk-derived antioxidative peptides. *Amino Acids* **2013**, *44*, 797–820. [CrossRef] [PubMed]
36. Ren, J.; Zhao, M.; Shi, J.; Wang, J.; Jiang, Y.; Cui, C.; Xue, S.J. Purification and identification of antioxidant peptides from grass carp muscle hydrolysates by consecutive chromatography and electrospray ionization-mass spectrometry. *Food Chem.* **2008**, *108*, 727–736. [CrossRef] [PubMed]
37. Xie, Z.; Huang, J.; Xu, X.; Jin, Z. Antioxidant activity of peptides isolated from alfalfa leaf protein hydrolysate. *Food Chem.* **2008**, *111*, 370–376. [CrossRef] [PubMed]
38. Peña-Ramos, E.A.; Xiong, Y.L.; Arteaga, G.E. Fractionation and characterisation for antioxidant activity of hydrolysed whey protein. *J. Sci. Food Agric.* **2004**, *84*, 1908–1918. [CrossRef]
39. Chen, H.M.; Muramoto, K.; Yamauchi, F.; Nokihara, K. Antioxidant activity of designed peptides based on the antioxidative peptide isolated from digests of a soybean protein. *J. Agr. Food Chem.* **1996**, *44*, 2619–2623. [CrossRef]
40. Hsu, K.C. Purification of antioxidative peptides prepared from enzymatic hydrolysates of tuna dark muscle by-product. *Food Chem.* **2010**, *122*, 42–48. [CrossRef]
41. Wójciak, K.M.; Dolatowski, Z.J.; Kołożyn-Krajewska, D.; Trząskowska, M. The effect of the *Lactobacillus casei* LOCK 0900 probiotic strain on the quality of dry-fermented sausage during chilling storage. *J. Food Qual.* **2012**, *355*, 353–365. [CrossRef]
42. Molina, I.; Toldrá, F. Detection of proteolytic activity in microorganisms isolated from dry-cured ham. *J. Food Sci.* **1992**, *57*, 1308–1310. [CrossRef]

43. Fadda, S.; Sanz, Y.; Vignolo, G.; Aristoy, M.C.; Oliver, G.; Toldrá, F. Characterization of muscle sarcoplasmic and myofibrillar protein hydrolysis caused by *Lactobacillus plantarum*. *Appl. Environ. Microbiol.* **1999**, *65*, 3540–3546. [PubMed]
44. Gornall, A.G.; Bardawill, C.J.; David, M.M. Determination of serum proteins by means of the biuret reaction. *J. Biol. Chem.* **1949**, *177*, 751–766. [PubMed]
45. Adler-Nissen, J. Determination of the degree of hydrolysis of food protein hydrolysates by trinitrobenzenesulfonic acid. *J. Agric. Food Chem.* **1979**, *27*, 1256–1262. [CrossRef] [PubMed]
46. Re, R.; Pellegrini, N.; Proteggente, A.; Pannala, A.; Yang, M.; Rice-Evans, C. Antioxidant activity applying an improved ABTS radical cation decolorization assay. *Free Radic. Biol. Med.* **1999**, *26*, 1231–1237. [CrossRef]
47. Minkiewicz, P.; Dziuba, J.; Iwaniak, A.; Dziuba, M.; Darewicz, M. BIOPEP database and other programs for processing bioactive peptide sequences. *J. AOAC Int.* **2008**, *91*, 965–980. [PubMed]
48. ProtParam. Available online: https://web.expasy.org/protparam/ (accessed on 14 February 2018).

nutrients

MDPI

Review

Egg and Soy-Derived Peptides and Hydrolysates: A Review of Their Physiological Actions against Diabetes and Obesity

Stephenу C. de Campos Zani [1], Jianping Wu [2,*] and Catherine B. Chan [1,2,*]

[1] Department of Physiology, University of Alberta, Edmonton, AB T6G 2R3, Canada; zani@ualberta.ca
[2] Department of Agricultural, Food & Nutritional Science, University of Alberta, Edmonton, AB T6G 2R3, Canada
* Correspondence: jwu3@ualberta.ca (J.W.); cbchan@ualberta.ca (C.B.C.); Tel.: +1-780-492-6885 (J.W.); +1-780-492-9964 (C.B.C.)

Received: 23 March 2018; Accepted: 26 April 2018; Published: 28 April 2018

Abstract: Type 2 diabetes and obesity are two chronic conditions associated with the metabolic syndrome and their prevalences are increasing worldwide. The investigation of food protein-derived bioactive peptides that can improve the pathophysiology of diabetes or obesity while causing minimal side effects is desired. Egg and soy proteins generate bioactive peptides with multiple biological effects, exerting nutritional and physiological benefits. This review focuses on the anti-diabetic and anti-obesity effects of egg- and soy-derived peptides and hydrolysates in vivo and in vitro relevant to these conditions. Studies using the intact protein were considered only when comparing the results with the hydrolysate or peptides. In vivo evidence suggests that bioactive peptides from egg and soy can potentially be used to manage elements of glucose homeostasis in metabolic syndrome; however, the mechanisms of action on glucose and insulin metabolism, and the interaction between peptides and their molecular targets remain unclear. Optimizing the production of egg- and soy-derived peptides and standardizing the physiological models to study their effects on diabetes and obesity could help to clarify the effects of these bioactive peptides in metabolic syndrome-related conditions.

Keywords: diabetes; obesity; egg; soy; peptides; hydrolysate; bioactive peptides

1. Introduction

Diabetes is a chronic disease marked by the presence of hyperglycemia that occurs when the pancreas cannot produce enough insulin, or the body cannot effectively use the insulin that is produced. Uncontrolled diabetes can lead to several serious complications such as cardiovascular disease, nephropathy, retinopathy, amputation and nerve damage [1,2]. Well-managed diabetes can reduce the risk of these complications and increase life expectancy [1]. The treatment of diabetes requires long-term self-management and adherence to therapy, but several commonly used drugs can cause side-effects, which could negatively impact adherence [3].

Identifying natural products that can improve the disease state while exerting fewer side-effects is a current research trend. Many studies have explored the potential of biologically active peptides derived from food sources, which could be referred to as functional food ingredients. In the absence of a common definition, The European Commission Concerted Action on Functional Food Science in Europe together with The International Life Sciences Institute Europe published a consensus document and defined functional foods as those that beyond their nutritional value can exert one or more physiological effects in the body in a manner that can improve health/well-being or reduce the risk of diseases [4]. These peptides are produced enzymatically or using fermentation under controlled conditions of pH and temperature.

Two interesting sources of bioactive peptides are hen egg and soy. Egg is relatively cheap, found in almost every country and is nutrient-dense, which means it could be affordable and beneficial to a broad range of the world's population. Although the physiological effects of egg hydrolysates (EH) and peptides have been tested, the majority of publications investigated the angiotensin converting enzyme (ACE)-inhibitory, antioxidant or anti-inflammatory effects as reviewed by Liu et al. [5]. Soy, which is also protein-dense and broadly available, has been mostly studied regarding its antioxidant and anti-inflammatory actions as reviewed by Masilamani et al. [6]. Since an upregulated renin angiotensin system, inflammation and oxidative stress are observed in obesity and diabetes, which in turn are components of the metabolic syndrome (MetS) along with hypertension, it is of interest to study egg and soy in terms of their anti-diabetic and anti-obesity properties.

This review focuses on the effects of EH and soy hydrolysate (SH) or peptides in improving or preventing type 2 diabetes (T2D) and obesity in vivo or relevant in vitro endpoints such as insulin signaling pathways. The inclusion criteria were studies using egg, egg white (EW), egg yolk or soy in the form of hydrolysate or peptides. Studies where the results of intact protein were compared to the hydrolysate were also included. Only studies using oral administration of the hydrolysate or peptides in vivo were considered.

2. Diversity of Bioactive Peptides

Although several processes can be used to generate bioactive peptides, the most common method is enzymatic hydrolysis. Substrate specificity of enzymes generates peptides of different amino acid sequences and can be used to optimize the production of peptides with desired biological effects, as can be seen in Tables 1–4. Nevertheless, the peptides are complex and the use of a purification step following hydrolysis is common [7–9]. Alternatively, synthetic production of peptides [10,11] can be used to obtain specific peptides and study their physiological action.

Several groups have used the whole hydrolysate instead of individual peptides when studying their effects [12–18]. In those cases, effects cannot be attributed to a specific peptide, because the enzymatic hydrolysis can generate a myriad bioactive peptides, raising the possibility that the effect observed could be due to a combination of numerous peptides presented in the hydrolysate. Another variable of enzymatic hydrolysis process is the processing duration, which can impact both the peptide sequences and concentration in the hydrolysate [19].

It is worth mentioning that some of the enzymes used in hydrolysate production are not naturally produced by the human body, such as thermoase [20], flavourzyme [8,19] and neutrase [19], which means the peptides produced may not replicate those generated by the natural digestion process in the human body. Even though some studies used enzymes that are naturally produced in humans, such as pepsin and pancreatin [7,11,15,17] there is also no guarantee that the desired peptides would be produced or stable after further gastrointestinal digestion.

Due to the diversity of peptides obtained after enzymatic hydrolysis, multiple mechanisms of action of the peptides may influence outcomes. The length of the peptides can influence the absorption process in the gut as reviewed by Miner-Williams et al. [21] and specific amino acids can have a greater influence in the interaction with enzymes, for example the regions of interaction between a soy peptide and the enzyme dipeptidyl peptidase-IV (DPP-IV) correlated with the presence of the amino acids glutamine and arginine [11].

There is little evidence that accounts for the mechanisms of action of the peptides and important questions remain unanswered. For instance, are the peptides absorbed intact? Or can they initiate a cascade reaction by binding to receptors in the gut cells? Is the integrity and stability of the peptides after gastrointestinal digestion a requirement for them to exert their physiological effects?

3. In Vitro Study of Egg Hydrolysate (EH)/Peptides

A summary of in vitro studies and identified peptide sequences are provided in Table 1. Multiple metabolic pathways in several organs are involved in glucoregulation. One possibility to help manage diabetes is inhibition of intestinal α-glucosidase, which is an effective method to delay carbohydrate absorption [22] and reduce blood glucose concentrations. Peptides obtained after pepsin hydrolysis of egg white (EW) exhibited α-glucosidase IC_{50} values ranging from 365 to 1694 μg/mL [7], while peptides obtained from alcalase hydrolysis of egg yolk yielded IC_{50} values ranging from 23 to 40 μmol/L [22]. Beside α-glucosidase inhibition, the peptides from EW exerted multiple activities, for instance, ACE-inhibitory capacity with IC_{50} ranging from 9 to 27 μg/mL and DPP-IV- inhibitory activity with IC50 from 223 to 1402 μg/mL. The only exception was the peptide YIEAVNKVSPRAGQPF, which did not present either α-glucosidase or DPP-IV inhibitory activity [7]. The results suggest that egg peptides can potentially exert more than one physiological effect. Multiple activities exerted by the egg white hydrolysate (EWH) were found in other studies using cell lines as well [19,20]. EWH obtained with different enzymes (Table 2) exerted concomitantly anti-inflammatory, antioxidant, hypocholesterolemic, DPP-IV- and ACE-inhibitory activity [19]. The EWH derived from pepsin and peptidase-mediated hydrolysis had the highest potential against disorders associated with MetS such as hypertension, obesity and T2D, presenting IC_{50} against DPP-IV of <10 mg protein/mL and against ACE ranging from 47 to 151 μg/mL [19].

In the 3T3-L1 adipocyte cell line, thermoase + pepsin-prepared EWH not only sensitized the cells to insulin action but also mimicked insulin signaling. The EWH stimulated adipocyte differentiation by enhancing peroxisome proliferator associated receptor gamma (PPAR-γ) and CAAT/enhancer binding protein alpha (C/EBPα) expression, which led to enhanced adiponectin release and intracellular lipid accumulation. Moreover, these EWH enhanced the phosphorylation of proteins involved in the insulin signaling pathway, such as extracellular signal regulated kinase 1/2 (ERK 1/2), insulin receptor substrate 1 (IRS-1) and insulin receptor and protein kinase B (AKT) [20]. In adipocytes, the same EWH also presented anti-inflammatory properties by reducing cyclooxygenase-2 (COX-2) expression and C-Jun phosphorylation induced by tumor necrosis factor-α (TNF-α) [20]. Thus, the effect of thermoase + pepsin-prepared EWH in 3T3-L1 cells is exerted via insulin receptor and downstream proteins in the insulin signaling pathway. The adipogenic effect observed was partially mediated by PPAR-γ, because peptides identified in the hydrolysate upregulated PPAR-γ expression in vitro [20]. In macrophages, no effects were observed regarding TNF-α using peptidase or pepsin or flavourzyme EWH, but peptidase-prepared EWH reduced IL-6 after lipopolysaccharides stimulation [19].

An improvement in insulin sensitivity was also observed in a muscle cell line exposed to EW peptides. IRW, a peptide from egg ovotransferrin improved insulin resistance induced by angiotensin-II in skeletal muscle cells [10]. The peptide reversed the impaired insulin signaling and glucose uptake by normalizing phosphorylation of the serine residue in IRS and increasing AKT phosphorylation, which contributed to increased translocation of glucose transporter 4 (GLUT4) to the plasma membrane. It was shown that these effects were exerted partly by reducing angiotensin II type 1 receptor expression and reactive oxygen species (ROS) production [10]. In contrast, IQW and LPK egg white-derived peptides only exhibited antioxidant activity [10].

Although anti-diabetic activity is exerted by specific peptides, others presented low or no activity as antidiabetic agents [7,10,19,22], a fact that was attributed to their different amino acid sequences once they all were tested under the same conditions [10,19]. This fact indicates that the effects observed were due to the presence of specific peptides; however, there is a lack of experiments studying the relationship between the amino acid sequence in the peptides and their actions.

In summary, in vitro studies show that EWH or peptides derived from EW and egg yolk can exert multiple biological activities, including antidiabetic, by inhibiting enzymes such as DDP-IV and α-glucosidase or improving insulin sensitivity or signaling. However, the peptide amino acid sequence is important in determining the peptides' ability to act as antidiabetic agents. Therefore, there is a need for more in vitro experiments to specifically identify the interaction between the peptides, their amino acid sequence and the targets involved in the insulin signaling pathway.

Table 1. In vitro studies of egg-derived hydrolysates/peptides and their effects related to diabetes and obesity.

	Aims	Hydrolysis	Main Findings	Additional Assays	Peptides
			Egg yolk specific peptides **Enzymatic activity**		
Zambrowicz et al. 2015 [7]	Investigate multiple biological properties of peptides	Pepsin (120 min)	Three out of four peptides ↓ ACE, α-glucosidase and DPP-IV activity. The peptides presented antioxidant and ion chelating activity.	**DPPH - radical scavenging** All peptides tested presented radical scavenging properties (from 1.5 to 2.3 μMTroloxeq/mg)	YINQMPQKSRE YINQMPQKSREA VTGRFAGHPAAQ YIEAVNKVSPRAGQPF
Egg white specific peptides **Enzymatic activity**					
Yu et al. 2011 [22]	Investigate the inhibitory activity of hydrolysates against α-glucosidase and α-amylase and identify peptides	Alcalase (180 min)	Peptides from EW ↓ α-glucosidase but not α-amylase.	N/A	**Ovotransferrin** RVPSLM TPSPR DLQGK AGLAPY **Ovalbumin** RVPSL DHPFLF HAGN WIGLF
Egg white specific peptides **Cell culture**					
Garcés-Rimon et al. 2016 [19] 264.7 RAW macrophages	Investigate multiple biological properties of related to the metabolic syndrome	Alcalase Flavourzyme Neutrase Trypsin Pepsin Pancreatin Peptidase Promod 144P (0, 2, 4, 8, 12, 24, 36 and 48 h)	Pepsin hydrolysate: ↓ACE. Peptidase hydrolysate: ↓ ROS, CHOL and IL-6.	**Peptidase hydrolysate (24 h)** **Hypocholesterolemic activity** 0.259 ± 0.01 (mmol bound/mg protein) **ORAC test** 1099.9 ± 0.6 (μmol Trolox/g protein) **Pepsin hydrolysate (8 h)** **Hypocholesterolemic activity** 0.154 ± 0.011 (mmol bound/mg protein) **ORAC test** 574.2 ± 4.0 (μmol Trolox/g protein)	**Peptidase hydrolysate (24 h)** LPDEVSG DDNKVED GVDTKSD IESGSVEQA GGLVVT **Pepsin hydrolysate (8 h)** FRADHPPL FSL SALAM YQIGL RADHPFL IVF YAEERYPIL YRGGLEPINF RDILNQ ESIINF
Jahandideh et al., 2017 [20] 3T3-F442A Preadipocyte cell culture	Investigate the effect of hydrolysate on differentiation, insulin signaling and inflammation markers in pre-adipocytes	Thermoase (90 min) + Pepsin (180 min)	↑ intracellular lipid accumulation, adiponectin levels. ↑PPAR-γ and C/EBPα. ↑ p-ERK 1/2, p-IRβ and p-IRS-1. ↓ COX-2 and TNF-α -mediated C-Jun phosphorylation.↑ p-AKT after insulin treatment.	↑ PPAR-γ expression in dose-dependent manner with EWH at 2.5, 5 and 10 mg/mL	ERYPIL VFKGL WEKAFKDED QAMPFRVTEQE
Son et al., 2017 [10] Rat L6 myoblasts	Study the effect of specific ACE inhibitory peptides on insulin resistance induced by Ang-II and their mechanisms of action in muscular cells	N/A	IRW prevented the decrease in glucose uptake induced by Ang-II, normalized serine phosphorylation of IRS and GLUT4 expression and ↑ p-AKT. IRW ↓ AT1R, no effect on AT2R; ↓ ROS and NADPH activity. IQW and LPK peptides had anti-oxidant but no other actions.	N/A	**Ovotransferrin** IRW IQW LPK

Abbreviations: ACE, angiotensin converting enzyme; Ang-II, Angiotensin II; DPP IV, Dipeptidyl peptidase IV; EW, Egg white; IRS-1, Insulin receptor substrate 1; IRS, Insulin receptor; IRβ, Insulin receptor β; COX-2, cyclooxygenase 2; PPARγ, peroxisome proliferator associated receptor gamma; C/EBP-α, CAAT/enhancer binding protein alpha; AKT, protein kinase B; ERK1/2, Extracellular signal regulated kinase 1/2; TNF-α, Tumor necrosis factor alpha; DPPH, 1,1-diphenyl-2-picrylhydrazyl; ROS, Reactive oxygen species; CHOL, Cholesterol; IL-6, Interleukin 6; GLUT4, Glucose transporter 4; AT1R, Angiotensin II type 1 receptor; AT2R, Angiotensin II type 2 receptor; ↑ enhanced/stimulated; ↓ reduced/inhibited.

4. In Vivo Studies of Egg White Hydrolysate (EWH)/Peptides

In vivo EWH presents multiple biological activities as demonstrated in Table 2. All these in vivo studies were done in rodents and the specific peptides in EWH were not reported. Although no changes were found in circulating insulin, one study observed a reduction in blood glucose concentration and reduced homeostasis model assessment of insulin resistance (HOMA-IR) with protease-prepared EWH treatment [12]. Another three studies reported no changes in blood glucose levels with EWH obtained from protease and alcalase hydrolysis [13,23,24]. Serum leptin concentrations were not statistically different [23,24], and reduction or no changes were observed in plasma adiponectin levels [12,14].

Alongside enlarged adipose tissue, ectopic fat accumulation can lead to insulin resistance (IR) and consequently T2D. Analysis of the lipid content in liver and muscle, and total body fat percentage in rats showed reduced values after protease- and pepsin-prepared EWH treatment [12–14,23]. The steatotic state was improved (reduced size and number of fat vesicles), but no histological changes were seen in the adipose tissue with the pepsin-prepared EWH groups presenting similar adipocyte size as the obese control [14]. Stearoyl-CoA desaturase (SCD) is an enzyme involved in fat synthesis and responsible for converting a saturated fatty acid to its respective unsaturated fatty acid [12]. The SCD index is the ratio between those fatty acids and is related to obesity and insulin resistance. Dietary supplementation with protease-prepared EWH decreased SCD index in serum, muscle and liver in rodents [12,13,23]. Several hypotheses were tested in an attempt to elucidate the mechanisms responsible for reducing fat accumulation; for instance, SCD-1 is an enzyme essential in fat synthesis and because the abundance of lipogenic enzymes such as lipoprotein lipase (LPL) and fatty acids synthase (FAS) were not altered by EWH, the decrease in non-adipose tissue lipid content was attributed to the reduced SCD index [3]. Garcés-Rimon et al. postulate that the reduction in liver fat accumulation could be due to the ability of pepsin-prepared EWH to stimulate FFA oxidation in the hepatocytes but this hypothesis has not been tested [14]. Another possibility is that the reduction in fat accumulation occurred due to increased fat excretion. Indeed, two studies reported increased excretion of cholesterol (CHOL) and/or triglyceride (TG) and total bile acids in feces after protease-prepared EWH treatment [12,23]. In serum, reduction of CHOL or TG and/or free fatty acids (FFA) was observed [13,14,23]. However, no improvement in serum lipid profile was seen in another two studies [12,24]. An interesting corollary finding was that protease-prepared EWH increased muscular mass while decreasing fat accumulation, although the mechanism by which the hydrolysate acts remains unclear [13].

A study of the gut microbiota revealed that pepsin-prepared EWH treatment improved dysbiosis in obese rats; furthermore, short chain fatty acid (SCFA) and lactate concentrations in feces were lower compared to the obese group [15]. SCFAs are produced by gut microbiota through fermentation of dietary fiber, carbohydrates and peptides and are shown to improve glucose homeostasis and insulin sensitivity in rodents [25]; in addition, increased fecal SCFA content is found in obese human subjects [26]. Mechanisms that could explain the lower fecal SCFA in the pepsin-prepared EWH-fed group include maintenance of intestinal microbiota homeostasis or prevention of absorptive dysfunction by EWH; nevertheless, Requena et al. hypothesized that the change in microbiota occurred secondary to peptide absorption, with their actions on target tissues as antioxidant and anti-inflammatory agents leading to modulation of the gut microbiota [15] but there is as yet no evidence for this hypothesis.

Anti-inflammatory and antioxidant activity can contribute towards obesity and diabetes management [15]. In two studies in vivo, treatment with pepsin- and alcalase-prepared EWH reduced TNF-α in plasma and kidney and reduced malondialdehyde levels in plasma and urine indicating antioxidant properties [14,24]; these results are compatible with those observed in vitro previously mentioned in Table 1.

Table 2. In vivo studies of egg-derived hydrolysates/peptides and their effects related to diabetes and obesity in rodents.

	Aims	Hydrolysis	Treatment Details	Food Intake and Body Weight (BW)	Blood/Feces/Urine Analysis	Tissue Analysis	Main Findings
Egg white hydrolysate Studies in rodents							
Wang et al., 2012 [24] Zucker obese rats	Measure effect of hydrolysate NWT-03 on renovascular damage	Alcalase (6 h)	Aqueous NWT-03 (1 g/kg/day) 15 weeks	Food intake—not given BW—no effect	No effect on blood glucose, insulin, HBA1C, cholesterol and FFA levels. ↑ GLP-1 only by VIL URINE: Reduced MDA levels and decreased albuminuria	KIDNEY - ↓ inflammatory interleukins (IL-1β, IL-13) and TNF-α. Improved FGS, ↓ expression of α-SMA and ↑ TXA2R expression.	No changes in the diabetic profile of the rats; renovascular damage ↓ by NWT-03 treatment.
Ochiai and Matsuo 2014 [13] Wistar rats	Investigate the effect of EW and EWH on fat metabolism and TG content in non-adipose tissues	Protease (duration not specified)	Casein (297 g/kg) EWH (394 g/kg) EW (286 g/kg) 8 weeks	Food intake EWH ↓, EW ↓↓ BW EW ↓	EWH vs. casein- ↓ TG, ALP activity and FFA by EWH. EW vs. EWH- ↓ HDL-CHOL, FFA and ↑ total- CHOL by EWH. FECES EWH vs. casein - ↑CHOL excretion by EWH. EW vs. EWH- ↑ TG, TBA and CHOL excretion by EW.	EWH vs. Casein - Similar results in all parameters, except for ↓ fat mass. MUSCLE- ↑ mass; ↓ SCD index, TG content and G6PDH activity. LIVER- ↓CHOL, TG and SCD index (LIVER). EW vs. EWH - Similar results in all parameters, except for ↑ mass and ↓ SCD (MUSCLE) ↓ SCD (LIVER) by EW.	EW and protease EWH ↓ fat in adipose and non-adipose tissues Inhibited enzymes involved in lipogenesis and ↑ muscular mass and lipid excretion.
Ochiai et al., 2014 [12] Goto-Kakizaki rats	Feeding trial with EWH to study fat and glucose diabetic or normal rats	Protease (duration not specified)	Casein (200 g/kg) And EWH (267 g/kg) 6 weeks	Food intake Not different BW ↓ by EWH	Glucose, HOMA-IR, SCD Index - ↓ No difference between any other parameters tested.	MUSCLE - ↓ TG and SCD. LPL, FAS and G6PDH similar. LIVER - TG similar, ↓ SCD index. Liver, adipose tissue and muscle similar weight.	improved blood glucose levels and HOMA-IR, but not insulin secretion. ↓ TG in muscle and ↓ lipid accumulation in tissues.
Wistar rats			Casein (200 g/kg) And EWH (267 g/kg) 6 weeks	Food intake and BW not different	No difference in any of the parameters tested. (glucose, insulin, HOMA-R, HOMA-P, TG, NEFA, TC, HDL-CHOL, non-HDL-CHOL, adiponectin and SCD index)	MUSCLE - ↓ SCD but LPL, FAS and G6PDH similar LIVER - TG similar, ↓ SCD index. Liver, adipose tissue and muscle similar weight	↓ lipid content in muscle.
Garcés-Rimon et al., 2016 [14] Zucker obese rats	Demonstrate the effects of EWH related to obesity, lipid metabolism, inflammation and oxidative stress	Pepsin (8 or 14 h)	Aqueous EWH (750 mg/kg/day) 12 weeks	No difference in food intake and BW regardless of the hydrolysate	↓TNF-α, FFA and adiponectin, MDA. No changes in blood TG and CHOL.	ADIPOSE TISSUE - ↓weight but no changes in histology. LIVER - ↓ steatosis, ↑ GSH. Similar kidney and liver weight. Longer duration of hydrolysis negated effects.	↓ fat accumulation, improved hepatic steatosis and dyslipidemia. ↓ inflammatory and oxidative stress markers in plasma.
Ochiai et al., 2017 [23] Wistar rats	Study the effect of EW and low allergenic EWH on fat accumulation	Protease (duration not specified)	Equicaloric Diets Casein (297 g/kg) EWH (394 g/kg) EW (286 g/kg) 8 weeks	No difference in food intake and body weight between the three groups.	EWH vs. Casein ↓, total CHOL, ALP. Similar glucose, TG, NEFA, HDL-CHOL, non-HDL-CHOL, HOMA-β and insulin. EW vs. EWH Similar results in all parameters. FECES EWH & EW vs. Casein ↑ TG, CHO and TBA	EWH vs. Casein- Similar results in all parameters, except for ↓ weight, TG and NEFA, SCD index (LIVER). ↓ TG (MUSCLE) EWH vs. EW- Similar results in all parameters, except for ↑ G6PDH activity (muscle), SCD (adipose tissue) ↓ FAS (liver) in EWH.	↓ fat accumulation non- adipose tissues, ↓ intestinal absorption of lipid by increasing lipid excretion. Similar results as EW, however EWH was less allergenic
Requena et al., 2017 [15] Zucker obese rats	Observe the effect of EWH on the gut microbiota of rats	Pepsin (8 h)	Aqueous EWH (750 mg/kg/day) 12 weeks	Food intake N/A BW no difference.	FECES ↓ lactate and SCFA. *Lactobacillus/Enterococcus* and *C. leptum* similar to lean control.	N/A	Partially reverted dysbiosis present in Zucker obese rats.

Abbreviations: EWH, Egg white hydrolysate; FFA, free fatty acids; MDA, Malondialdehyde; EW, Egg white; TG, Triglyceride; CHO, Cholesterol; ALP, Alkaline phosphatase; TBA, Total bile acids; SCD, Stearoyl CoA desaturase; NEFA, Non esterified fatty acids; FGS, Focal glomerulosclerosis; AST, Aspartate aminotransferase; ALT, Alanine aminotransferase; G6PDH, Glucose 6-phosphate dehydrogenase; LPL, Lipoprotein lipase; FAS, Fatty acid synthase; TNF-α, Tumor necrosis factor alpha; α-SMA, Anti-a-smooth muscle actin; VIL, Vildagliptin; HOMA-R, homeostasis model assessment of insulin resistance; HOMA-β, Homeostasis model assessment of insulin secretion; GSH, Reduced Glutathione; HBA1C, Glycated hemoglobin A1C; GLP-1, Glucagon like peptide-1; TXA2R, Thromboxane A2 receptor; SCFA, Short chain fatty acids; WK, week; ↑ enhanced/stimulated; ↓ reduced/inhibited.

When not treated, diabetes can lead to several complications including nephropathy. Although NWT-03, an alcalase-prepared EWH, exerted in vitro DPP IV-inhibitory activity, in vivo it was not efficient in improving the diabetic state; however, the treatment reduced renal injury development and albuminuria in T2D rats [24]. When compared with vildagliptin (VIL), a currently used DPP-IV inhibitor, both NWT-03 and VIL exerted renal protection effects but only VIL increased GLP-1 levels. Therefore, it is believed that NWT-03 and VIL can act via similar mechanisms but independently of their DPP-IV inhibitory activity [24].

It is worth noting that when administered in a single dose, protease-prepared EWH did not alter lipid profile, inhibit pancreatic lipase or slow food transit [23]. Interestingly, when compared, protease-prepared EWH and EW, both prevented fat accumulation and increased muscle mass, but EW increased fat excretion compared to EWH [13,23].

To summarize, EWH presented antidiabetic properties in vivo, reducing ectopic fat accumulation in liver and muscle, which can enhance insulin sensitivity, and increasing fat excretion, which reduces absorption of calories and could contribute to weight loss. It also protected against diabetes complications (nephropathy), but little or no change was observed regarding blood glucose, adiponectin or insulin levels and regarding inhibition of DPP-IV. The discrepancies in the results observed in vivo could be attributed to the difference in the physiological background of the animals used but is more likely due to variation in the mixture of peptides present in the hydrolysates. Furthermore, the studies suggest that bioactive peptides present in the EWH were responsible for at least part of the effects observed; nevertheless, no measurement of the peptides in plasma, identification of those peptides or any other specific assay was conducted. There is a gap in the literature to explain the mechanism of absorption and action of these peptides.

5. In Vitro Studies of Soy Hydrolysates (SH)/Peptides

Soybean also contains bioactive peptides, and eight studies evaluating the in vitro effects of SH or peptides against diabetes and obesity are summarized in Table 3. Similarly to EH, during adipocyte differentiation SH obtained from pepsin hydrolysis increased lipid accumulation, expression of PPAR-γ and the expression and secretion of adiponectin in a dose dependent manner in 3T3-L1 pre-adipocytes; furthermore, this SH enhanced glucose uptake and expression of GLUT4, which could contribute to improve insulin sensitivity [16]. It is believed that this SH stimulated pre-adipocyte differentiation through PPAR-γ activation, although the SH did not present PPAR- γ ligand activity [16]. Interestingly, a study found that compared to pepsin + pancreatin-prepared SH from ungerminated soybeans, using germinated soybean hydrolysate reduced the number of adipocytes during the differentiation process and increased lipolysis in mature adipocytes, which could lead to less fat accumulation [17].

Higher lipolysis in 3T3-L1 mature cells was observed after treatment with flavourzyme-prepared SH even after gastrointestinal (GI)-simulated digestion as well [8]. Along similar lines, SH prepared with alcalase lowered lipid accumulation and downregulated LPL and FAS gene expression (enzymes involved in the lipid uptake and de novo fatty acid synthesis) in the absence of or following GI-simulated digestion [18]. A hydrolysate obtained only with naturally-occurring GI enzymes (pepsin + pancreatin) exerted similar effects, although to a lesser extent. It suggests that GI digestion in vivo may not markedly affect the bioavailability of that SH [18] although whether that is true for all hydrolysates remains to be determined. β-conglycin is a storage protein naturally found in soybean and it is interesting to note that the higher the β-conglycin concentration in the hydrolysate, the higher the inhibition of LPL and FAS [18].

IR in skeletal muscle and liver is a prominent state found in T2D. Pepsin + pancreatin- prepared SH and its fractions (peptides not identified) enhanced glucose uptake in L6-muscle cells; in addition, the fractions, but not the SH, were able to activate AMPK pathway in those cells [9]. Glucose uptake in C2C12 skeletal muscle cells was also enhanced by another soy peptide, named aglycin [27]. In HepG2 cells soy peptides previously known to modulate cholesterol metabolism by activating AMPK and ERK1/2 pathway [28], affected glucose metabolism by enhancing AKT phosphorylation, which in turn inactivated glycogen synthase kinase 3 (GSK3) by phosphorylating its serine residue, which can lead to higher glucose storage [29]. Moreover, the peptides increased glucose uptake and enhanced the expression GLUT4 and GLUT1 in liver cells [28]. One of these peptides (IAVPTGVA) also presented DPP-IV inhibitory activity with an IC_{50} value of 106 μM, and the regions of interaction between IAVPTGVA and DPP-IV were identified as the amino terminal Glu205 and Glu206 and carboxyl terminal Arg358 residues [11].

Inflammation is not the focus of this review, but it is linked with obesity and diabetes. Two studies reported changes in inflammatory markers by SH [18] or soy peptide [30] in co-cultured adipocytes and macrophages such as, reduced COX-2 and inducible nitric oxide synthase protein and lowered nitric oxide and prostaglandin E2 production [18]. The treatment with synthetized soy peptide FLV reduced the production and effect of inflammatory molecules and improved insulin sensitivity in adipocytes (higher IRS-1 and AKT phosphorylation) [30]. The authors showed evidence that peptide transport into 3T3-L1 cells occurred mainly via the peptide transporter PepT2 [30].

Taken together, the in vitro results show that SH obtained after hydrolysis by specific enzymes and some identified peptides can improve insulin sensitivity, inhibit DPP-IV, increase glucose uptake in muscle and liver, and reduce lipid accumulation and inflammation in adipose tissue (Table 3). Some of the studies suggest that the soy peptides can act through AMPK and AKT pathways to modulate glucose metabolism and via PPAR-γ to stimulate adipocyte differentiation. Although one peptide transporter in adipocytes and regions of interaction between soy peptide and DPP-IV was identified [30], there is still a lack of studies regarding the specific interactions between the peptides and enzymes involved in the glucoregulation process and the mechanism of absorption of those peptides.

Table 3. In vitro studies of soy-derived hydrolysates (SH)/peptides and their effects related to diabetes and obesity.

	Aims	Hydrolysis	Outcomes	Main Findings	Peptides
Soy specific peptides **Enzymatic activity**					
Lammi et al., 2016 [11]	Verify that soy peptide inhibits DPP-IV in vitro and identify the regions of interactions	Pepsin and/or Pancreatin synthetized peptides	Only IAVPTGVA ↓ DPP-IV activity. Regions of interaction were n-terminus Glu205 and Glu206 and c-terminus Arg358; the peptide has a proline flanked by valine in the fourth n-terminal residue, predicts interaction with DPP-IV.	Soy peptide IAVPTGVA ↓ DPP-IV activity in vitro. YVVNPDNDEN and YVVNPDNNEN were inactive against DPP-IV.	IAVPTGVA YVVNPDNDEN YVVNPDNNEN
Soy specific peptides **Cell culture**					
Tsou et al., 2013 [8] 3T3-L1 adipocytes	Isolate and identify peptides from soy hydrolysate with lipolytic activity	Flavourzyme 1% (125 min)	Three peptides ↑ glycerol release. After in vitro GI simulated digestion, VHVV capacity was not affected; ILL and LLL had attenuated lipolytic activity.	Soy peptides ↑ lipolysis in 3T3-L1 adipocytes and were little or not affected by GI enzymes.	ILL LLL VHVV
Lammi et al., 2015 [29] Human HepG2 cells	Verify that soy peptides modulate glucose metabolism	Trypsin or pepsin - synthetized peptides	All three peptides ↑ p-AKT, ↓ GSK3 activation, ↑ GLUT 4 and GLUT 1 mRNA, ↑ glucose uptake. IAVPTVGVA > IAVPGEVA > LPYP). IAVPGEVA and IAVPTVGVA ↑ GLUT1 mRNA more; LPYP ↑ GLUT4 mRNA more.	Soy peptides modulate glucose metabolism and ↑ glucose uptake in liver cells by activation of AKT and AMPK pathways.	IAVPGEVA IAVPTGVA LPYP
Kuak et al., 2016 [30] RAW 264.7 macrophages and 3T3-L1 adipocytes	Demonstrate the mechanism of transport of soy peptide into adipocytes and evaluate TNF-α induced inflammation and insulin response	Synthetized peptide	FLV peptide ↓ TNF-α, MCP-1 and IL-6 in co-cultured cell line (macrophages + adipocytes). FLV ↓ TNF-α-induced p- JNK and p-IKK and ↓ degradation of IκBα. TNF-α induced insulin resistance in adipocytes was ameliorated by FLV (↑ p-IRS-1, p-AKT). PepT2 > PepT1 expressed in adipocytes, ↑ by LPS and TNF-α.	FLV is transported into adipocyte cells mainly through PepT2 action and FLV can ↓ the inflammatory and insulin resistant states linked to obesity mainly by ↓ TNF-α induced inflammatory pathways.	FLV
Soy Hydrolysate **Cell culture**					
Martinez-Villaluenga et al., 2009 [18] 3T3-L1 adipocytes and RAW 264.7 macrophages	Study the effect of SH on lipid accumulation and inflammation	Alcalase (3 h) **or** Pepsin + Pancreatin (3 h each)	**Alcalase SH** in 3T3-L1 cells: ↓ lipid accumulation, LPL and FAS mRNA. Further GI simulated digestion did not reduce the bioavailability of Alcalase SH; Compared to Pepsin + pancreatin SH, Alcalase SH ↓ LPL and FAS mRNA in a higher extension, before and after GI digestion. **Alcalase SH** in RAW cells: ↓ LPL-induced nitrite formation, iNOS and COX-2 protein expression, PGE2 production. **Pepsin + pancreatin SH** in 3T3-L1 cells: ↓ lipid accumulation, LPL mRNA, but not FAS mRNA.	SH ↓ lipid accumulation and inflammatory marker expression, even after GI simulated digestion. Downregulation of LPL and FAS partially explain mechanism of action. Higher concentration of β-conglycin in the hydrolysate related to higher activity in vitro.	N/A

Table 3. *Cont.*

	Aims	Hydrolysis	Outcomes	Main Findings	Peptides
Soy specific peptides Enzymatic activity					
González-Espinosa de los Monteros et al., 2011 [17] 3T3-L1 adipocytes	Investigate the effect of germinated vs. ungerminated soybean hydrolysate on fat metabolism in adipocytes. Assess the interaction with soy phytochemicals.	Pepsin + Pancreatin (duration not specified)	Concentration > 1 mg/mL ↓ cell viability during differentiation process (10 days incubation), but not during 24 h of exposure. SH with and without phytochemicals ↓ lipogenesis, with higher germination time correlated to greater lipogenesis reduction. Lipolysis were present in a dose-dependent manner only with SH without phytochemicals treatment.	Germination changed the amino acids composition in the SH and interfered with the responses. Overall, SH ↓ the number of adipocytes during the differentiation process and ↑ lipolysis in mature adipocytes.	N/A
Goto et al., 2013 [16] 3T3-L1 pre-adipocytes	Observe effects of soybean peptic hydrolysate on adipocyte differentiation	Peptic hydrolysate (duration and enzymes not specified)	**During adipocyte differentiation** SH dose-dependently ↑ lipid accumulation, aP2 mRNA, adiponectin mRNA and secretion, PPAR-γ mRNA and protein expression, glucose uptake, GLUT4 mRNA.	SH ↑ adipocyte differentiation via PPAR-γ pathway and ↑ glucose uptake during differentiation process.	N/A
Roblet et al., 2014 [9] L6-skeletal muscle cells	Verify the potential of EDUF to concentrate soy peptides and identify the mechanism of action of those peptides	Pepsin (45 min) + Pancreatin (120 min)	The initial hydrolysate, anionic and cationic peptides ↑ glucose uptake. Only the peptides ↑ p-AMPK.	Anionic and cationic soy ↑ glucose uptake and AMPK phosphorylation in L6- skeletal muscle cells in vitro.	N/A

Abbreviations: SH, Soy hydrolysate; Ap2, adipocyte fatty acid-binding protein; IRS-1, Insulin receptor substrate 1; COX-2, Cyclooxygenase 2; PPARγ, Peroxisome proliferator associated receptor gamma; AKT, protein kinase B; TNF-α, Tumor necrosis factor alpha; LPL, Lipoprotein lipase; FAS, Fatty acid synthase; GLUT4, Glucose transporter 4; GLUT1,glucose transporter 1; SH, Soy hydrolysate; GI- gastrointestinal; iNOS, Inducible nitric oxide synthase; PGE2, Prostaglandin E2; AMPK, Activated protein kinase; JNK, c-Jun N-terminal kinase; IKK, IκB kinase; PepT2, Peptide transporter 2; PepT1, Peptide transporter 1; IL-6, Interleukin 6; DPP-IV, Dipeptidyl peptidase IV; MCP-1, Monocyte chemoattractant protein-1; LPS, Lipopolysaccharide; GSK3, Glycogen synthase kinase 3; ↑ enhanced/stimulated; ↓ reduced/inhibited.

6. In Vivo Studies of Soy Hydrolysate (SH)/Peptides

The tests in vivo described in Table 4 show that SH can modulate glucose metabolism and reduce body weight. Two studies reported reduced blood glucose levels by SH or peptides [27,31]. Similarly to in vitro studies (Table 3), a 37-amino acid soy peptide named aglycin improved muscle glucose uptake by increasing the phosphorylation of insulin receptor, IRS-1 and AKT, and enhancing membrane GLUT4 levels, which contribute to improved insulin sensitivity in T2D mice [27]. In fact, treatment with aglycin led to similar results as those exerted by metformin in oral glucose tolerance (OGTT) and insulin tolerance tests [27]; furthermore, the release of insulin during OGTT was normal in the treated animals and, as expected, abnormal in T2D mouse controls, suggesting that the effect on glucose tolerance was primarily due to enhanced glucose uptake and insulin sensitivity [27]. It is noteworthy that intact aglycin-37 amino acids were found in blood samples from mice, indicating that it is stable after GI digestion and probably absorbed intact [27].

With regards to serum lipid profile and lipid excretion, protease-prepared SH reduced fat accumulation in genetically obese mice, enhanced lipid excretion and improved plasma CHOL levels in diet obese rats [31]. The reduction in fat accumulation could be due to the higher postprandial energy expenditure observed after intake of protease-prepared SH compared to casein [32]; furthermore, the major contributor to enhanced postprandial energy expenditure was increased exogenous carbohydrate oxidation. Although the effect on energy expenditure was not sustained after 24 h, total carbohydrate oxidation continued to be higher in the SH-treated group, perhaps due to higher plasma insulin levels and lower glucose concentrations during the postprandial period or due to lower lipid absorption and increased carbohydrate absorption [32]. No experiments were conducted to substantiate these hypotheses.

Tests in humans have only been done with respect to glucagon and insulin responses after intake of SH or intact soy protein. SH induced a slower response of insulin and glucagon compared to its intact protein and no effect in plasma glucose was observed. The concentration of soy protein or SH administered did not correlate with the increase in plasma levels of insulin but, interestingly, glucagon was sensitive to protein concentration in a dose-dependent manner for both soy groups [33]. Another comparison, in rodents, showed that SH reduced body weight compared to whey isolate (WI) and whey isolate hydrolysate (WIH). In addition, soy intact protein and SH reduced liver and fat pad weight and maintained body protein percentage compared to WIH and WI, respectively [34].

The results in vivo herein, although scarce show that SH and soy peptides can potentially reduce tissue fat accumulation and increase fat excretion. Moreover, the soy peptide aglycin is resistant to GI digestion and can be absorbed intact by mice [27]. SH may also facilitate metabolic flexibility by shifting to carbohydrate utilization [32]. Nevertheless, only a few studies were done to test SH and peptides as antidiabetic agents in vivo and only one identified the peptide responsible for the effects.

7. Conclusions

In conclusion, the research so far shows that both egg and soybean can be rich sources of bioactive peptides; furthermore, they can potentially exert multiple physiological activities, including anti-obesity and anti-diabetic effects, which is relevant in the management of MetS. Bioactive peptides can be produced by different methods such as, enzymatically, chemically or by molecular biology. However, there is a huge variability in the methods, consequently generating many different hydrolysates and peptides, as shown in Tables 1–4. The duration of the hydrolysis process and the enzymes used generate different amino acid sequences, which influence the type and intensity of activity exerted by the peptides. Although an in silico approach may help to investigate the predictability of peptide generation [11], the predictability, purity and cost-effectiveness of each method vary [35]; therefore, optimization of the production process and the identification of amino acid sequences that can potentially act as anti-diabetic agents are still in need.

Table 4. In vivo studies of soy-derived hydrolysates/peptides and their effects related to diabetes and obesity.

	Aims	Hydrolysis	Treatment Details	Food Intake and Body Weight (BW)	Blood/Feces/Urine Analysis	Tissue Analysis	Main Findings	Peptides
Soy Specific peptide Studies in rodents								
Lu et al., 2011 [27] BALB/c mice	Investigate effects of soy peptide aglycin as antidiabetic agent	Not specified	HFD + aglycin (50 mg/g) or Metformin (100 mg/kg/d) orally daily for 28 days	No difference in **BW or food intake** (compared with diabetic model control)	Intact peptide detected in plasma after oral administration. **Glucose after 28 days** ↓ by Aglycin. **OGTT and ITT**- Aglycin similar effect as metformin. Insulin release not affected during OGTT.	**Skeletal Muscle** ↑ mRNA and total protein of IR and IRS-1. Total AKT and GLUT 4 mRNA not different. ↑ p-IR, p-IRS-1, p-AKT and GLUT4 on membrane.	Aglycin ameliorated glucose intolerance and insulin resistance in T2D mice mainly by ↑ glucose utilization and insulin sensitivity after long-term treatment. **In vitro** -glucose uptake ↑ in C2C12 skeletal muscle by aglycin in normal and insulin resistant cells.	Aglycin (37 aa)
Soy hydrolysate Studies in rodents								
Aoyama et al., 2000 [31] Sprague-Dawley rats	Study the effect of soy isolate hydrolysate on weight reduction	Protease (duration not specified)	HFD for 12 weeks + SH (40.4%) or SPI or Casein (39.1%) for 4 weeks	Similar **BW**, **food intake** and body composition in all 3 groups	**SP XSH**- SPIH ↓Glucose, total CHOL and HDL. **SH X Casein**- SH ↓Glucose total CHOL and HDL. **SP X SH**- similar **SH X Casein**- SH ↑ protein and fat % and ↓ apparent fat digestibility	**Liver** SH ↓weight. **fat pad** similar weight	SH ↓ fat accumulation and blood lipid profile levels by ↑ fat excretion. SH ↓ blood glucose in rats.	Mixture of peptides within five to six amino acids in length
Yellow KK mice			HFD for 31 days + SH (40.4%) or Casein (39.1%) for 4 weeks	No difference in **BW**. SH ↓ % fat and ↑ % protein (body composition).	N/A	**Liver** similar weight. **Fat pad** SPIH ↓ weight	SH ↓ fat accumulation and ↑ total protein % in genetically obese KK mice.	
Aoyama et al., 2000 [34] Yellow KK mice	Study the effect of intact soy protein and hydrolysate as anti-obesity agents	Protease (duration not specified)	HFD for 4 weeks + SPI or SPIH or WI or WIH for 2 weeks (energy restricted diet)	SH ↓ **BW** and carcass weight than WI and WIH. **SP and SH** ↓ fat %. **Food intake** similar.	Glucose and TG similar between four groups. SP ↓ total-CHOL than WIH	SP and SH ↓ liver weigh than WIH and WI and ↓ fat pad than WI	No differences were observed between the SP and SH groups; however, compared to WI and WIH. SH ↓weight gain, liver and fat pad weight while maintaining body protein.	N/A
Ishihara et al., 2003 [32] Yellow KK mice	Investigate the effect of soy isolate hydrolysate on energy expenditure	Protease (duration not specified)	HFD for 28 days + high protein diet SH (404 g/kg) or Casein (391 g/kg) for 4 weeks	No difference in **BW or food intake**	SH ↑ lipid content	SH ↓ kidney weight. No difference in liver, muscle, fat pad, heart or spleen weights.	SH- ↑ postprandial energy expenditure, ↑ exogenous carbohydrate oxidation. No difference in postprandial exogenous lipid oxidation. 24-h energy expenditure similar; ↑ 24-h carbohydrate oxidation. SH excreted more TG in feces than casein group.	Mixture of peptides within five to six amino acids in length
Soy hydrolysate Studies in Humans								
Claessens et al., 2008 [33] Male, non-obese human (average 28 years, BMI 24 kg/m^2)	Compare glucagon and insulin response after ingestion of soy protein and SH	Not specified	Cross-over trial: consumed drinks containing 0.3, 0.4 or 0.6 g/kg BW of soy protein or SH	N/A	Intact soy protein > SH for insulin and glucagon response. Blood glucose not different. Enhanced effect on glucagon response with increased protein load during intact and SH ingestion than on insulin response.	N/A	Intact soy protein induced a more rapid insulin and glucagon response than the SH. Glucagon was more sensitive to protein load than insulin and responded in a dose dependent manner. No effects in blood glucose were observed.	N/A

Abbreviations: IRS, Insulin receptor; IRS-1, Insulin receptor substrate 1; AKT, protein kinase B; GLUT4, Glucose transporter 4; SPIH, Soy hydrolysate; SP, intact soy protein; HFD, High fat diet; CHOL-cholesterol; TG, Triglyceride; OGTT, Oral glucose tolerance test; ITT, Insulin tolerance test; T2D, Type 2 diabetes; BW, Body weight; BMI, Body mass index; WK, week; ↑ enhanced/stimulated; ↓ reduced/inhibited.

In addition, the treatment length and the use of animals with different physiological and genetic backgrounds, such as obesity, diabetes and normal physiology contributed to the discrepancies in the results observed in vivo, which indicates the need of a standardized physiological model to better evaluate the activity of the peptides in diabetic states. Despite these limitations, it is clear that a wide variety of peptides from egg and soybean have overlapping biological activities that may be useful in the treatment of diabetes or obesity.

A weak correlation between the studies mentioned in this review and clinical trials could be drawn. Only one clinical trial using egg peptides was identified and it showed that NWT-03, an egg peptide previously mentioned in this review [24], reduced blood pressure in mild-hypertensive subjects [36]. In terms of soy, only data from clinical trials using black soy peptides were found. Black soy peptides reduced 2h-OGTT, weight, fat mass, leptin levels, blood pressure and oxidative stress in Korean subjects [37–39]. At this time, no data from clinical trials associating egg hydrolysate/peptides and glucose metabolism were found.

Even though some investigation of the effects of EH and SH on markers of diabetes and obesity have been done, there is still a lack of studies with focus on the mechanisms of absorption and action of the peptides, especially related to their interaction with cellular and molecular targets involved in insulin and glucose metabolism. Therefore, more studies are necessary to elucidate the effect of EH and SH and their real potential as functional food ingredients to be implemented in the management of obesity and T2D.

Author Contributions: S.C.d.C.Z. wrote the paper; J.W. and C.B.C. edited the paper.

Acknowledgments: This work is supported by research grants from the Alberta Livestock and Meat Agency, Egg Farmers of Canada, and the Natural Sciences and Engineering Research Council of Canada.

Conflicts of Interest: The authors declare no conflict of interest.

References

1. World Health Organization (WHO). *Definition and Diagnosis of Diabetes Mellitus and Intermediate Hyperglycemia: Report of a WHO/IDF Consultation*; WHO Press: Geneva, Switzerland, 2006; p. 5. ISBN 92-4-1594934.
2. World Health Organization (WHO). *Global Report on Diabetes*; WHO Press: Geneva, Switzerland, 2016; p. 13, ISBN 978-92-4-156525.
3. García-Pérez, L.-E.; Álvarez, M.; Dilla, T.; Gil-Guillén, V.; Orozco-Beltrán, D. Adherence to therapies in patients with type 2 diabetes. *Diabetes Ther.* **2013**, *4*, 175–194. [CrossRef] [PubMed]
4. European Commission Concerted Action on Functional Food Science in Europe (FUFOSE). *Scientific concepts of functional foods in Europe consensus document. Br. J. Nutr.* **1999**, *81*, S1–S27. [CrossRef]
5. Liu, Y.; Oey, I.; Bremer, P.; Carne, A.; Silcock, P. Bioactive peptides derived from egg proteins: A review. *Crit. Rev. Food Sci. Nutr.* **2017**, 1–23. [CrossRef] [PubMed]
6. Masilamani, M.; Wei, J.; Sampson, H.A. Regulation of the immune response by soybean isoflavones. *Immunol. Res.* **2012**, *54*, 95–110. [CrossRef] [PubMed]
7. Zambrowicz, A.; Pokora, M.; Setner, B.; Dąbrowska, A.; Szołtysik, M.; Babij, K.; Szewczuk, Z.; Trziszka, T.; Lubec, G.; Chrzanowska, J. Multifunctional peptides derived from an egg yolk protein hydrolysate: Isolation and characterization. *Amino Acids* **2015**, *47*, 369–380. [CrossRef] [PubMed]
8. Tsou, M.J.; Kao, F.J.; Lu, H.C.; Kao, H.C.; Chiang, W.D. Purification and identification of lipolysis-stimulating peptides derived from enzymatic hydrolysis of soy protein. *Food Chem.* **2013**, *138*, 1454–1460. [CrossRef] [PubMed]
9. Roblet, C.; Doyen, A.; Amiot, J.; Pilon, G.; Marette, A.; Bazinet, L. Enhancement of glucose uptake in muscular cell by soybean charged peptides isolated by electrodialysis with ultrafiltration membranes (EDUF): Activation of the AMPK pathway. *Food Chem.* **2014**, *147*, 124–130. [CrossRef] [PubMed]
10. Son, M.; Chan, C.B.; Wu, J. Egg white ovotransferrin-derived ACE inhibitory peptide ameliorates angiotensin II-stimulated insulin resistance in skeletal muscle cells. *Mol. Nutr. Food Res.* 2017. [CrossRef] [PubMed]

11. Lammi, C.; Zanoni, C.; Arnoldi, A.; Vistoli, G. Peptides derived from soy and lupin protein as dipeptidyl-peptidase IV inhibitors: In vitro biochemical screening and in silico molecular modeling study. *J. Agric. Food Chem.* **2016**, *64*, 9601–9606. [CrossRef] [PubMed]
12. Ochiai, M.; Kuroda, T.; Matsuo, T. Increased muscular triglyceride content and hyperglycemia in Goto-Kakizaki rat are decreased by egg white hydrolysate. *Int. J. Food Sci. Nutr.* **2014**, *65*, 495–501. [CrossRef] [PubMed]
13. Ochiai, M.; Matsuo, T. Effect of egg white and its hydrolysate on stearoyl-CoA desaturase index and fat accumulation in rat tissues. *Int. J. Food Sci. Nutr.* **2014**, *65*, 948–952. [CrossRef] [PubMed]
14. Garcés-Rimón, M.; González, C.; Uranga, J.A.; López-Miranda, V.; López-Fandiño, R.; Miguel, M. Pepsin egg white hydrolysate ameliorates obesity-related oxidative stress, inflammation and steatosis in Zucker fatty rats. *PLoS ONE* **2016**, *11*, e0151193. [CrossRef] [PubMed]
15. Requena, T.; Miguel, M.; Garcés-Rimón, M.; Martínez-Cuesta, M.C.; López-Fandiño, R.; Peláez, C. Pepsin egg white hydrolysate modulates gut microbiota in Zucker obese rats. *Food Funct.* **2017**, *8*, 437–443. [CrossRef] [PubMed]
16. Goto, T.; Mori, A.; Nagaoka, S. Soluble soy protein peptic hydrolysate stimulates adipocyte differentiation in 3T3-L1 cells. *Mol. Nutr. Food Res.* **2013**, *57*, 1435–1445. [CrossRef] [PubMed]
17. González Espinosa de los Monteros, L.A.; Ramón-Gallegos, E.; Torres-Torres, N.; Mora-Escobedo, R. Effect of germinated soybean protein hydrolysates on adipogenesis and adipolysis in 3T3-L1 cells. *Plant Foods Hum. Nutr.* **2011**, *66*, 355–362. [CrossRef] [PubMed]
18. Martinez-Villaluenga, C.; Dia, V.P.; Berhow, M.; Bringe, N.A.; de Mejia, E.G. Protein hydrolysates from β-conglycinin enriched soybean genotypes inhibit lipid accumulation and inflammation in vitro. *Mol. Nutr. Food Res.* **2009**, *53*, 1007–1018. [CrossRef] [PubMed]
19. Garcés-Rimón, M.; López-Expósito, I.; López-Fandiño, R.; Miguel, M. Egg white hydrolysates with in vitro biological multiactivities to control complications associated with the metabolic syndrome. *Eur. Food Res. Technol.* **2016**, *242*, 61–69. [CrossRef]
20. Jahandideh, F.; Chakrabarti, S.; Davidge, S.T.; Wu, J. Egg white hydrolysate shows insulin mimetic and sensitizing effects in 3T3-F442A pre-adipocytes. *PLoS ONE* **2017**, *12*. [CrossRef] [PubMed]
21. Miner-Williams, W.M.; Stevens, B.R.; Moughan, P.J. Are intact peptides absorbed from the healthy gut in the adult human? *Nutr. Res. Rev.* **2014**, *27*, 308–329. [CrossRef] [PubMed]
22. Yu, Z.; Yin, Y.; Zhao, W.; Yu, Y.; Liu, B.; Liu, J.; Chen, F. Novel peptides derived from egg white protein inhibiting alpha-glucosidase. *Food Chem.* **2011**, *129*, 1376–1382. [CrossRef]
23. Ochiai, M.; Misaki, K.; Takeuchi, T.; Narumi, R.; Azuma, Y.; Matsuo, T. Egg white hydrolysate can be a low-allergenic food material to suppress ectopic fat accumulation in rats fed an equicaloric diet. *J. Nutr. Sci. Vitaminol.* **2017**, *63*, 111–119. [CrossRef] [PubMed]
24. Wang, Y.; Landheer, S.; van Gilst, W.H.; van Amerongen, A.; Hammes, H.P.; Henning, R.H.; Deelman, L.E.; Buikema, H. Attenuation of renovascular damage in Zucker diabetic fatty rat by NWT-03, an egg protein hydrolysate with ACE- and DPP4-inhibitory activity. *PLoS ONE* **2012**, *7*, 1–11. [CrossRef] [PubMed]
25. Gao, Z.; Yin, J.; Zhang, J.; Ward, R.E.; Martin, R.J.; Lefevre, M.; Cefallu, W.T.; Ye, J. Butyrate Improves Insulin Sensitivity and Increases Energy Expenditure in Mice. *Diabetes* **2010**, *58*, 1–14. [CrossRef] [PubMed]
26. Schwiertz, A.; Taras, D.; Schäfer, K.; Beijer, S.; Bos, N.A.; Donus, C.; Hardt, P.D. Microbiota and SCFA in lean and overweight healthy subjects. *Obesity* **2010**, *18*, 190–195. [CrossRef] [PubMed]
27. Lu, J.; Zeng, Y.; Hou, W.; Zhang, S.; Li, L.; Luo, X.; Xi, W.; Chen, Z.; Xiang, M. The soybean peptide aglycin regulates glucose homeostasis in type 2 diabetic mice via IR/IRS1 pathway. *J. Nutr. Biochem.* **2012**, *23*, 1449–1457. [CrossRef] [PubMed]
28. Lammi, C.; Zanoni, C.; Arnoldi, A. IAVPGEVA, IAVPTGVA, and LPYP, three peptides from soy glycinin, modulate cholesterol metabolism in HepG2 cells through the activation of the LDLR-SREBP2 pathway. *J. Funct. Foods* **2015**, *14*, 469–478. [CrossRef]
29. Lammi, C.; Zanoni, C.; Arnoldi, A. Three peptides from soy glycinin modulate glucose metabolism in human hepatic HepG2 cells. *Int. J. Mol. Sci.* **2015**, *16*, 27362–27370. [CrossRef] [PubMed]
30. Kwak, S.-J.; Kim, C.-S.; Choi, M.-S.; Park, T.; Sung, M.-K.; Yun, J.W.; Yoo, H.; Mine, Y.; Yu, R. The soy peptide Phe–Leu–Val reduces TNFα-induced inflammatory response and insulin resistance in adipocytes. *J. Med. Food* **2016**, *19*, 678–685. [CrossRef] [PubMed]

31. Aoyama, T.; Fukui, K.; Takamatsu, K.; Hashimoto, Y.; Yamamoto, T. Soy protein and its hydrolysate reduce body fat of dietary obese rats and generically obese mice (yellow KK). *Nutrition* **2000**, *16*, 349–354. [CrossRef]
32. Ishihara, K.; Oyaizu, S.; Fukuchi, Y.; Mizunoya, W.; Segawa, K.; Takahashi, M.; Mita, Y.; Fukuya, Y.; Fushiki, T.; Yasumoto, K. A soybean peptide isolate diet promotes postprandial carbohydrate oxidation and energy expenditure in type II diabetic mice. *J. Nutr.* **2003**, *133*, 752–757. [CrossRef] [PubMed]
33. Claessens, M.; Saris, W.H.; van Baak, M.A. Glucagon and insulin responses after ingestion of different amounts of intact and hydrolyzed proteins. *Br. J. Nutr.* **2008**, *100*, 61–69. [CrossRef] [PubMed]
34. Aoyama, T.; Fukui, K.; Nakamori, T.; Hashimoto, Y.; Yamamoto, T.; Takamatsu, K.; Sugano, M. Effect of soy and milk whey protein isolates and their hydrolysates on weight reduction in genetically obese mice. *Biosci. Biotechnol. Biochem.* **2000**, *64*, 2594–2600. [CrossRef] [PubMed]
35. Zambrowicz, A.; Timmer, M.; Polanowski, A.; Lubec, G.; Trziszka, T. Manufacturing of peptides exhibiting biological activity. *Amino Acids* **2013**, *44*, 315–320. [CrossRef] [PubMed]
36. Plat, J.; Severins, N.; Morrison, S.; Mensink, R.P. Effects of NWT-03, an egg-protein hydrolysate, on blood pressure in normotensive, high-normotensive and mild-hypertensive men and women: A dose-finding study. *Br. J. Nutr.* **2017**, *117*, 942–950. [CrossRef] [PubMed]
37. Kwak, J.H.; Lee, J.H.; Ahn, C.W.; Park, S.H.; Shim, S.T.; Song, Y.D.; Han, E.N.; Lee, K.H.; Chae, J.S. Black Soy Peptide Supplementation Improves Glucose Control in Subjects with Prediabetes and Newly Diagnosed Type 2 Diabetes Mellitus. *J. Med. Food* **2010**, *13*, 1307–1312. [CrossRef] [PubMed]
38. Kwak, J.H.; Ahn, C.W.; Park, S.H.; Jung, S.U.; Min, B.J.; Kim, O.Y.; Lee, J.H. Weight reduction effects of a black soy peptide supplement in overweight and obese subjects: Double blind, randomized, controlled study. *Food Funct.* **2012**, *3*, 1019. [CrossRef] [PubMed]
39. Kwak, J.H.; Kim, M.; Lee, E.; Lee, S.H.; Ahn, C.W.; Lee, J.H. Effects of black soy peptide supplementation on blood pressure and oxidative stress: A randomized controlled trial. *Hypertens. Res.* **2013**, *36*, 1060–1066. [CrossRef] [PubMed]

nutrients

Article

Amelioration of Ethanol-Induced Gastric Ulcers in Rats Pretreated with Phycobiliproteins of *Arthrospira (Spirulina) Maxima*

Oscar Guzmán-Gómez [1], Rosa Virginia García-Rodríguez [2], Lucía Quevedo-Corona [3], Ricardo Pérez-Pastén-Borja [1], Nora Lilia Rivero-Ramírez [4], Emmanuel Ríos-Castro [5], Salud Pérez-Gutiérrez [6], Julia Pérez-Ramos [6] and Germán Alberto Chamorro-Cevallos [1,*]

1 Departamento de Farmacia, Escuela Nacional de Ciencias Biológicas, Instituto Politécnico Nacional, 07738 Ciudad de México, Mexico; oguz1985@live.com.mx (O.G.-G.); pastenrich@yahoo.com.mx (R.P.-P.-B.)
2 Unidad de Servicios de Apoyo en Resolución Analítica, Universidad Veracruzana, Xalapa, 91190 Veracruz, Mexico; rosga74@hotmail.com
3 Departamento de Fisiología, Escuela Nacional de Ciencias Biológicas, Instituto Politécnico Nacional, 07738 Ciudad de México, Mexico; quevedocorona@hotmail.com
4 Departamento de Morfología, Escuela Nacional de Ciencias Biológicas, Instituto Politécnico Nacional, 11350 Ciudad de México, Mexico; jazzband19@hotmail.com
5 Unidad de Genómica, Proteómica y Metabolómica, LaNSE, Cinvestav-IPN, 07360 Ciudad de México, Mexico; eriosc@cinvestav.mx
6 Departamento de Sistemas Biológicos, Universidad Autónoma Metropolitana-Xochimilco, Calzada del Hueso 1100, Col. Villa Quietud, Coyoacán, Ciudad de México 04960, Mexico; msperez@correo.xoc.uam.mx (S.P.-G.); jperez@correo.xoc.uam.mx (J.P.-R.)
* Correspondence: gchamcev@yahoo.com.mx; Tel.: + 52-57296300 (ext. 52398)

Received: 19 April 2018; Accepted: 8 June 2018; Published: 13 June 2018

Abstract: Phycobiliproteins of *Arthrospira* (*Spirulina*) *maxima* have attracted attention because of their potential therapeutic antioxidant properties. The aim of this study was to assess the possible antiulcerogenic activity of these phycobiliproteins (ExPhy) against ethanol-induced gastric ulcers in rats. To explore the possible mechanisms of action, we examined antioxidant defense enzymes (e.g., catalase, superoxide dismutase, and glutathione peroxidase), as well as the level of lipid peroxidation (MDA) and the histopathological changes in the gastric mucosa. Intragastric administration of ExPhy (100, 200, and 400 mg/kg body weight) significantly lowered the ulcer index value compared to the ulcer control group ($p < 0.05$). The greatest protection was provided by the concentration of 400 mg/kg. The histological study supported the observed gastroprotective activity of ExPhy, showing a reduced inflammatory response. Moreover, the alcohol-induced decrease in stomach antioxidant enzyme activity found in the ulcer control group was prevented by ExPhy pretreatment. Furthermore, ExPhy reversed the ethanol-induced increase in lipid peroxidation. In summary, the antiulcerogenic potential of ExPhy may be due, at least in part, to its anti-oxidant and anti-inflammatory effects.

Keywords: antiulcerogenic; *Arthrospira* (*Spirulina*) *maxima*; phycobiliproteins; ethanol

1. Introduction

Stomach ulcers, one of the most common gastrointestinal disorders, affect people of all ages around the world [1]. Under normal conditions, the integrity of the stomach mucosal barrier is maintained by an equilibrium between irritation and defensive factors [2]. When the gastric mucosa is continuously exposed to extremely aggressive agents, such as non-steroid anti-inflammatory drugs

(NSAIDs), nutritional deficiencies, smoking, stress, and excessive ingestion of ethanol, this equilibrium can be jeopardized and the risk of developing a gastric ulcer increases [3–6].

In the gastrointestinal tract, exposure to alcohol can damage the motility of the esophagus, stomach, and gut as well as the capacity of gut absorption. It can generate mucosal damage and even carcinogenesis [7,8]. Ethanol is a harmful agent associated with multiple pathologies and is applied orally in experimental animals to cause acute gastric lesions and ulcers [9,10]. The mechanism of ethanol-induced damage is complex and not fully understood. Ethanol produces a disruption in the integrity of the gastric mucosal barrier through exfoliation of cells, thus increasing mucosal permeability and in some cases provoking bleeding [3,11]. The extravasation of neutrophils to the site of injury triggers elevated concentrations of reactive oxygen species (ROS) and other mediators of inflammation, causing oxidative damage with deleterious effects on cells. Oxidative stress has been shown to play a role in alcohol-induced gastric mucosal damage [12,13].

Spirulina maxima is a blue-green alga, now given the name *Arthrospira maxima* (Am). This cyanobacterium has been used as food since antiquity, with some of the first historical records coming from the Aztec civilization and the early inhabitants of Central Africa [14,15]. Due to its high content of proteins (mainly phycocyanin and allophycocyanin), vitamins, amino acids, minerals, and essential fatty acids, it has been the object of several pharmacological studies [16]. Am has been reported as having anti-inflammatory, immunostimulatory, antiviral, and antioxidant activity [17–20], as well as producing anti-hepatotoxic and anti-nephrotoxic effects and improving vascular reactivity [21–23]. These effects have been related to the antioxidant activity of Am, while others are attributed to some of its active ingredients, such as phycobiliproteins, which decrease oxidative stress [19,24]. Various studies have shown that extracts of Am rich in phycobiliproteins exhibit relevant pharmacological properties, including anti-teratogenic and neuroprotective effects, antigenotoxic properties, anti-inflammatory, and antioxidant activities, and protection against colitis [19,25–28]. However, to our knowledge, there are no reports on the anti-ulcerative activities of phycobiliproteins from Am.

Hence, the aim of the present study was to assess the gastroprotective effects of an extract of Am rich in phycobiliproteins (ExPhy) on ethanol-induced gastric ulcers in rats. Accordingly, evaluation was made of some antioxidant and oxidative markers as well as histopathological damage.

2. Materials and Methods

2.1. Preparation of the Phycobiliprotein Extract (ExPhy)

ExPhy was prepared as described by Cruz de Jesús et al. [29], with some modifications. Three grams of Am powder (AEH Spiral Spring, Mexico City) were suspended in 12 g of phosphate buffer (20 mM, pH 7) and stirred at room temperature (r.t.) for 5 min. The solution was then subjected to three cycles of freezing and thawing, being frozen at −70 °C and thawed at r.t. Subsequently, the mixture was shaken for 1 h at r.t., followed by centrifuging the crude extract of phycobiliproteins at 18,000 rpm for 30 min at 4 ° C in a Beckman Coulter Avanti j-30I centrifugue (Beckman Coulter, Brea, CA, USA). The blue supernatant obtained was separated and again centrifuged at 22,000 rpm, discarding the green precipitate after each centrifugation step. Finally, the supernatant was lyophilized and stored (protected from light) at −20 °C.

The phycobiliprotein concentration in the supernatant was calculated from absorption measurements at 562, 620, and 652 nm. Equation (1) was used for estimating C-phycocyanin (C-PC) and Equation (2) for allophycocyanin (APC) [30]:

$$\text{C-PC (mg/mL)} = [\text{A620} - 0.474\ (\text{A652})]/5.34 \quad (1)$$

$$\text{APC (mg/mL)} = [\text{A652} - 0.208\ (\text{A620})]/5.09 \quad (2)$$

The purity of C-PC and APC extracts was also evaluated, finding C-PC with an A620/A280 absorbance ratio and APC with an A652/A280 ratio [31].

2.2. LC-MALDI-MS/MS and Data Analysis

Sodium dodecyl sulfate–polyacrylamide gel electrophoresis (SDS–PAGE) was performed according to the Gallagher method [32], with a separating gel of 12% and a stacking gel of 5% acrylamide. An electrophoresis was run with 50 μg/mL ExPhy at 120 V for 90 min. Resolved proteins were visualized with Coomassie Brilliant Blue (G250) staining. Four fragments from SDS-PAGE were enzymatically digested according to the modified protocol of Shevchenko et al. [33]. The resulting tryptic peptides were concentrated at an approximate volume of 10 μL. Then, 9 μL were loaded into a ChromXP Trap Column C18-CL precolumn (Eksigent, Redwood City, CA, USA), with 350 μm × 0.5 mm, a 120 A° pore size and a 3 μm particle size, desalted with 0.1% TFA in H_2O at a flow rate of 5 μL/min for 10 min. Then, peptides were loaded and separated on a Waters BEH130 C18 column (Waters, Milford, MA, USA), with 75 μm × 150 mm, a 130 A° pore size and a 1.7 μm particle size, using an HPLC Ekspert nanoLC 425 (Eksigent, Redwood City, CA, USA). Mobile phase A was 0.1% trifluoroacetic acid (TFA) in H_2O and mobile phase B 0.1% TFA in acetonitrile (ACN) at a flow rate of 300 nL/min, with the following gradient: 0–3 min, 10% B (90% A); 35 min, 60% B (40% A); 36–45 min, 90% B (10% A); 46–120 min, 10% B (90% A). Eluted fractions were automatically mixed with a solution of 2 mg/mL of α-Cyano-4-hydroxycinnamic acid (CHCA) in 0.1% TFA and 50% ACN as a matrix, spotted in a stainless-steel plate of 384 spots with a MALDI Ekspot (Eksigent, Redwood City, CA, USA), with a spotting velocity of 30 s per spot at a matrix flow of 1.6 μL/min. The spots generated were analyzed by a MALDI-TOF/TOF 4800 Plus mass spectrometer (ABSciex, Framingham, MA, USA). Each MS spectrum was acquired by accumulating 1000 shots in a range of m/z 850–4000 with a laser intensity of 3100. The 100 most intense ions with a minimum signal-noise (S/N) of 20 were programmed to fragment. The MS/MS spectra were obtained after fragmentation of selected precursor ions by using collision-induced dissociation (CID), acquired by 3000 shots with a laser intensity of 3800. The MS/MS spectra were compared to the Am CS-328 database (downloaded from Uniprot, 5505 protein sequences) with Protein Pilot software v. 2.0.1 (ABSciex, Framingham, MA, USA) and Paragon algorithm [34]. Search parameters were: carbamidomethylated cysteine, trypsin as a cut enzyme, all biological modifications and amino acid substitutions set by the algorithm, and phosphorylation emphasis and gel-based ID as special factors. The detection threshold was considered at 1.3 to acquire 95% confidence, and the identified proteins observed a local FDR of 5% or less. These proteins were grouped by the ProGroup algorithm in the software to minimize redundancy.

2.3. Animals

Male Wistar rats (170–250 g) were supplied from the breeding colony of the Autonomous University of Hidalgo State (UAEH). The animals were maintained in cages with raised floors and wide mesh (to prevent coprophagy), in a separate animal room under standard conditions of temperature (22 ± 1 °C) and a 12 h light/dark cycle. They were fed a standard diet, with water provided ad libitum throughout the experiment. Prior to inducing ulcers, the rats were fasted for 22 h. After each experiment, the animals were euthanized in a carbon dioxide euthanasia chamber. The current protocol was accepted by the Ethics Committee of the National School of Biological Sciences (CEI-ENCB-08-2016). All procedures and handling of the animals were in accordance with the Mexican Official Regulation (NOM ZOO–062-200-1999) entitled "Technical Specifications for Production, Care, and Use of Laboratory Animals".

2.4. Drugs and Chemicals

Omeprazole was acquired from Sigma-Aldrich (St. Louis, MO, USA). Thiobarbituric acid (TBA) and trichloro acetic acid (TCA) were purchased from Merck (Darmstadt, Germany). SOD and GPx were obtained from Randox, Mexico city. Other reagents and solvents, procured from local sources, were of analytical grade.

2.5. Antiulcer Activity and Experimental Design

The assay was carried out with the methodology described by Almasaudi et al. [35], with some modifications. The animals were randomly divided into six groups (n = 6). All treatments were administrated by intragastric gavage for eight consecutive days, with the gastric ulcer induced on the last day with 80% ethanol solution (1 mL/animal). Group I (vehicle control) received the vehicle only (10 mL/kg body weight (bw) of 1% Tween-80 aqueous solution). For all other groups, an ulcer was induced on the last day of treatment, one hour after administering the corresponding compound. Group II (ulcer control) was given the vehicle, group III 40 mg/kg bw omeprazole, group IV, V and VI the different concentrations of ExPhy (100, 200 and 400 mg/kg bw, respectively).

One hour after inducing an ulcer, animals were sacrificed. The stomachs were excised, filled by injecting 2.5 mL of a 4% formaldehyde solution, and put in a beaker with formaldehyde. After 10 min, the stomachs were opened over the greater curvature and rinsed with saline solution (0.9%) to remove the blood clots. Thereafter, each gastric sample was placed on a slide. The gastric damage area (mm^2) was determined with "Image J" image processing software. The Ulcer Index (UI) for each rat was calculated with the following formula:

$$UI = (TAML\ (mm^2) \times 100)/(TMA\ (mm^2))$$

where TMA is the total mucosal area and TAML the total area of mucosal lesion of each rat [36]. The protection percentage (PP) was calculated using the following formula:

$$UI = (TAML\ (mm^2) \times 100)/(TMA\ (mm^2))$$

$$PP = (UI\ control - UI\ treated)/(UI\ control) \times 100$$

where UI control is the ulcer index of the ulcer control (group II) and UI treated is the ulcer index of the treated group (groups III–VI) [37]. From the three concentrations tested for ExPhy, the one with the least UI was adopted for all other tests.

2.6. Stomach Tissue Preparation

In a second experiment, another series of four groups of rats were formed. After the eight days of the corresponding treatments, the ulcer was induced and the rats were sacrificed (see previous section). The stomachs were extracted, cut along the greater curvature, and gently rinsed with cold phosphate buffer (PBS) (pH 7.4). A portion of each stomach tissue (0.5 g) was cut into small pieces and 4.5 mL of cold PBS were added. The mixture was homogenized on ice with an Ultra-turrax homogenizer (T18, IKA, Staufen im Breisgau, Germany) and a Polytron (Newtown, CT, USA) handheld homogenizer, and then tissue homogenates were centrifuged for 12 min at 12,000 rpm (4 °C). The supernatants were divided into aliquots and conserved at −20 °C until the biochemical analysis.

2.7. Biochemical Analysis

Gastric activity of glutathione peroxidase (GPx) was determined with a commercial kit Ransel RS504 (Crumlim, Country Antrim, UK), based on the method developed by Plagia and Valentine [38]. GPx catalyzes the oxidation of glutathione by cumene hydroperoxide. In the presence of glutathione reductase (GR) and NADPH, the oxidized glutathione is immediately converted to the reduced form with concomitant oxidation of NADPH to NADP+. The decrease in absorbance was measured after 1 and 2 min at 340 nm, with enzyme activity being directly proportional to the rate of change.

Superoxide dismutase activity (SOD) was assessed according to the method of McCord and Fridovich [39] with a Ransod SD125 Kit (Crumlim, Country Antrim, UK). The method employs xanthine and xanthine oxidase to generate superoxide radicals, which react with 2-(4-iodophenyl)-3-(4-nitrophenol)-5-phenyltetrazolium chloride (INT) to form a red formazan dye. SOD inhibits the reaction by converting the superoxide radical to oxygen. The SOD activity was determined as the degree of inhibition of this reaction, measured by absorbance at 505 nm.

Catalase activity (CAT) in gastric tissue was evaluated by tracking the rate of decomposition of H_2O_2 in the presence of CAT at 240 nm [40].

The protein concentration in supernatants was established by the Bradford method [41], using bovine serum albumin as a standard. This assay involves the binding of Coomassie Brilliant Blue G-250 dye to proteins at r.t. When the dye binds to the protein, it is converted from an unstable form (red in color) to a stable unprotonated form (turning blue). The blue protein dye is detected at 595 nm.

Lipoperoxidation Assessment

The content of malondialdehyde (MDA) was determined in each of the supernatants by the thiobarbituric acid reactive substances (TBARS) assay, as described by Esterbauer and Cheeseman [42]. To 0.5 mL of gastric mucosal homogenates were added 1.0 mL of reactive mixture containing 0.375% of TBA and 15% of trichloroacetic acid (TCA) in 0.20 N HCl. After incubation for 15 min in boiling water, the samples were cooled and centrifuged at 1000 rpm for 10 min at 4 °C. The absorbance of the supernatant was measured at 532 nm and the concentration of MDA was calculated with an extinction coefficient of 156,000 M^{-1} cm^{-1}.

2.8. Histopathological Examination

After determination of the UI, the stomachs of each group were fixed in 10% formalin solution for 24 h. Subsequently, they were dehydrated by immersing them in ascending concentrations of alcohol solutions (70–100%) and in paraffin. Slides of stomach slices of 4–5 μm thickness were prepared and stained with hematoxylin and eosin (H&E) and then analyzed under light microscope at 20× and 40× for pathological changes, including necrosis, edema, vasocongestion, eosinophilic infiltration, and glandular damage. All slides were photographed with Zeiss Axiophot microscopy (Thornwood, NY, USA).

2.9. Statistical Analysis

Statistical analysis was carried out with SigmaPlot version 12.0 (Systat Software, San Jose, CA, USA). All data are expressed as the mean ± standard error of the mean (SEM). One-way analysis of variance (ANOVA) and Dunnett's post hoc test were applied, comparing the treated groups with the ulcer control group; statistical significance was attributed at $p < 0.05$.

3. Results

3.1. Evaluation of Phycobiliprotein Content and Purity of ExPhy

The phycobiliprotein (C-PC and APC) content and purity of ExPhy were evaluated (Table 1). C-PC purity was found to be 0.86 and APC purity 0.81. The content of C-PC was 0.40 mg/mL and of APC 0.56 mg/mL.

3.2. LC-MALDI-MS/MS Analysis

Liquid chromatography (HPLC) along with mass analysis by MALDI-MS/MS was carried out to identify and characterize the protein components of ExPhy, isolated from *Arthrospira maxima*. Nine different proteins were identified that belong to phycobilisomes, which is a light-harvesting macromolecular complex (Table 2). The spot number (band of gel), accession number, protein name, unused, % coverture (% Cov), and molecular weight are reported. Other proteins were also detected (their specific data are summarized in Table S1).

Table 1. Concentration and purity ratio of ExPhy.

Phycobiliprotein	Concentration (mg/mL)	Purity Ratio A620/A280 (C-PC) A652/A280 (APC)
C-PC	0.40	0.86
APC	0.56	0.81

C-PC, Phycocyanin C; APC, Allophycocyanin; ExPhy, extract rich in phycobiliproteins.

Table 2. Results of different protein spots identified by MALDI-MS/MS.

No.	Spot No.	Accession	Protein	Unused	% Cov	MW (Da)
1	1, 2, 3, 4	tr I Q8VRJ2	Phycocyanin alpha chain	16	69.75309	17,600
2	1, 2, 3, 4	tr I Q7BA94	Phycocyanin beta chain	10.44	78.48837	18,094
3	1, 2, 3, 4	tr I B5VUA2	Allophycocyanin, beta subunit	8	82.60869	17,330
4	1, 3, 4	tr I B5W3K3	Allophycocyanin, beta subunit	4.85	56.80473	18,442
5	1, 2, 3, 4	tr I B5W789	Phycobilisome linker polypeptide	2.8	52.7559	29,427
6	1, 2, 3	tr I B5VV49	Phycobilisome linker polypeptide	2.75	30.90278	32,509
7	2	tr I B5VV50	Phycobilisome linker polypeptide	3.67	59.77859	30,834
8	3, 4	tr I B5W2H7	Phycobilisome protein	8.72	55.90062	18,002
9	1, 2, 3, 4	tr I B5VUA1	Phycobilisome protein	9.49	80.12422	17,392

No, number; % Cov, % coverture; MW (Da), molecular weight (daltons); MALDI-MS/MS, matrix-assisted laser desorption/ionization mass spectrometry.

3.3. *Effect of ExPhy on Ethanol-Induced Gastric Lesions*

The gastroprotective effect of pretreatment with ExPhy on ethanol-induced gastric lesions was determined (Table 3). In the vehicle control group, no macroscopic lesions were found (Figure 1A). In the ulcer control group, severe gastric lesions were observed in the mucosa layer, such as gastric hyperemia and thick linear hemorrhages (Figure 1B), with a UI of 13.73 ± 1.50. Pretreatment with ExPhy (at 100, 200, and 400 mg/kg) and omeprazole (at 40 mg/kg) (Figure 1C–F, respectively) significantly reduced the ulcer index of lesions compared to the ulcer control group, with values of 8.91 ± 0.87, 6.61 ± 1.10, 5.13 ± 0.94, and 1.32 ± 0.96, respectively. The decrease in the ulcer index was also expressed as a percentage of protection, being 35.10%, 51.87%, 62.62%, and 90.36%, respectively.

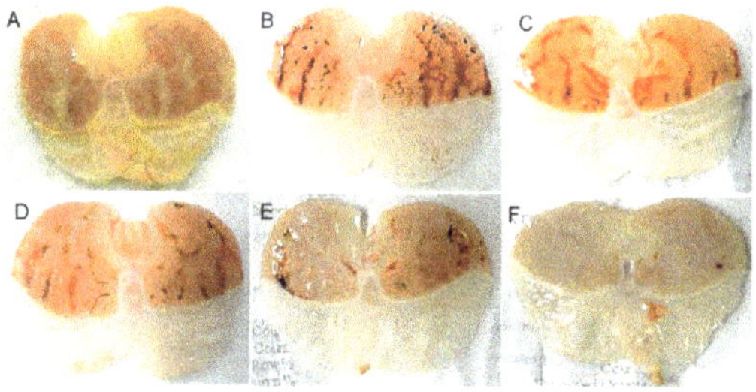

Figure 1. Gastric ulcer area of ethanol-induced ulceration in rats. (**A**) Vehicle control; (**B**) ulcer control; (**C**) ExPhy (100 mg/kg); (**D**) ExPhy (200 mg/kg); (**E**) ExPhy (400 mg/kg); (**F**) omeprazole (40 mg/kg).

3.4. *Histopathology*

The microscopic study of the vehicle control group (Figure 2A,a) shows typical gastric histoarchitecture with intact epithelium and glands. The ulcer control group, on the other hand, displayed several changes in the integrity of the gastric mucosa (Figure 2B,b), such as severe desquamation and loss of surface epithelial (mucous) cell, necrosis, vacuolization, edema and dilated gastric glands along with infiltration of inflammatory cells (neutrophils and eosinophils). Pretreatment with omeprazole decreased the gastric lesions compared to the ulcer control. The gastric mucosa exhibited focal loss of superficial gastric epithelium. The gastric glands were almost normal in appearance. There was mild edema with limited eosinophilic infiltration and minimal hemorrhage (Figure 2C,c). Pretreatment with ExPhy resulted in gastric lesions, characterized by focal areas of disruption in one-third of the mucosa, without a mucus layer in this zone. Nevertheless, the rest of the mucosa showed almost normal gastric glands, with mild edema and limited eosinophilic infiltration (Figure 2D,d) compared to the ulcer control.

Table 3. Effect of ExPhy and omeprazole on ulcer parameters in rats with ethanol-induced ulcers.

Groups	Pretreatment	Ulcer Index (mm^2)	Protection Percentage (%)
I	Vehicle control	0 *	0
II	Ulcer control	13.73 ± 1.50	0
III	Omeprazole (40 mg/kg)	1.32 ± 0.96 *	90.36
IV	ExPhy (100 mg/kg)	8.91 ± 0.87 *	35.10
V	ExPhy (200 mg/kg)	6.61 ± 1.10 *	51.87
VI	ExPhy (400 mg/kg)	5.13 ± 0.94 *	62.62

Data are expressed as the mean ± SEM; n = 6 rats per group; * indicates $p < 0.05$ compared to the ulcer control group; ExPhy = extract rich in phycobiliproteins.

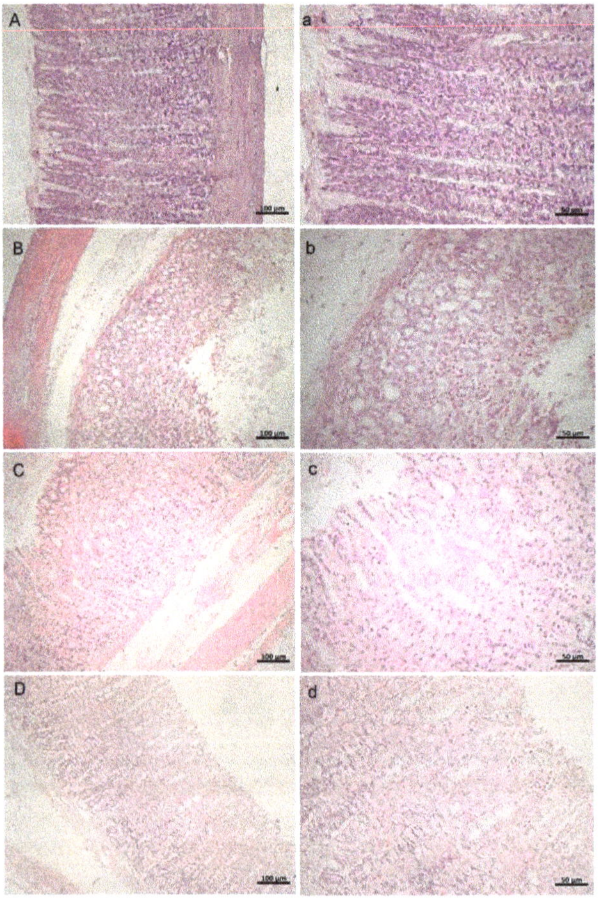

Figure 2. H&E staining of rat gastric mucosa in ethanol-induced gastric ulcers (magnification at 20× and 40×). (**A**,**a**) Vehicle control; (**B**,**b**) ulcer control; (**C**,**c**) omeprazole (40 mg/kg); (**D**,**d**) ExPhy (400 mg/kg).

3.5. MDA and Antioxidant Enzyme Determination

After ethanol administration, an evaluation was made of the effect of ExPhy on the activity of antioxidant enzymes (SOD, CAT, and GPx) and the level of MDA (as a lipoperoxidation index) in gastric tissue (Figure 3). The SOD enzyme activity in the ulcer control significantly decreased compared to the vehicle control. Pretreatment of rats with ExPhy (400 mg/kg) and omeprazole (40 mg/kg) significantly restored SOD activity in relation to the ulcer control. CAT activity in the stomach of the ulcer control was significantly lower than that of the vehicle control. In the groups treated with ExPhy (400 mg/kg) and omeprazole (40 mg/kg), CAT activity was significantly greater than in the ulcer control. The depletion of GPx activity observed in ulcer control was significantly reversed in rats pretreated with ExPhy (400 mg/kg) and omeprazole (40 mg/kg). Regarding gastric MDA, there was a significantly higher level in the ulcer control versus the vehicle control. Pretreatment with ExPhy (400 mg/kg) and omeprazole (40 mg/kg) protected against the damage found in the ulcer control and led to decreased concentrations of MDA.

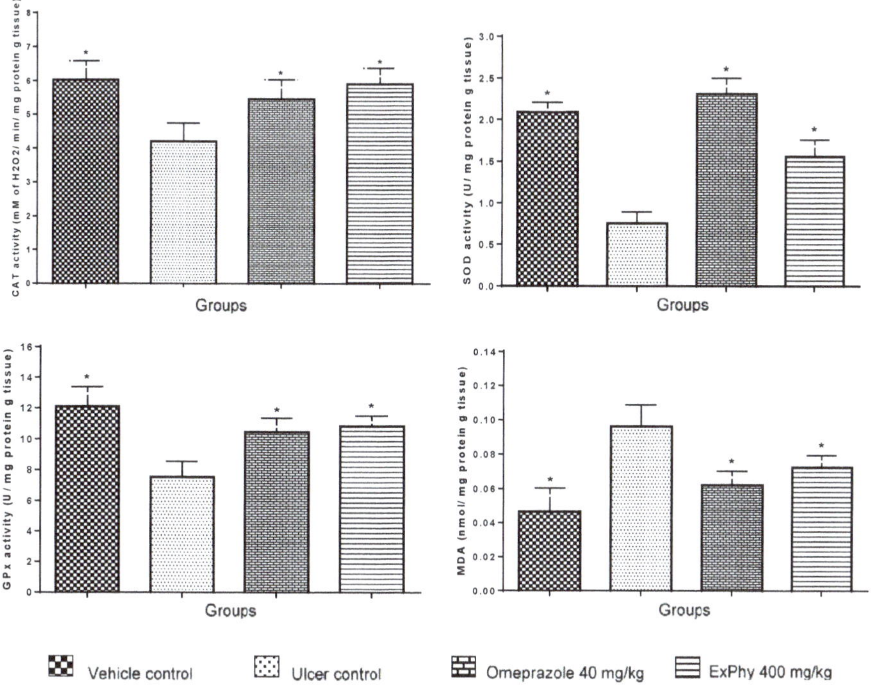

Figure 3. ExPhy and omeprazole pretreatments, followed by ethanol-induced gastric ulcers, produced protective effects on the gastric mucosal activity of GPx, SOD and CAT, as well as lowering the levels of MDA compared to the ulcer control. * Indicates $p < 0.05$. Data are expressed as the mean ± SEM. ExPhy, extract rich in phycobiliproteins.

4. Discussion

Considering the frequency of gastric ulcers in humans and the side effects and cost of some available synthetic drugs, the use of natural products represents an important alternative for many [43,44]. In this sense, *Spirulina maxima* and ExPhy have proven to be advantageous in the treatment of various ailments in lab animals and patients. Moreover, their absence of toxicity has been demonstrated by short- and long-term studies [45].

The current investigation evaluated the antiulcerogenic activity of ExPhy of Am on an ethanol-induced gastric ulcer model. A determination was made of the effects of ExPhy in relation to some antioxidant and oxidative markers, along with protection against histopathological damage. C-PC and APC in ExPhy were identified and characterized by standard analytical methods (UV–VIS spectroscopy and MALDI-MS/MS).

Phycobilisomes are supramolecular complexes on the stromal surface of the thylakoid membrane in cyanobacteria (e.g., Am). These complexes, which participate in trapping light energy and transferring it within the cell, can make up to 60% of the total protein [46,47]. The antioxidant potential reported for Am may be attributed to this major class of proteins. Phycobilisomes are constituted mainly by individual protein components denominated phycobiliproteins and linker polypeptides [48]. Phycobiliproteins consist of two different polypeptides (the α and β chains) that are covalently linked to bilin chromophores [49]. In this study, MALDI-MS/MS analysis corroborated that the protein bands excised from SDS-PAGE belonged to α and β subunits of C-PC and APC, the main photosynthetic accessory pigments present in cyanobacteria [47]. On the other hand, the values of purity achieved for C-PC and APC from ExPhy (Table 1) can be considered good, since a purity of 0.7 is accepted as food grade [50]. Interestingly, the analysis by mass spectrometry showed the presence of other cellular proteins (see the Supplementary Materials) that probably influenced the purity of phycobiliproteins in a minor way.

Phycobiliproteins have attracted attention due to their special structure and potential therapeutic properties, either in a pure state or in protein extract. C-PC and APC are known to exert several beneficial activities, including antioxidant (shown in vitro and in vivo) [19,51,52], anti-inflammatory, and immune-stimulatory [27,53–56]. The antioxidant mechanism of phycobiliproteins has been associated with various activities: (1) ROS scavenging [25,51,52]; (2) chelating [25]; (3) neutralizing free radicals through the sulfur atom of cysteine and methionine of apophycocyanin, which can transfer hydrogen atoms or electrons to free radicals [51,57]; and (4) influencing the activity of antioxidant enzymes [58–60].

Excessive ethanol consumption is considered one of the risk factors for gastric ulcers in humans [61,62]. Its use in experimental animals allows for the evaluation of cytoprotective activity of potentially active products [63]. Different mechanisms of gastric cytoprotection have been suggested, including increased gastric mucosal blood flow, free radical scavenging, and stimulation of cell growth and repair [64]. In the current study, consistent with previous findings, administration of 80% ethanol solution by intragastric gavage produced marked damage in the gastric mucosa of rats, characterized mainly by elongated macroscopic lesions with intense hemorrhaging and hyperemia, as well as loss of mucus [35,65,66]. Pre-treatment of rats for eight days with ExPhy markedly attenuated gastric damage and promoted healing of gastric mucosa lesions induced by ethanol, although to a lesser extent than the standard drug, omeprazole. ExPhy provided the best protection at the highest concentration tested. These results indicate that ExPhy may have a protective effect against the ulcerative lesions induced by ethanol on gastric mucosa.

Additionally, though it was not explored presently, direct contact of phycocyanin with injured gastric mucosa possibly contributes to the healing process. There is evidence that both Spirulina and C-phycocyanin are capable of stimulating cell growth and viability, both in human keratinocytes and in a rat model [67]. These properties underlie the use of Spirulina in the development of new biomaterials for the construction of scaffolds for cell growth in the field of tissue engineering [68].

After demonstrating that ExPhy provided a protective effect against the development of ethanol-induced ulcers, the next step was to confirm these findings through a histopathological analysis of gastric tissue. In accordance with previous studies, the ulcer control group showed typical histological damage 1 h after ethanol administration. This damage was characterized by vascular congestion, submucosal edema formation, loss of gastric mucosa integrity, and necrotic tissue injury, as well as an inflammatory response characterized by neutrophil and eosinophil infiltration [65,69,70]. The aggregation of neutrophils plays a fundamental role in the process of injury and inflammation in the gastric mucosa due to their release of tissue-disruptive substances like proteases, leukotrienes B4 (LTB4), and reactive oxygen species [71,72]. Via NADPH oxidase, neutrophils release superoxide anions, and these in turn are metabolized into the hydroxyl radical. The latter can mediate lipid peroxidation of polyunsaturated fatty acids and cause damage to cell membranes, leading to an alteration in the structural integrity and biochemical function of membranes [73,74].

Interestingly, the microscopic study revealed a lesser extent of inflammatory infiltrate in the group of rats treated with ExPhy. Moreover, the histopathological changes triggered by ethanol were significantly diminished. The gastric mucosa showed a more regular architecture and less hemorrhaging and submucosal edema. Previous reports have confirmed the anti-inflammatory properties of phycobiliproteins. In rats with colitis treated with phycocyanin, Gonzales et al. [27] described a substantial reduction in neutrophil infiltration in colonic mucosal injury. Remirez et al. [28] evaluated the protective effect of the phycocyanin extract in the zymosan-induced arthritis model in mice, finding that treatment with phycocyanin displayed an inhibition of cellular infiltration. Further studies carried out by Romay et al. [75,76] demonstrated that phycocyanin is able to inhibit the inflammatory response and edema triggered by 12-O tetradecanoyl phorbol 13-acetate in mice, as well as reduce the LTB4 levels in arachidonic acid-induced mouse ear edema. Inhibitors of cyclooxygenase (COX) and lipooxygenase (LOX) enzymes have proven to be active in this model [77], suggesting that the mechanism of action of ExPhy for diminishing inflammatory infiltrate and edema could be linked, at least in part, to their antioxidant properties (as previously described), an inhibitory effect on cyclooxygenase-2 (COX-2), and/or the biosynthesis of LTB4.

Currently, there is consensus that alcohol intake is noxious to gastric tissue. The generation of ROS and subsequent oxidative stress is one of the major mechanisms in the pathogenesis of gastric tissue damage and ulcerogenesis induced by ethanol [71,78]. It has been documented that the administration of alcohol not only has necrotizing effects but also gives rise to oxidative stress by provoking injury to the mitochondria. The latter occurs through a decrease in mitochondrial membrane potential, which leads to a perturbation of the mitochondrial electron transfer system and an overproduction of O_2—[79,80]. Oxidative stress is manifested as an abnormal elevation of reactive oxygen species, leading to the depletion of the antioxidant defense system (enzymatic and non-enzymatic), thus furthering damage to cell structures such as carbohydrates, nucleic acids, proteins and lipids (promoting lipid peroxidation) [12,81]. Potent antioxidants and free radical scavengers have been shown to inhibit oxidative stress and consequently the progression of lipid peroxidation [82,83]. Molecules with this capability include flavonoids, phenolic compounds, vitamins (tocopherol), and phycocyanin [53]. The latter is a powerful antioxidant that removes free radicals, including peroxynitrite radicals, nitric oxide radicals, peroxyl radicals, hydroxyl radicals, superoxide anion, hypochlorous oxygen, hydrogen peroxide, and synthetic radicals DPPH and ABTS. This action is given by its structure, rich in amino acids such as methionine, cysteine, and the tetrapyrolic prosthetic group, which can stabilize highly reactive species such as free radicals [60]. In addition, in vivo and in vitro models have been shown to exert antioxidant action within the cells [84]. Therefore, the administration of ExPhy in this study probably improves cellular antioxidant defenses.

In the current study, we corroborated that intragastric administration of ethanol causes severe oxidative stress in stomach tissue (ulcer control group) by significant inhibition of the activity of antioxidant enzymes such as CAT, GPx, and SOD compared to the vehicle control group. Additionally, there was a significant increase in the level of MDA, as previously reported [66,85]. MDA is commonly measured as a biomarker to assess lipid peroxidation levels in tissues [86]. ExPhy pretreatment exhibited antioxidant properties by decreasing the levels of MDA, suggesting its potential to protect against ethanol-induced lipid peroxidation in rats. Furthermore, ExPhy preserved the antioxidant activity of GPx, CAT, and SOD enzymes after ethanol administration, thus protecting the gastric mucosa.

Normally, these antioxidant enzymes provide cells with mechanisms for defending themselves against ROS damage. SOD represents the first line of defense against ROS by catalyzing the conversion of O_2—to oxygen and H_2O_2, the latter of which is catalyzed to H_2O by CAT or GPx [83]. The possibility of this protective effect being fostered by ExPhy is consistent with previous findings that phycobiliproteins engender a significant decrease in oxidative stress by increasing the antioxidant defense system and reducing the levels of lipid peroxidation in different pathologic conditions. Fernandez-Rojas et al. [60] reported the protective effect of C-PC against cisplatin-induced nephrotoxicity in CD-1 mice through the attenuation of oxidative stress and an enhancement of the activity of antioxidant enzymes. This effect was associated with the ROS-scavenging ability of C-PC. Additionally, Rodríguez-Sánchez et al. [87] found that phycobiliproteins protect renal cells against mercury-induced oxidative stress in mice. The mechanism of action suggested involves the reduction of oxidative markers and the chelating properties of phycobiliproteins. More recently, Kumari and Anbarusa [59] documented the protective action of C-PC in the rat selenite cataract model, which might be a consequence of its ability to scavenge the free radicals generated and exert an anti-apoptotic function.

In conclusion, the current results suggest a significant gastroprotective effect of ExPhy against ethanol-induced gastric damage. This protection may be related to the antioxidant properties of ExPhy by activating some enzymatic antioxidant mechanisms (SOD, CAT, and GPx), diminishing lipid peroxidation, and attenuating the inflammatory response, improving defenses against the erosive lesion that characterize the development of gastric ulcers produced by ethanol. However, further detailed studies are needed to clarify the mechanisms underlying the gastroprotective effect shown by ExPhy.

Supplementary Materials: The following are available online at http://www.mdpi.com/2072-6643/10/6/763/s1, Table S1: Additional proteins identified by MALDI-MS/MS.

Author Contributions: O.G.-G., G.A.C.-C. and R.V.G.-R. conceived and designed the experiments; O.G.-G., N.L.R.-R. and E.R.-C. performed the experiments; O.G.-G., E.R.-C., N.L.R.-R., L.Q.-C. and R.P.-P.-B. analyzed the data; R.P.-P.-B., G.A.C.-C., S.P.-G. and J.P.-R. contributed reagents/materials; O.G.-G. and G.A.C.-C. wrote the paper.

Acknowledgments: We thank Gloria Mercado for reviewing the use of English in this manuscript. This work was supported in part by the grant SIP 20160763X, I.P.N., Mexico.

Conflicts of Interest: The authors declare no conflict of interest.

References

1. Brucker, M.; Faucher, M. Pharmacologic Management of Common Gastrointestinal Health Problems in Women. *J. Nurse. Midwifery* **1997**, *42*, 145–162. [CrossRef]
2. Dimaline, R.; Varro, A. Attack and Defence in the Gastric Epithelium—A Delicate Balance. *Exp. Physiol.* **2007**, *92*, 591–601. [CrossRef] [PubMed]
3. Guslandi, M. Effects of Ethanol on the Gastric Mucosa. *Dig. Dis.* **1987**, *5*, 21–32. [CrossRef] [PubMed]
4. Maity, P.; Biswas, K.; Roy, S.; Banerjee, R.K.; Bandyopadhyay, U. Smoking and the Pathogenesis of Gastroduodenal Ulcer—Recent Mechanistic Update. *Mol. Cell. Biochem.* **2003**, *253*, 329–338. [CrossRef] [PubMed]
5. Spirt, M.J. Stress-Related Mucosal Disease: Risk Factors and Prophylactic Therapy. *Clin. Ther.* **2017**, *26*, 197–213. [CrossRef]
6. Vonkeman, H.E.; Klok, R.M.; Postma, M.J.; Brouwers, J.R.B.J.; van de Laar, M.A.F.J. Direct Medical Costs of Serious Gastrointestinal Ulcers among Users of NSAIDs. *Drugs Aging* **2007**, *24*, 681–690. [CrossRef] [PubMed]
7. Bujanda, L. The Effects of Alcohol Consumption upon the Gastrointestinal Tract. *Am. J. Gastroenterol.* **2000**, *95*, 3374–3382. [CrossRef] [PubMed]
8. Bode, C.; Bode, J.C. Alcohol's Role in Gastrointestinal Tract Disorders. *Alcohol. Health Res. World* **1997**, *21*, 76–83. [PubMed]
9. Cadirci, E.; Suleyman, H.; Aksoy, H.; Halici, Z.; Ozgen, U.; Koc, A.; Ozturk, N. Effects of Onosma Armeniacum Root Extract on Ethanol-Induced Oxidative Stress in Stomach Tissue of Rats. *Chem. Biol. Interact.* **2007**, *170*, 40–48. [CrossRef] [PubMed]

10. Alimi, H.; Hfaiedh, N.; Bouoni, Z.; Sakly, M.; Ben Rhouma, K. Evaluation of Antioxidant and Antiulcerogenic Activities of Opuntia Ficus Indica F. Inermis Flowers Extract in Rats. *Environ. Toxicol. Pharmacol.* **2011**, *32*, 406–416. [CrossRef] [PubMed]
11. Melchiorri, D.; Sewerynek, E.; Reiter, R.J.; Ortiz, G.G.; Poeggeler, B.; Nisticò, G. Suppressive Effect of Melatonin Administration on Ethanol-Induced Gastroduodenal Injury in Rats in Vivo. *Br. J. Pharmacol.* **1997**, *121*, 264–270. [CrossRef] [PubMed]
12. Pan, J.-S.; He, S.-Z.; Xu, H.-Z.; Zhan, X.-J.; Yang, X.-N.; Xiao, H.-M.; Shi, H.-X.; Ren, J.-L. Oxidative Stress Disturbs Energy Metabolism of Mitochondria in Ethanol-Induced Gastric Mucosa Injury. *World J. Gastroenterol.* **2008**, *14*, 5857–5867. [CrossRef] [PubMed]
13. Arda-Pirincci, P.; Bolkent, S.; Yanardag, R. The Role of Zinc Sulfate and Metallothionein in Protection Against Ethanol-Induced Gastric Damage in Rats. *Dig. Dis. Sci.* **2006**, *51*, 2353–2360. [CrossRef] [PubMed]
14. Vonshak, A. *Spirulina Platensis Arthrospira: Physiology, Cell-Biology and Biotechnology*; Taylor Francis Press: London, UK, 1997; p. 151.
15. Al-Dhabi, N.A. Heavy Metal Analysis in Commercial Spirulina Products for Human Consumption. *Saudi J. Biol. Sci.* **2013**, *20*, 383–388. [CrossRef] [PubMed]
16. Campanella, L.; Crescentini, G.; Avino, P. Chemical Composition and Nutritional Evaluation of Some Natural and Commercial Food Products Based on Spirulina. *Analusis* **1999**, *27*, 533–540. [CrossRef]
17. Mao, T.K.; van de Water, J.; Gershwin, M.E. Effect of Spirulina on the Secretion of Cytokines from Peripheral Blood Mononuclear Cells. *J. Med. Food* **2000**, *3*, 135–140. [CrossRef] [PubMed]
18. Hernández-Corona, A.; Nieves, I.; Meckes, M.; Chamorro, G.; Barron, B.L. Antiviral Activity of Spirulina Maxima against Herpes Simplex Virus Type 2. *Antivir. Res.* **2002**, *56*, 279–285. [CrossRef]
19. Piñero Estrada, J. Antioxidant Activity of Different Fractions of Spirulina Platensis Protean Extract. *Farmaco* **2001**, *56*, 497–500. [CrossRef]
20. Chamorro-Cevallos, G.; Garduño-Siciliano, L.; Barrón, B.L.; Madrigal-Bujaidar, E.; Cruz-Vega, D.E.; Pages, N. Chemoprotective Effect of *Spirulina* (*Arthrospira*) against Cyclophosphamide-Induced Mutagenicity in Mice. *Food Chem. Toxicol.* **2008**, *46*, 567–574. [CrossRef] [PubMed]
21. Juárez-Oropeza, M.A.; Mascher, D.; Torres-Durán, P.V.; Farias, J.M.; Paredes-Carbajal, M.C. Effects of Dietary Spirulina on Vascular Reactivity. *J. Med. Food* **2009**, *12*, 15–20. [CrossRef] [PubMed]
22. Jatav, S.K.; Kulshrestha, A.; Zacharia, A.; Singh, N.; Tejovathi, G.; Bisen, P.S.; Prasad, G.B.K.S. Spirulina Maxima Protects Liver From Isoniazid and Rifampicin Drug Toxicity. *J. Evid. Based. Complement. Altern. Med.* **2014**, *19*, 189–194. [CrossRef] [PubMed]
23. Sinanoglu, O.; Yener, A.N.; Ekici, S.; Midi, A.; Aksungar, F.B. The Protective Effects of Spirulina in Cyclophosphamide Induced Nephrotoxicity and Urotoxicity in Rats. *Urology* **2012**, *80*, 1392.e1–1392.e6. [CrossRef] [PubMed]
24. Miranda, M.S.; Cintra, R.G.; Barros, S.B.M.; Mancini-Filho, J. Antioxidant Activity of the Microalga Spirulina Maxima. *Braz. J. Med. Biol. Res.* **1998**, *31*, 1075–1079. [CrossRef] [PubMed]
25. Bermejo-Bescós, P.; Piñero-Estrada, E.; Villar del Fresno, Á.M. Neuroprotection by Spirulina Platensis Protean Extract and Phycocyanin against Iron-Induced Toxicity in SH-SY5Y Neuroblastoma Cells. *Toxicol. Vitr.* **2008**, *22*, 1496–1502. [CrossRef] [PubMed]
26. Romay, C.; Delgado, R.; Remirez, D.; Gonzalez, R.; Rojas, A. Effects of Phycocyanin Extract on Tumor Necrosis Factor-α and Nitrite Levels in Serum of Mice Treated with Endotoxin. *Arzneimittelforschung* **2001**, *51*, 733–736. [CrossRef] [PubMed]
27. González, R.; Rodríguez, S.; Romay, C.; Ancheta, O.; González, A.; Armesto, J.; Remirez, D.; Merino, N. Anti-Inflammatory Activity of Phycocyanin Extract in Acetic Acid-Induced Colitis in Rats. *Pharmacol. Res.* **1999**, *39*, 55–59. [CrossRef] [PubMed]
28. Remirez, D.; González, A.; Merino, N.; González, R.; Ancheta, O.; Romay, C.; Rodríguez, S. Effect of Phycocyanin in Zymosan-Induced Arthritis in Mice—Phycocyanin as an Antiarthritic Compound. *Drug Dev. Res.* **1999**, *48*, 70–75. [CrossRef]
29. Cruz de Jesús, V. Methods for Extraction, Isolation and Purification of C-Phycocyanin: 50 Years of Research in Review. *Int. J. Food Nutr. Sci.* **2016**, *3*, 1–10.
30. Bennett, A.; Bogorad, L. Complementary Chromatic Adaption in a Filamentous Blue-Green Alga. *J. Cell. Biol.* **1973**, *58*, 419–435.

31. Boussiba, S.; Richmond, A.E. Isolation and Characterization of Phycocyanins from the Blue-Green Alga Spirulina Platensis. *Arch. Microbiol.* **1979**, *120*, 155–159. [CrossRef]
32. Gallagher, S.R. One-Dimensional SDS Gel Electrophoresis of Proteins. *Curr. Protoc. Protein Sci.* **2012**, *1*, 1–44.
33. Shevchenko, A.; Tomas, H.; Havli, J.; Olsen, J.V.; Mann, M. In-Gel Digestion for Mass Spectrometric Characterization of Proteins and Proteomes. *Nat. Protoc.* **2007**, *1*, 2856. [CrossRef] [PubMed]
34. Shilov, I.V.; Seymour, S.L.; Patel, A.A.; Loboda, A.; Tang, W.H.; Keating, S.P.; Hunter, C.L.; Nuwaysir, L.M.; Schaeffer, D.A. The Paragon Algorithm, a Next Generation Search Engine That Uses Sequence Temperature Values and Feature Probabilities to Identify Peptides from Tandem Mass Spectra. *Mol. Cell. Proteom.* **2007**, *6*, 1638–1655. [CrossRef] [PubMed]
35. Almasaudi, S.B.; El-Shitany, N.A.; Abbas, A.T.; Abdel-Dayem, U.A.; Ali, S.S.; Al Jaouni, S.K.; Harakeh, S. Antioxidant, Anti-Inflammatory, and Antiulcer Potential of Manuka Honey against Gastric Ulcer in Rats. *Oxid. Med. Cell. Longev.* **2016**, *2016*, 1–10. [CrossRef] [PubMed]
36. Alirezaei, M.; Dezfoulian, O.; Neamati, S.; Rashidipour, M.; Tanideh, N.; Kheradmand, A. Oleuropein Prevents Ethanol-Induced Gastric Ulcers via Elevation of Antioxidant Enzyme Activities in Rats. *J. Physiol. Biochem.* **2012**, *68*, 583–592. [CrossRef] [PubMed]
37. Adinortey, M.B.; Ansah, C.; Galyuon, I.; Nyarko, A. In Vivo Models Used for Evaluation of Potential Antigastroduodenal Ulcer Agents. *Ulcers* **2013**, *2013*, 1–12. [CrossRef]
38. Paglia, D.E.; Valentine, W.N. Studies on the Quantitative and Qualitative Characterization of Erytrocyte Glutathione Peroxidase. *J. Lab. Clin. Med.* **1967**, *70*, 158–169. [PubMed]
39. Mccord, J.; Fridovich, I.; McCOrd, J.M.; Fridovich, I. Superoxide Dismutase. An Enzymic Function for Erythrocuprein (Hemocuprein). *J. Biol. Chem. J. Biol. Chem.* **1969**, *244*, 6049–6055. [PubMed]
40. Aebi, H. Catalase in vitro. In *Oxygen Radicals in Biological Systems*; Academic Press: Cambridge, MA, USA, 1984; Volume 105, pp. 121–126.
41. Bradford, M.M. A Rapid and Sensitive Method for the Quantitation of Microgram Quantities of Protein Utilizing the Principle of Protein-Dye Binding. *Anal. Biochem.* **1976**, *72*, 248–254. [CrossRef]
42. Esterbauer, H.; Cheeseman, K.H. Determination of Aldehydic Lipid Peroxidation Products: Malonaldehyde and 4-Hydroxynonenal. In *Oxygen Radicals in Biological Systems Part B: Oxygen Radicals and Antioxidants*; Academic Press: Cambridge, MA, USA, 1990; Volume 186, pp. 407–421.
43. Vimala, G.; Gricilda Shoba, F. A Review on Antiulcer Activity of Few Indian Medicinal Plants. *Int. J. Microbiol.* **2014**, *2014*, 1–14. [CrossRef] [PubMed]
44. Al-Wajeeh, N.S.; Halabi, M.F.; Hajrezaie, M.; Dhiyaaldeen, S.M.; Bardi, D.A.; Salama, S.M.; Rouhollahi, E.; Karimian, H.; Abdolmalaki, R.; Azizan, A.H.S.; et al. The Gastroprotective Effect of Vitex Pubescens Leaf Extract against Ethanol-Provoked Gastric Mucosal Damage in Sprague-Dawley Rats. *PLoS ONE* **2016**, *11*, 179072. [CrossRef] [PubMed]
45. Gutiérrez-Salmeán, G.; Fabila-Castillo, L.; Chamorro-Cevallos, G. Aspectos Nutricionales Y Toxicológicos de *Spirulina* (*Arthrospira*). *Nutr. Hosp.* **2015**, *32*, 34–40. [PubMed]
46. Viskari, P.J.; Colyer, C.L. Separation and Quantitation of Phycobiliproteins Using Phytic Acid in Capillary Electrophoresis with Laser-Induced Fluorescence Detection. *J. Chromatogr. A* **2002**, *972*, 269–276. [CrossRef]
47. Bryant, D.A.; Guglielmi, G.; de Marsac, N.T.; Castets, A.M.; Cohen-Bazire, G. The Structure of Cyanobacterial Phycobilisomes: A Model. *Arch. Microbiol.* **1979**, *123*, 113–127. [CrossRef]
48. Singh, N.K.; Sonani, R.R.; Prasad Rastogi, R.; Madamwar, D. The Phycobilisomes: An Early Requisite for Efficient Photosynthesis in Cyanobacteria. *EXCLI J.* **2015**, *14*, 268–289. [PubMed]
49. Scheer, H.; Zhao, K.H. Biliprotein Maturation: The Chromophore Attachment. *Mol. Microbiol.* **2008**, *68*, 263–276. [CrossRef] [PubMed]
50. Rito-Palomares, M.; Nuez, L.; Amador, D. Practical Application of Aqueous Two-Phase Systems for the Development of a Prototype Process for c-Phycocyanin Recovery from Spirulina Maxima. *J. Chem. Technol. Biotechnol.* **2001**, *76*, 1273–1280. [CrossRef]
51. Cherdkiatikul, T.; Suwanwong, Y. Production of the α and β Subunits of Spirulina Allophycocyanin and C-Phycocyanin in *Escherichia Coli*: A Comparative Study of Their Antioxidant Activities. *J. Biomol. Screen.* **2014**, *19*, 959–965. [CrossRef] [PubMed]
52. Romay, C.; Armesto, J.; Remirez, D.; González, R.; Ledon, N.; García, I. Antioxidant and Anti-Inflammatory Properties of C-Phycocyanin from Blue-Green Algae. *Inflamm. Res.* **1998**, *47*, 36–41. [CrossRef] [PubMed]

53. Romay, C.; Gonzalez, R.; Ledon, N.; Remirez, D.; Rimbau, V. C-Phycocyanin: A Biliprotein with Antioxidant, Anti-Inflammatory and Neuroprotective Effects. *Curr. Protein Pept. Sci.* **2003**, *4*, 207–216. [CrossRef] [PubMed]
54. Reddy, M.C.; Subhashini, J.; Mahipal, S.V.; Bhat, V.B.; Srinivas Reddy, P.; Kiranmai, G.; Madyastha, K.; Reddanna, P. C-Phycocyanin, a Selective Cyclooxygenase-2 Inhibitor, Induces Apoptosis in Lipopolysaccharide-Stimulated RAW 264.7 Macrophages. *Biochem. Biophys. Res. Commun.* **2003**, *304*, 385–392. [CrossRef]
55. Belay, A. The Potential Application of *Spirulina* (*Arthrospira*) as a Nutritional Health and Therapeutic Supplement in Health Management. *J. Am. Nutr. Assoc.* **2002**, *5*, 27–48.
56. El Sheikh, S.M.; Shalaby, M.A.M.; Hafez, R.A.; Metwally, W.S.A.; El-Ayoty, Y.M. The Immunomodulatory Effects of Probiotic Bacteria on Peripheral Blood Mononuclear Cells (PBMCS) of Allergic Patients. *Am. J. Immunol.* **2014**, *10*, 116–130. [CrossRef]
57. Atmaca, G. Antioxidant Effects of Sulfur-Containing Amino Acids. *Yonsei Med. J.* **2004**, *45*, 776–788. [CrossRef] [PubMed]
58. Ou, Y.; Zheng, S.; Lin, L.; Jiang, Q.; Yang, X. Chemico-Biological Interactions Protective Effect of C-Phycocyanin against Carbon Tetrachloride-Induced Hepatocyte Damage in Vitro and in Vivo. *Chem. Biol. Interact.* **2010**, *185*, 94–100. [CrossRef] [PubMed]
59. Kumari, R.P.; Anbarasu, K. Protective Role of C-Phycocyanin Against Secondary Changes During Sodium Selenite Mediated Cataractogenesis. *Nat. Products Bioprospect.* **2014**, *4*, 81–89. [CrossRef] [PubMed]
60. Fernandez-Rojas, B.; Medina-Campos, O.N.; Hernandez-Pando, R.; Negrette-Guzman, M.; Huerta-Yepez, S.; Pedraza-Chaverri, J. C-Phycocyanin Prevents Cisplatin-Induced Nephrotoxicity through Inhibition of Oxidative Stress. *Food Funct.* **2014**, *5*, 480–490. [CrossRef] [PubMed]
61. Lulu, D.J.; Dragstedt, L.R. Massive Bleeding Due to Acute Hemorrhagic Gastritis. *Arch. Surg.* **1970**, *101*, 550–554. [CrossRef] [PubMed]
62. Søreide, K.; Thorsen, K.; Harrison, E.M.; Bingener, J.; Møller, M.H.; Ohene-Yeboah, M.; Søreide, J.A. Perforated Peptic Ulcer. *Lancet* **2015**, *386*, 1288–1298. [CrossRef]
63. Bighetti, A.E.; Antônio, M.A.; Kohn, L.K.; Rehder, V.L.G.; Foglio, M.A.; Possenti, A.; Vilela, L.; Carvalho, J.E. Antiulcerogenic Activity of a Crude Hydroalcoholic Extract and Coumarin Isolated from Mikania Laevigata Schultz Bip. *Phytomedicine* **2005**, *12*, 72–77. [CrossRef] [PubMed]
64. Diniz D'Souza, R.S.; Dhume, V.G. Gastric Cytoprotection. *Indian J. Physiol. Pharmacol.* **1991**, *35*, 88–98.
65. Ben Barka, Z.; Tlili, M.; Alimi, H.; Ben Miled, H.; Ben Rhouma, K.; Sakly, M.; Ksouri, R.; Schneider, Y.J.; Tebourbi, O. Protective Effects of Edible Rhus Tripartita (Ucria) Stem Extract against Ethanol-Induced Gastric Ulcer in Rats. *J. Funct. Foods* **2017**, *30*, 260–269. [CrossRef]
66. Antonisamy, P.; Duraipandiyan, V.; Aravinthan, A.; Al-Dhabi, N.A.; Ignacimuthu, S.; Choi, K.C.; Kim, J.H. Protective Effects of Friedelin Isolated from Azima Tetracantha Lam. against Ethanol-Induced Gastric Ulcer in Rats and Possible Underlying Mechanisms. *Eur. J. Pharmacol.* **2015**, *750*, 167–175. [CrossRef] [PubMed]
67. Sevimli Gur, C.; Erdogan, D.K.; Onbasılar, I.; Atilla, P.; Cakar, N.; Deliloglu Gurhan, I. In Vitro and in Vivo Investigations of the Wound Healing Effect of Crude Spirulina Extract and C-Phycocyanin. *J. Med. Plants Res.* **2013**, *7*, 425–433.
68. Morais, M.; da Silva Vaz, B.; Morais, E.; Costa, J.A. Biological Effects of *Spirulina* (*Arthrospira*) Biopolymers and Biomass in the Development of Nanostructured Scaffolds. *BioMed Res. Int.* **2014**, *2014*, 1–9. [CrossRef] [PubMed]
69. Zakaria, Z.A.; Abdul Hisam, E.E.; Rofiee, M.S.; Norhafizah, M.; Somchit, M.N.; Teh, L.K.; Salleh, M.Z. In Vivo Antiulcer Activity of the Aqueous Extract of Bauhinia Purpurea Leaf. *J. Ethnopharmacol.* **2011**, *137*, 1047–1054. [CrossRef] [PubMed]
70. Rozza, A.L.; Hiruma-Lima, C.A.; Takahira, R.K.; Padovani, C.R.; Pellizzon, C.H. Effect of Menthol in Experimentally Induced Ulcers: Pathways of Gastroprotection. *Chem. Biol. Interact.* **2013**, *206*, 272–278. [CrossRef] [PubMed]
71. Yao, J. Tiao He Yi Wei Granule, a Traditional Chinese Medicine, against Ethanol-Induced Gastric Ulcer in Mice. Evidence-based Complement. *Altern. Med.* **2015**, *2015*, 1–8.
72. Hamauzu, Y.; Forest, F.; Hiramatsu, K.; Sugimoto, M. Effect of Pear (*Pyrus Communis* L.) Procyanidins on Gastric Lesions Induced by HCl/ethanol in Rats. *Food Chem.* **2007**, *100*, 255–263. [CrossRef]

73. Naito, Y.; Yoshikawa, T.; Matsuyama, K.; Yagi, N.; Arai, M.; Nakamura, Y.; Kaneko, T.; Nishimura, S.; Yoshida, N.; Kondo, M. Role of Lipid Peroxidation and Neutrophil Accumulation in the Gastric Mucosal Injury Induced by Aspirin-HCl in Rats Effect of Roxatidine, a Histamine H2receptor Antagonist with Antioxidative Properties. *Pathophysiology* **1995**, *2*, 1–8. [CrossRef]
74. Kobayashi, T.; Ohta, Y.; Yoshino, J.; Nakazawa, S. Teprenone Promotes the Healing of Acetic Acid-Induced Chronic Gastric Ulcers in Rats by Inhibiting Neutrophil Infiltration and Lipid Peroxidation in Ulcerated Gastric Tissues. *Pharmacol. Res.* **2001**, *43*, 23–30. [CrossRef] [PubMed]
75. Romay, C.; Ledón, N.; González, R. Further Studies on Anti-Inflammatory Activity of Phycocyanin in Some Animal Models of Inflammation. *Inflamm. Res.* **1998**, *47*, 334–338. [CrossRef] [PubMed]
76. Romay, C.; Ledón, N.; González, R. Phycocyanin Extract Reduces Leukotriene B4 Levels in Arachidonic Acid-Induced Mouse-Ear Inflammation Test. *J. Pharm. Pharmacol.* **1999**, *51*, 641–642. [CrossRef] [PubMed]
77. Carlson, R.P.; Lynn, O.-D.; Chang, J.; Lewis, A.J. Modulation of Mouse Ear Edema by Cyclooxygenase and Lipoxygenase Inhibitors and other Pharmacologic Agents. *Agents Actions* **1985**, *17*, 197–204. [CrossRef] [PubMed]
78. El-Naga, R.N. Apocynin Protects against Ethanol-Induced Gastric Ulcer in Rats by Attenuating the Upregulation of NADPH Oxidases 1 and 4. *Chem. Biol. Interact.* **2015**, *242*, 317–326. [CrossRef] [PubMed]
79. Sun, Q.; Zhong, W.; Zhang, W.; Zhou, Z. Defect of Mitochondrial Respiratory Chain Is a Mechanism of ROS Overproduction in a Rat Model of Alcoholic Liver Disease: Role of Zinc Deficiency. *Am. J. Physiol. Gastrointest. Liver Physiol.* **2016**, *310*, G205–G214. [CrossRef] [PubMed]
80. Tamura, M.; Matsui, H.; Kaneko, T.; Hyodo, I. Alcohol Is an Oxidative Stressor for Gastric Epithelial Cells: Detection of Superoxide in Living Cells. *J. Clin. Biochem. Nutr.* **2013**, *53*, 75–80. [CrossRef] [PubMed]
81. Mittal, M.; Siddiqui, M.R.; Tran, K.; Reddy, S.P.; Malik, A.B. Reactive Oxygen Species in Inflammation and Tissue Injury. *Antioxid. Redox Signal.* **2014**, *20*, 1126–1167. [CrossRef] [PubMed]
82. Ligumsky, M.; Sestieri, M.; Okon, E.; Ginsburg, I. Antioxidants Inhibit Ethanol-Induced Gastric Injury in the Rat: Role of Manganese, Glycine, and Carotene. *Scand. J. Gastroenterol.* **1995**, *30*, 854–860. [CrossRef]
83. Neamati, S.; Alirezaei, M.; Kheradmand, A. Ghrelin Acts as an Antioxidant Agent in the Rat Kidney. *Int. J. Pept. Res. Ther.* **2011**, *17*, 239. [CrossRef]
84. Li, X.L.; Xu, G.; Chen, T.; Wong, Y.S.; Zhao, H.L.; Fan, R.R.; Gu, X.M.; Tong, P.C.Y.; Chan, J.C.N. Phycocyanin Protects INS-1E Pancreatic Beta Cells against Human Islet Amyloid Polypeptide-Induced Apoptosis through Attenuating Oxidative Stress and Modulating JNK and P38 Mitogen-Activated Protein Kinase Pathways. *Int. J. Biochem. Cell Biol.* **2009**, *41*, 1526–1535. [CrossRef] [PubMed]
85. Jeon, W.-Y.; Shin, I.-S.; Shin, H.-K.; Lee, M.-Y. Gastroprotective Effect of the Traditional Herbal Medicine, Sipjeondaebo-Tang Water Extract, against Ethanol-Induced Gastric Mucosal Injury. *BMC Complement. Altern. Med.* **2014**, *14*, 373. [CrossRef] [PubMed]
86. Dursun, H.; Bilici, M.; Albayrak, F.; Ozturk, C.; Saglam, M.B.; Alp, H.H.; Suleyman, H. Antiulcer Activity of Fluvoxamine in Rats and Its Effect on Oxidant and Antioxidant Parameters in Stomach Tissue. *BMC Gastroenterol.* **2009**, *9*, 1–10. [CrossRef] [PubMed]
87. Rodriguez-Sanchez, R.; Ortiz-Butron, R.; Blas-Valdivia, V.; Hernandez-Garcia, A.; Cano-Europa, E. Phycobiliproteins or C-Phycocyanin of *Arthrospira* (*Spirulina*) *Maxima* Protect against $HgCl_2$-Caused Oxidative Stress and Renal Damage. *Food Chem.* **2012**, *135*, 2359–2365. [CrossRef] [PubMed]

nutrients

MDPI

Article

Whey Protein Concentrate WPC-80 Intensifies Glycoconjugate Catabolism and Induces Oxidative Stress in the Liver of Rats

Marta Żebrowska-Gamdzyk [1,2,*,†], Mateusz Maciejczyk [2,3,*,†], Anna Zalewska [4], Katarzyna Guzińska-Ustymowicz [5], Anna Tokajuk [2] and Halina Car [2]

1 Lomza State University of Applied Sciences, 14 Akademicka Street, 18-400 Lomza, Poland
2 Department of Experimental Pharmacology, Medical University of Bialystok, 37 Szpitalna Street, 15-767 Bialystok, Poland; ania.tokajuk@gmail.com (A.T.); halina.car@umb.edu.pl (H.C.)
3 Department of Physiology, Medical University of Bialystok, 2c Mickiewicza Street, 15-233 Bialystok, Poland
4 Department of Conservative Dentistry, Medical University of Bialystok, 24a M. Sklodowskiej-Curie Street, 15-274 Bialystok, Poland; azalewska426@gmail.com
5 Department of General Pathomorphology, Medical University of Bialystok, 24a M. Sklodowskiej-Curie Street, 15-274 Bialystok, Poland; kguzinska74@gmail.com
* Correspondence: mzebrowska@pwsip.edu.pl or zfarmdosw@umb.edu.pl (M.Ż.-G.); mat.maciejczyk@gmail.com (M.M.); Tel.: +48 692609749 (M.Ż.-G.); +48 604998854 (M.M.)
† The authors had equal participation.

Received: 29 July 2018; Accepted: 27 August 2018; Published: 28 August 2018

Abstract: The aim of this study was to evaluate the effect of whey protein concentrate (WPC-80) on glycoconjugate catabolism, selected markers of oxidative stress and liver inflammation. The experiment was conducted on male Wistar rats (n = 63). The animals from the study group were administered WPC-80 at a dose of 0.3 or 0.5 g/kg body weight for 7, 14 or 21 days, while rats from the control group received only 0.9% NaCl. In liver homogenates, we assayed the activity of N-acetyl-β-D-hexosaminidase (HEX), β-glucuronidase (GLU), β-galactosidase (GAL), α-mannosidase (MAN), α-fucosidase (FUC), as well as the level of reduced glutathione (GSH), malondialdehyde (MDA), interleukin-1β (IL-1β) and transforming growth factor-β1 (TGF-β1). A significantly higher activity of HEX, GLU, MAN and FUC were found in the livers of rats receiving WPC-80 compared to controls. Serum ALT and AST were significantly higher in the animals supplemented with WPC-80 at a dose of 0.5 g/kg body weight for 21 days. In the same group of animals, enhanced level of GSH, MDA, IL-1β and TGF-β1 were also observed. WPC-80 is responsible for intensive remodelling of liver tissue and induction of oxidative stress especially at a dose of 0.5 g/kg body weight.

Keywords: exoglycosidases; liver; oxidative stress; whey

1. Introduction

In recent years, there has been an increase in interest in whey [1]. It is a by-product of cheese production and a rich source of exogenous amino acids and biologically active proteins. It has been proven that α-lactalbumin and β-lactoglobulin are the main whey proteins, forming up to 80% of the protein mass [2,3]. Other whey peptides include: immunoglobulins, albumins, lactoferrin and lactoperoxidase [3]. Due to its varied composition, whey is commonly supplemented to emaciated patients (e.g., during convalescence or cancer cachexia), children with cow's milk protein allergy and sportsmen to increase their muscle mass [1,4]. Whey proteins are also a valuable source of sulphuric amino acids: cysteine and methionine, crucial for the synthesis of reduced glutathione (GSH) [5].

GSH reveals strong antioxidant properties, which affects the proper functioning of the body, both healthy and ill [5].

Excess protein in the diet (including whey proteins) can adversely affect the activity of the organs participating in its metabolism [6]. One of such organs is the liver. It has been demonstrated that high-protein diet may result in a positive nitrogen balance, which causes increased production of urea and ammonia in the urea cycle [7]. This situation may lead to a significant overload of the liver [6,8]. One of the markers used to assess liver function are lysosomal exoglycosidases: N-acetyl-β-D-hexosaminidase (HEX, EC 3.2.1.52), β-glucuronidase (GLU, EC 3.2.1.31), β-galactosidase (GAL, EC 3.2.1.23), α-mannosidase (MAN, EC 3.2.1.24) and α-fucosidase (FUC, EC 3.2.1.51) [9–11]. These enzymes are responsible for the degradation of individual monosaccharide residues from the non-reducing end in the oligosaccharide chain of glycoconjugates [12].

Increased protein supply in the diet (above the current needs of the body) may also induce oxidative stress [13]. This process involves increased production of reactive oxygen species (ROS) and impairment of enzymatic and non-enzymatic antioxidant mechanisms [14]. As a result, oxidative stress disrupts cell metabolism and can even lead to cell death by apoptosis or necrosis [15]. Lipids are the first to suffer oxidative damage, as they are the most susceptible to oxygen free radicals [16,17]. Although increased production of ROS under the influence of rich protein diet has been demonstrated in numerous organs (brain [18], pancreas [19], salivary glands [20] and liver [6]), the effect of whey on liver oxidative damage is still unknown. Whey reveals documented antioxidant properties [21] but it has not been established yet whether whey-induced boost in GSH synthesis can prevent oxidative stress in the conditions of increased protein supply. The existing literature on the subject also lacks data on the effect of whey protein concentrate (WPC-80) on liver function. Therefore, the aim of this study was to evaluate the activity of lysosomal exoglycosidases and selected markers of oxidative stress and inflammation of liver homogenates in rats fed with whey protein concentrate WPC-80.

2. Materials and Methods

The experiment had been approved by the Local Ethical Committee on Animal Testing: No. 106/2015 (Medical University of Bialystok, Poland).

2.1. WPC-80 Composition

Whey protein concentrate used in the study was produced by Dairy Cooperative in Mońki, Poland. WPC-80 was analysed in the accredited laboratory at SJ Hamilton Poland LTD (Gdynia, Poland) and Rtech laboratory at Land O'Lakes Laboratories (St. Paul, MN, USA). The content of proteins, carbohydrates, fat, ash, dietary fibre, amino acids, fatty acids, vitamins, as well as minerals was assayed. The humidity and calorific values of WPC-80 were also evaluated.

2.2. Animals

The experiment was conducted on 6–7-week-old outbreed male Wistar rats with an initial body weight of 180–250 g. The animals were provided with 12-h light/dark cycle, constant air temperature (20–21 °C ± 2 °C) and unlimited access to food (standard granulated food for rats: Agropol, Motycz, Poland; 10.3 kcal% fat, 24.2 kcal% protein, 65.5 kcal% carbohydrates) and drinking water. Upon arrival at the animal quarters and after 1 week of adaptation to the new surroundings, the animals were randomly divided into 9 groups of 7 ($n = 7$):

1. C7—control group receiving 0.9% NaCl for 7 days
2. C14—control group receiving 0.9% NaCl for 14 days
3. C21—control group receiving 0.9% NaCl for 21 days
4. 0.3 WPC 7—a group receiving WPC-80 at a dose of 0.3 g/kg body weight for 7 days
5. 0.3 WPC 14—a group receiving WPC-80 at a dose of 0.3 g/kg body weight for 14 days
6. 0.3 WPC 21—a group receiving WPC-80 at a dose of 0.3 g/kg body weight for 21 days

7. 0.5 WPC 7—a group receiving WPC-80 at a dose of 0.5 g/kg body weight for 7 days
8. 0.5 WPC 14—a group receiving WPC-80 at a dose of 0.5 g/kg body weight for 14 days
9. 0.5 WPC 21—a group receiving WPC-80 at a dose of 0.5 g/kg body weight for 21 days

The dose of WPC-80 was selected on the basis of the literature analysis [3,22,23]. Immediately prior to administration, an appropriate amount of WPC-80 was dissolved in 0.9% solution of NaCl (saline solution). WPC-80 was administered intragastrically every day, always at the same time, in the volume of 2 mL/kg body weight. At the same time, rats from the control group received saline solution intragastrically in the amount of 2 mL/kg body weight [3].

After 7, 14 or 21 days, sodium pentobarbital was administered intraperitoneally at a dose of 45 mg/kg body weight to rats of the respective groups (before pentobarbital administration, rats were denied food for 12 h). The rats had abdominal aortic blood collected and then their tissues were collected for further examination. The liver tissue was rinsed with cold phosphate buffered saline (PBS; 0.02 M, pH 7.4) and dried, then frozen in liquid nitrogen and stored at −80 °C until the day of assay. The liver specimen was also fixed with 10% buffered formalin.

The blood was collected for a test tube with EDTA (ethylenediaminetetraacetic acid) and a test tube with a clot activator. Complete blood counts (WBC, leukocytes; RBC, erythrocytes; HCT, haematocrit; HGB, haemoglobin; MCV, Mean Corpuscular Volume; MCH, Mean Corpuscular Haemoglobin; MCHC, Mean Corpuscular Haemoglobin Concentration; PLT, platelets) were analysed in the whole blood. Immediately after centrifugation (10 min, 1500× *g*, 4 °C; MPW-351, Mechanika Precyzyjna S.C., Warsaw, Poland), the obtained serum was tested for biochemical parameters (ALT, alanine aminotransferase; AST, aspartate aminotransferase; bilirubin; albumin; Cr, creatinine; UA, uric acid; urea; TC, total cholesterol). All determinations were performed using ABX Pentra 400 (Horiba, Northampton, UK). Plasma glucose level was determined using colorimetric kit. The liver index was calculated using the formula: liver index = liver weight/body weight × 100%.

2.3. Preparation of Homogenates

On the day of assays, the livers were slowly thawed in 4 °C, weighed and divided into two equal parts, one of which was diluted in 0.15 M potassium chloride solution with 0.2% Triton X-100 at a ratio of 1:10 (i.e., 1 g of tissue per 1 mL of solvent) to assess the activity of lysosomal exoglycosidases [12]. The other part of the tissue material was diluted in 0.02 M phosphate-buffered saline (pH 7.4) at a ratio of 1:10—to evaluate the concentration of total protein, reduced glutathione and malondialdehyde [24]. In order to prevent sample oxidation and proteolysis, butylated hydroxytoluene (BHT; 10 µL 0.5 M BHT in acetonitrile/1 mL buffer) and proteolysis inhibitor (1 tablet/10 mL buffer; Complete Mini Roche, France) were added [25,26]. The obtained tissue suspensions were homogenized with a glass homogenizer (Omni TH, Omni International, Kennesaw, GA, USA) and then centrifuged (30 min, 12,000× *g*, 4 °C). For further studies, a supernatant fluid was retained to be used immediately to perform the assays.

2.4. Evaluation of the Activity of Lysosomal Exoglycosidases

The activity of the selected lysosomal exoglycosidases (HEX, GLU, GAL, MAN, FUC) was determined by colorimetric micro methods. All assays were performed in triplicate samples and standardized to 100 mg of total protein. Absorbance was measured with the microplate reader Mindray MR-96-A, Hamburg, Germany.

2.4.1. Evaluation of HEX Activity

The activity of HEX was evaluated according to the method described by Marciniak et al. [27]. 40 µL citrate-phosphate buffer (0.1 M, pH 4.7) and 30 µL 20 mM substrate solution (p-nitrophenyl-2-acetamido-2-deoxy-β-D-glucopyranoside, Sigma-Aldrich, Steinheim, Germany) were added to 10 µL supernatant fluid. The reaction mixture was incubated on a shaker (DTS-4 Sky-Line,

Elmi, Riga, Latvia) for 60 min at 37 °C. The reaction was stopped by adding 200 μL borate buffer (0.2 M, pH 9.8). The absorbance of the released p-NP was measured at 405 nm wavelength.

2.4.2. Evaluation of GLU Activity

GLU activity was determined by the Marciniak et al. [27] method. 40 μL acetate buffer (0.1 M, pH 4.5) and 30 μL 20 mM substrate solution (p-nitrophenyl-β-D-glucopyranoside, Sigma-Aldrich; Steinheim, Germany) were added to 10 μL supernatant fluid. The reaction mixture was incubated on a shaker for 60 min at 37 °C. The reaction was stopped by adding 200 μL borate buffer (0.2 M, pH 9.8). The absorbance of the released p-NP was measured at 405 nm.

2.4.3. Evaluation of GAL Activity

The activity of GAL was determined according to the method described by Chojnowska et al. [28]. 40 μL citrate-phosphate buffer (0.1 M, pH 4.3) and 30 μL 1.6 mM substrate solution (p-nitrophenyl-β-D-galactopyranoside, Sigma-Aldrich; Steinheim, Germany) were added to 10 μL supernatant fluid. The reaction mixture was incubated on a shaker for 60 min at 37 °C. The reaction was stopped by adding 200 μL borate buffer (0.2 M, pH 9.8). The absorbance of the released p-NP was measured at 405 nm wavelength.

2.4.4. Evaluation of MAN Activity

MAN activity was determined by Chojnowska et al. [28] method. 40 μL citrate-phosphate buffer (0.1 M, pH 4.3) and 30 μL 0.8 mM substrate solution (p-nitrophenyl-α-mannopyranoside, Sigma-Aldrich; Steinheim, Germany) were added to 10 μL supernatant fluid. The reaction mixture was incubated on a shaker for 60 min at 37 °C. The reaction was stopped by adding 200 μL borate buffer (0.2 M, pH 9.8). The absorbance of the released p-NP was measured at 405 nm.

2.4.5. Evaluation of FUC Activity

FUC activity was determined by Chojnowska et al. [28] method. 40 μL citrate-phosphate buffer (0.1 M, pH 4.3) and 30 μL 2.3 mM substrate solution (p-nitro-α-fucopyranoside, Sigma-Aldrich; Steinheim, Germany) were added to 10 μL supernatant fluid. The reaction mixture was incubated on a shaker for 60 min at 37 °C. The reaction was stopped by adding 200 μL borate buffer (0.2 M, pH 9.8). The absorbance of the released p-NP was measured at 405 nm wavelength.

2.5. Evaluation of Oxidative Stress Markers

The concentrations of reduced glutathione (GSH) and lipid peroxidation products (malondialdehyde, MDA) were determined using the colorimetric micro methods. All assays were performed in triplicate samples and standardized to 100 mg of total protein.

2.5.1. Evaluation of GSH Concentration

GSH concentration was assayed by the Ellman method using 5,5′-dithiobis-2-nitrobenzoic acid (DTNB) [29]. 100 μL 10% TCA and 100 μL 10 mM EDTA were added to 100 μL of supernatant. The samples were placed in a refrigerator (4 °C, 10 min) and then centrifuged for 5 min (5000× *g*, 4 °C). Next, 20 μL of deproteinised supernatant was collected and 180 μL of distilled water, 15 μL of 10 mM EDTA, 20 μL of 3.2 M TRIS buffer from HCl at pH = 8.1 and 10 μL DTNB were added. The absorbance of the supernatant was measured at 412 nm wavelength.

2.5.2. Evaluation of MDA Concentration

The concentration of MDA was measured with the colorimetric method using thiobarbituric acid (TBA) [30]. 250 μL distilled water, 500 μL 15% trichloroacetic acid (TCA) and 500 μL 0.37% TBA were added to 250 µL of the sample. The samples were water bath-heated for 10 min and then centrifuged for 10 min (10,000× g, 4 °C). The absorbance of the supernatant was measured at 535 nm wavelength.

2.6. Assessment of Pro-Inflammatory Cytokines

Levels of pro-inflammatory cytokines, IL-1β (interleukin-1β) and TGF-β1 (transforming growth factor), were determined by ELISA method using ready-made kits (R&D Systems, Canada, Minneapolis, MN, USA). The absorbance was measured at 450 nm. All assays were performed in duplicate samples and standardized to 100 mg of total protein.

2.7. Assessment of Total Protein Concentration

Total protein concentration was determined by means of the commercial BCA™ Protein Assay Kit (Pierce, Thermo Fisher Scientific, Rockfold, IL, USA). The principle of the method used is the reaction of Cu^{+} ions (formed upon the reduction of Cu^{2+} copper ions by protein molecules in the alkaline environment) with BCA bicinchoninic acid, resulting in a purple complex with a maximum absorbance at 562 nm wavelength.

2.8. Histological Examination

Histopathological examinations were performed by an experienced pathologist (K. G. U.). The liver sections were stained with haematoxylin and eosin (H&E) and examined under a light microscope (OPLYMPUS BX 51-P, OLYMPUS, Center Valley, PA, USA) at 10×, 20× and 40× magnification.

2.9. Statistical Analysis

The statistical analysis of the obtained results was performed using Statistica 12.0 statistical package (StatSoft, Tulsa, OK, USA) and GraphPad Prism 5.0 (GraphPad Software, Inc., La Jolla, CA, USA), with nonparametric tests: the ANOVA Kruskal-Wallis test and the Mann-Whitney test. Multiplicity adjusted p value was also calculated. The relationship between the quantitative data was assessed according to Spearman rank correlation. The results are presented as a median, minimum, maximum and percentiles. The threshold for statistical significance was $p < 0.05$. The sample size was set based on a previously conducted pilot study. The power of the test was set at 0.9.

3. Results

3.1. WPC-80 Composition

According to the analyses, the main component of WPC-80 is protein, which accounts for 78.2% of the concentrate mass. The preparation also contains fats, carbohydrates and small amounts of dietary fibre (Table 1). The remaining components of WPC-80 (endogenous and exogenous amino acids, fatty acids, vitamins and minerals) are listed in the Supplementary Material.

Table 1. General composition of whey protein concentrate (WPC-80).

General Composition	%
Protein	78.2
Fat	6.72
Carbohydrates	7.9
Ash	2.7
Dietary fibre	<0.5
Humidity	4.5
The calorific value	1712 kJ/100 g

3.2. Characteristics of the Animals

No significant differences were found in the body weight, liver weight and liver index of the animals from different groups (Figure 1). Similarly, complete blood counts were not significantly different between the study group and control (Table 2).

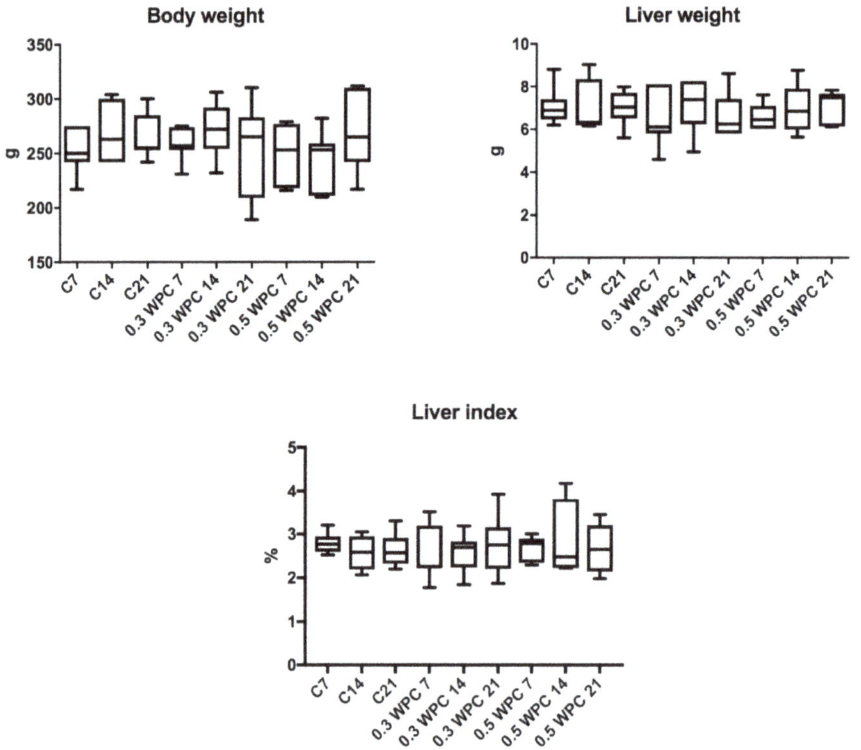

Figure 1. Body weight, liver weight and liver index of rats. C7, C14, C21, control groups; 0.3 WPC 7, 0.3 WPC 14, 0.3 WPC 21, 0.5 WPC 7, 0.5 WPC 14, 0.5 WPC 21, experimental groups.

Serum and plasma biochemical parameters did not differ significantly between the study and control rats (Table 3). Only serum ALT and AST level were statistically higher in the animals receiving WPC-80 at a dose of 0.5 g/kg body weight for 21 days versus control group (C21) ($p = 0.0079$; $p = 0.0317$ respectively). Similarly, only plasma creatinine and urea were significantly higher in the animals receiving higher dose of WPC-80 (0.5 g/kg body weight) for 21 days ($p = 0.05$; $p = 0.0079$) (Table 3).

Table 2. Complete blood counts in rats fed with WPC-80 and the controls [median (minimum-maximum)].

	WBC (× 10^{12}/L)	RBC (M/µL)	HGB (g/dL)	HTC (%)	MCV (fL)	MCH (pg)	MCHC (g/dL)	PLT (× 10^9/L)
C7	3.3 (2.8–3.7)	7.1 (6.6–9.9)	13.8 (13.6–13.9)	40.0 (38.9–43.0)	58.5 (58.0–59.0)	20.5 (18.3–21.1)	35.2 (34.8–35.6)	781.5 (635.0–928.0)
C14	2.9 (2.5–3.8)	7.0 (6.7–7.4)	14.0 (12.8–15.0)	41.6 (39.4–45.2)	59.0 (57.0–62.00)	19.9 (19.0–21.2)	33.2 (31.1–34.5)	825.0 (747.0–881.0)
C21	3.5 (2.5–4.8)	7.4 (6.8–8.9)	15.3 (12.3–17.4)	49.2 (36.2–52.2)	58.5 (56.0–59.0)	19.5 (18.2–20.5)	33.2 (31.1–33.3)	713.5 (406.0–821.0)
0.3 WPC 7	3.6 (2.8–4.9)	7.3 (6.3–7.9)	14.9 (12.9–15.8)	43.0 (26.5–46.0)	58.5 (57.0–59.0)	20.2 (19.8–20.8)	34.7 (34.4–35.4)	751.5 (627.0–914.0)
0.3 WPC 14	3.3 (2.4–4.0)	7.1 (6.4–8.1)	14.1 (12.7–15.3)	42.1 (37.2–44.8)	57.5 (54.0–62.0)	19.6 (18.0–20.5)	34.2 (31.8–34.7)	743.5 (462.0–920.0)
0.3 WPC 21	3.2 (2.5–4.8)	7.4 (6.5–8.7)	14.8 (13.2–16.4)	42.6 (36.7–49.5)	58.0 (55.0–60.0)	20.0 (18.0–21.0)	35.1 (33.0–36.4)	751.0 (667.0–855.0)
0.5 WPC 7	3.9 (3.2–5.0)	6.9 (6.4–8.9)	14.2 (13.0–17.8)	40.9 (37.3–50.8)	58.0 (57.0–61.0)	20.4 (20.0–20.6)	35.0 (33.8–35.7)	760.0 (589.0–930.0)
0.5 WPC 14	3.2 (2.6–3.9)	7.5 (6.6–8.0)	13.9 (13.3–16.0)	44.0 (39.8–54.0)	59.0 (42.9–60.0)	19.8 (14.2–20.0)	33.5 (18.0–35.6)	720.0 (331.0–778.0)
0.5 WPC 21	3.7 (2.8–5.4)	7.8 (6.6–8.9)	15.1 (13.7–16.6)	45.0 (38.7–49.7)	57.5 (50.0–61.0)	19.8 (17.9–20.9)	33.7 (32.0–35.3)	709.5 (599.0–880.0)

C7, C14, C21, control groups; 0.3 WPC 7, 0.3 WPC 14, 0.3 WPC 21, 0.5 WPC 7, 0.5 WPC 14, 0.5 WPC 21, experimental groups. HCT, haematocrit; HGB, haemoglobin; MCH, Mean Corpuscular Haemoglobin; MCHC, Mean Corpuscular Haemoglobin Concentration; MCV, Mean Corpuscular Volume; PLT, platelets; RBC, erythrocytes; WBC, leukocytes.

Table 3. Serum and plasma biochemical parameters in rats fed with WPC-80 and the controls [median (minimum-maximum)].

	ALT (U/L)	AST (U/L)	Bilirubin (mg/dL)	Albumin (µmol/L)	Cr (mg/dL)	UA (µmol/L)	Urea (mmol/L)	TC (mmol/L)	Glucose (mg/dL)
C7	52.6 (34.1–64.7)	100.3 (65.9–133.1)	1.6 (1.5–1.7)	419.9 (416.5–432.8)	0.5 (0.4–0.6)	27.0 (26.0–36.0)	6.4 (4.3–6.7)	80.7 (61.2–98.7)	94.2 (68.0–102.5)
C14	52.0 (42.8–66.6)	88.0 (76.0–117.7)	1.7 (1.0–2.0)	420.4 (337.0–435.8)	0.4 (0.4–0.5)	27.0 (24.0–34.0)	6.3 (5.6–8.6)	83.3 (51.3–97.0)	89.0 (83.0–92.0)
C21	47.2 (38.1–73.8)	91.5 (75.9–116.8)	2.0 (1.8–2.3)	417.2 (385.3–435.4)	0.5 (0.4–0.7)	26.0 (16.0–34.0)	8.2 (6.5–8.5)	84.0 (78.6–95.6)	89.0 (71.3–100.0)
0.3 WPC 7	59.0 (35.5–88.4)	122.2 (93.6–132.4)	1.2 (1.0–1.3)	418.7 (368.2–447.8)	0.4 (0.3–0.5)	24.0 (17.0–43.0)	5.8 (4.6–6.1)	70.4 (40.9–98.5)	89.0 (78.0–104.0)
0.3 WPC 14	55.2 (50.8–61.6)	115.1 (106.0–135.9)	1.1 (0.9–1.9)	461.3 (432.3–500.8)	0.5 (0.4–0.6)	29.0 (24.0–45.0)	7.8 (5.8–8.6)	88.7 (62.7–101.4)	85.0 (72.0–105.5)
0.3 WPC 21	57.0 (49.1–76.8)	103.3 (80.0–141.0)	1.2 (0.9–2.0)	419.7 (384.0–471.6)	0.5 (0.5–0.6)	36.0 (27.0–39.0)	8.1 (7.2–9.2)	90.1 (69.1–95.0)	82.5 (68.0–96.00)
0.5 WPC 7	57.5 (42.7–81.2)	86.0 (73.0–158.7)	2.0 (1.6–2.4)	460.4 (445.3–486.4)	0.6 (0.5–0.8)	29.0 (21.0–45.0)	6.0 (5.3–7.2)	79.7 (63.7–82.1)	90.5 (83.0–97.0)
0.5 WPC 14	57.9 (49.6–99.8)	109.4 (107.6–148.4)	1.7 (1.4–2.1)	430.0 (401.7–442.7)	0.5 (0.5–0.7)	33.0 (24.0–45.0)	6.9 (5.7–7.8)	88.8 (70.3–89.7)	78.0 (74.0–98.00)
0.5 WPC 21	101.1 (77.5–126.0)^c	173.0 (164.6–216.2)^c	1.3 (0.8–2.4)	464.7 (388.6–469.7)	0.7 (06–0.9)^c	33.0 (23.0–36.0)	9.7 (8.9–10.4)^c	78.0 (58.4–95.2)	85.5 (73.0–101.0)

C7, C14, C21, control groups; 0.3 WPC 7, 0.3 WPC 14, 0.3 WPC 21, 0.5 WPC 7, 0.5 WPC 14, 0.5 WPC 21, experimental groups. ALT, alanine aminotransferase; AST, aspartate aminotransferase; Cr, creatinine; TC, total cholesterol; UA, uric acid. Differences statistically important: c vs C21 ($p < 0.05$).

The content of total protein in rat liver did not differ significantly between the study and control group rats (Figure 2).

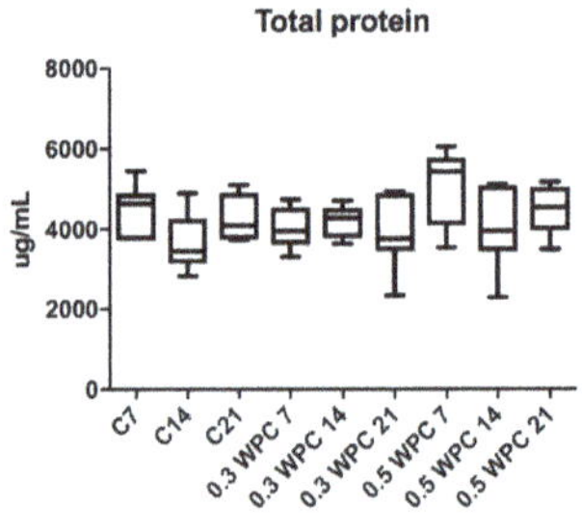

Figure 2. Total protein content in liver of rats fed with WPC-80 and the controls; C7, C14, C21, control groups; 0.3 WPC 7, 0.3 WPC 14, 0.3 WPC 21, 0.5 WPC 7, 0.5 WPC 14, 0.5 WPC 21, experimental groups.

3.3. Activity of Lysosomal Exoglycosidases

Specific activity of HEX and GLU in liver homogenates of rats receiving WPC-80 at a dose of 0.3 and 0.5 g/kg body weight for 7 days was significantly higher compared to control group rats receiving physiological saline (C7) (HEX: 0.3 WPC 7 versus C7 $p = 0.0012$, 0.5 WPC 7 versus C7 $p = 0.0006$; GLU: 0.3 WPC 7 versus C7 $p = 0.0700$, 0.5 WPC 7 versus C7 $p = 0.0210$). GLU activity was considerably higher in the group supplemented with WPC-80 at a dose of 0.3 g/kg body weight for 14 days than in the control group (C14) ($p = 0.011$). Both HEX ($p = 0.0006$) and GLU ($p = 0.0006$) activity was significantly higher in the group of animals fed with whey at a dose of 0.3 g/kg body weight for 21 days (0.3 WPC 21) compared to WPC 7 and WPC 21 control groups and HEX activity in the group of 0.3 WPC 21 rats was considerably higher compared to the group receiving WPC-80 at the same dose for 14 days (0.3 WPC 14) ($p = 0.0041$) (Figure 3).

The specific activity of HEX in the group of rats receiving WPC-80 at a dose of 0.5 g/kg body weight for 14 days was significantly higher in comparison with both the control group (C14) ($p = 0.0070$) and group supplemented with a lower dose of whey (0.3 WPC 14) ($p = 0.0175$). The activity of HEX and GLU in the group of animals receiving WPC-80 supplementation at a dose of 0.5 g/kg body weight for 21 days was by far higher than in the 21-day control group ($p = 0.0070$, $p = 0.0006$ respectively). Similar changes were observed in the group of rats supplemented with the same dose of WPC-80 for 7 days. The specific activity of GLU in the group of 0.5 WPC 21 was also significantly higher compared to the group of animals fed with the same dose of the supplement for 14 days ($p = 0.011$) (0.5 WPC 14) (Figure 3).

The specific activity of GAL was significantly higher in the liver of rats fed with WPC-80 at a dose of 0.3 g/kg body weight for 21 days compared to the group receiving whey for 7 days (0.3 WPC 7) ($p = 0.0379$). Similar relation has been observed in rats receiving the supplement at a dose of 0.5 g/kg body weight: GAL activity was considerably higher in animals fed with WPC-80 for 21 days compared to those supplemented for 7 days ($p = 0.0379$) (Figure 4).

The specific activity of MAN in the liver of rodents fed with WPC-80 at a dose of 0.3 g/kg body weight for 21 days was significantly higher than in those receiving the same supplementation both for 7 ($p = 0.0060$) and 14 days ($p = 0.0060$) (Figure 4).

We demonstrated a significantly higher MAN activity in the liver of rats supplemented with WPC-80 at a dose of 0.5 g/kg body weight for 7 days (0.5 WPC 7) compared to the control group (C7) ($p = 0.0041$). Similarly, a considerably higher activity of the enzyme was observed in the group 0.5 WPC 7 compared to animals receiving WPC-80 at a dose of 0.3 g/kg body weight for the same period ($p = 0.0041$). In the group of rats receiving WPC-80 at a dose of 0.5 g/kg body weight for 14 days we observed significantly lower MAN activity than in the group fed with WPC-80 at the same dose for 7 days ($p = 0.0379$) (Figure 4).

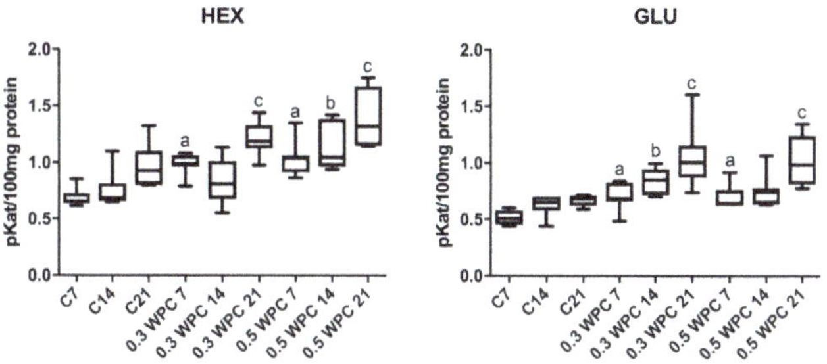

Figure 3. Activity of N-acetyl-β-D-hexosaminidase (HEX) and β-glucuronidase (GLU) in the liver of WPC-80-fed rats and the controls. C7, C14, C21, control groups; 0.3 WPC 7, 0.3 WPC 14, 0.3 WPC 21, 0.5 WPC 7, 0.5 WPC 14, 0.5 WPC 21, experimental groups. Differences statistically important: a vs C7; b vs C14; c vs C21 ($p < 0.05$).

The specific activity of FUC was significantly higher in the group of rats receiving WPC-80 at a dose of 0.3 g/kg body weight for 21 days compared to the control group (C21) ($p = 0.0379$) and the rats supplemented with WPC-80 at the same dose for 7 ($p = 0.0060$) and 14 ($p = 0.011$) days (Figure 4).

The specific activity of FUC was notably lower in the liver of rats fed with whey for 21 days at a dose of 0.5 g/kg body weight compared to the group of animals supplemented with WPC-80 at a dose of 0.3 g/kg body weight for 21 days. A significantly higher activity of the enzyme was also observed in the WPC-80-supplemented group receiving a dose of 0.5 g/kg body weight for 21 days than in the animals fed the same dose of the concentrate for 7 ($p = 0.0175$) and 14 days ($p = 0.0379$) (Figure 4).

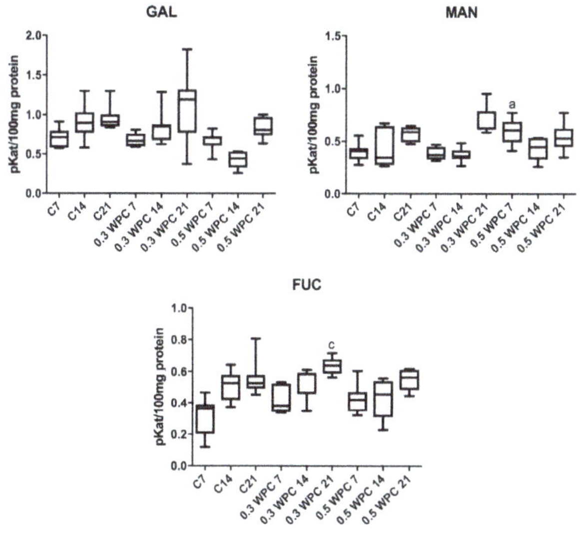

Figure 4. Activity of β-galactosidase (GAL), α-mannosidase (MAN) and α-fucosidase (FUC) in the liver of WPC-80-supplemented rats and the control group. C7, C14, C21, control groups; 0.3 WPC 7, 0.3 WPC 14, 0.3 WPC 21, 0.5 WPC 7, 0.5 WPC 14, 0.5 WPC 21, experimental groups. Differences statistically important: a vs C7; c vs C21 ($p < 0.05$).

3.4. Oxidative stress Markers

Significantly higher GSH concentration was obtained in the group of rats receiving WPC-80 at a dose of 0.3 g/kg body weight compared to the 21-day control group ($p = 0.0260$) and the group receiving whey at a dose of 0.3 g/kg body weight for 7 ($p = 0.0152$) and 14 ($p = 0.0152$) days (Figure 5).

The concentration of GSH was considerably higher in the group supplemented with WPC-80 at a dose of 0.5 g/kg body weight for 7 days in comparison with the controls (C7) ($p = 0.0152$). In the group of animals receiving WPC-80 at a dose of 0.5 g/kg body weight for 14 days we observed significantly higher concentration of GSH compared to both the group supplemented with a lower dose of whey ($p = 0.0087$) and the control group (C14) ($p = 0.0152$). Whey supplementation at a dose of 0.5 g/kg body weight for 21 days resulted in a significant increase in the concentration of GSH compared to the 21-day control group ($p = 0.0043$) (Figure 5).

The concentration of MDA was significantly higher in the group receiving 0.5 g/kg body weight of whey for 7 days compared to the control group (C7) ($p = 0.0023$) and the group receiving a lower dose of the supplement for the same period of time (0.3 WPC 7) ($p = 0.0041$). Significantly higher concentrations of malondialdehyde were observed in animals fed WPC-80 at a dose of 0.5 g/kg body weight for 14 days compared to both the control group ($p = 0.0006$) and the rats receiving 0.3 g/kg body weight of whey for 14 ($p = 0.0012$). The concentration of MDA was considerably higher in liver homogenates of rats receiving 0.5 g/kg body weight of WPC-80 for 21 days compared to the control group ($p = 0.0006$) as well as the rodents fed a lower dose of WPC-80 for 21 days ($p = 0.0006$) (Figure 5).

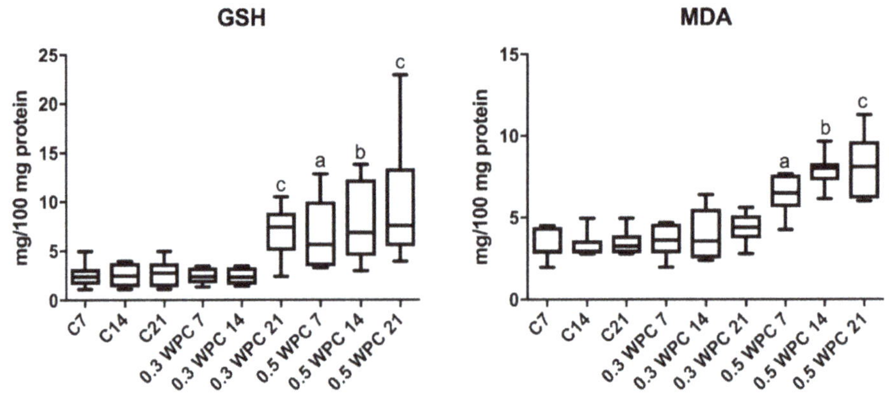

Figure 5. Reduced glutathione (GSH) and malondialdehyde (MDA) concentrations in the liver of WPC-80-fed rats and the control group. C7, C14, C21, control groups; 0.3 WPC 7, 0.3 WPC 14, 0.3 WPC 21, 0.5 WPC 7, 0.5 WPC 14, 0.5 WPC 21, experimental groups. Differences statistically important: a vs C7; b vs C14; c vs C21 ($p < 0.05$).

3.5. Pro-inflammatory Cytokines

The level of pro-inflammatory cytokines did not change between individual groups of rats. Only IL-1β and TGF-β1 levels were significantly higher in the liver of rats receiving WPC-80 at a dose of 0.5 g/kg body weight for 21 days ($p = 0.0070$; $p = 0.0012$ respectively) (Figure 6).

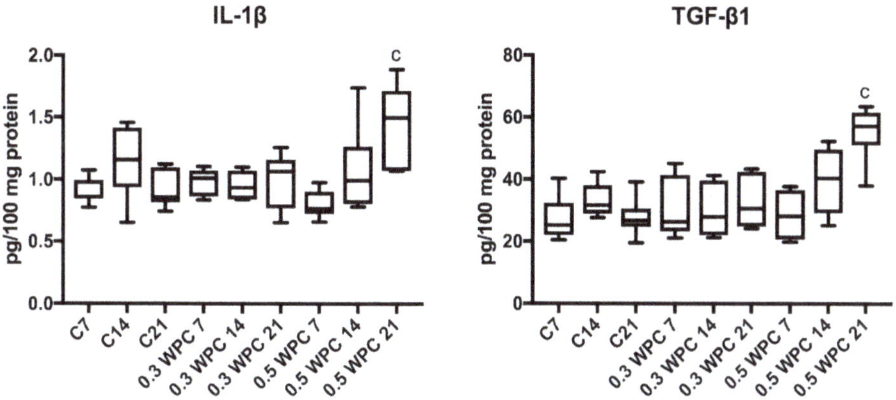

Figure 6. IL-1β and TGF-β1 levels in the liver of WPC-80-fed rats and the control group. C7, C14, C21, control groups; 0.3 WPC 7, 0.3 WPC 14, 0.3 WPC 21, 0.5 WPC 7, 0.5 WPC 14, 0.5 WPC 21, experimental groups. IL-1β, interleukin-1β; TGF-β1, transforming growth factor-β1. Differences statistically important: c vs C21 ($p < 0.05$).

3.6. Correlations

The results of statistically significant correlations between the activity of exoglycosidases and oxidative stress parameters are presented in Table 4. Importantly, in the group of rats supplemented with WPC-80 at a dose of 0.3 g/kg body weight for 14 days we observed a positive correlation between MAN activity and MDA concentration. A similar correlation between GLU and MDA was observed in the group of rats fed the whey concentrate at a dose of 0.5 g/kg body weight for 7 days. In the same group of animals (0.5 WPC 7) a positive correlation between HEX activity and MDA concentration was also observed. In addition, a positive correlation was found between GLU and IL-1β in the groups of rodents receiving WPC-80 at a dose of 0.5 g/kg body weight for 14 (0.5 WPC 14) and 21 days (0.5 WPC 21). Serum ALT correlated with HEX and GLU in the group of rats supplemented with WPC-80 at a dose of 0.5 g/kg body weight for 21 days. In the same group of animals (0.5 WPC 21) a positive correlation between HEX and AST was also observed (Table 4).

Table 4. Correlations between the profile of lysosomal exoglycosidases, oxidative stress and biochemical parameters in rats fed with WPC-80.

Pair of Variable	Group	*r*	*p*
MAN & MDA	0.3 WPC 14	0.886	0.003
GLU & MDA	0.5 WPC 7	0.812	0.005
HEX & MDA	0.5 WPC 7	0.607	0.05
HEX & Cr	0.5 WPC 7	0.650	0.05
GLU & GSH	0.5 WPC 14	0.771	0.04
GLU & IL-1β	0.5 WPC 14	0.650	0.05
GLU & IL-1β	0.5 WPC 21	0.810	0.005
HEX & ALT	0.5 WPC 21	0.741	0.001
HEX & AST	0.5 WPC 21	0.690	0.04
GLU & ALT	0.5 WPC 21	0.920	<0.0001

0.3 WPC 14, 0.5 WPC 7, 0.5 WPC 14, experimental groups; ALT, alanine aminotransferase; AST, aspartate aminotransferase; Cr, creatinine; GLU, β-glucuronidase; GSH, reduced glutathione; HEX, N-acetyl-β-D-hexosaminidase; IL-1β, interleukin-1β; MAN, α-mannosidase; MDA, malondialdehyde; MAN, α-mannosidase.

3.7. Histological Examination

In histological studies, we showed that WPC-80 leads to liver damage with the observed features of ischemic necrosis (Figure 7). In the liver of rats fed with WPC-80 at a dose of 0.3 g/kg body weight for 7 days, damage to single cells were demonstrated (Figure 7D). These changes were more pronounced in the liver of rats fed with WPC-80 at a dose of 0.5 g/kg body weight (0.5 WPC 7) (Figure 7G).

Feeding rats with WPC-80 at a dose of 0.3 g/kg body weight for 14 days caused focal lesions suggesting ischemic damage (Figure 7E), while increase of WPC-80 dose intensified these changes (Figure 7H). In addition, histological examination revealed the death of individual cell nuclei. In rats fed with a higher dose of whey protein concentrate (0.5 WPC 14), an increase in ischemic necrosis was observed by approx. 20% in relation to the dose of 0.3 g/kg body weight (0.3 WPC 14) (Figure 7E,H).

In rats fed with WPC-80 for 21 days at a dose of 0.3 g/kg body weight, hepatocellular damage was demonstrated with a loss of nuclei and obliteration of cell membranes (Figure 7F). More extensive changes were observed in the rats fed with a higher dose of WPC-80 (0.5 WPC 21) (Figure 7I). However, no signs of inflammation and liver fibrosis were confirmed in the histological examination (Figure 7).

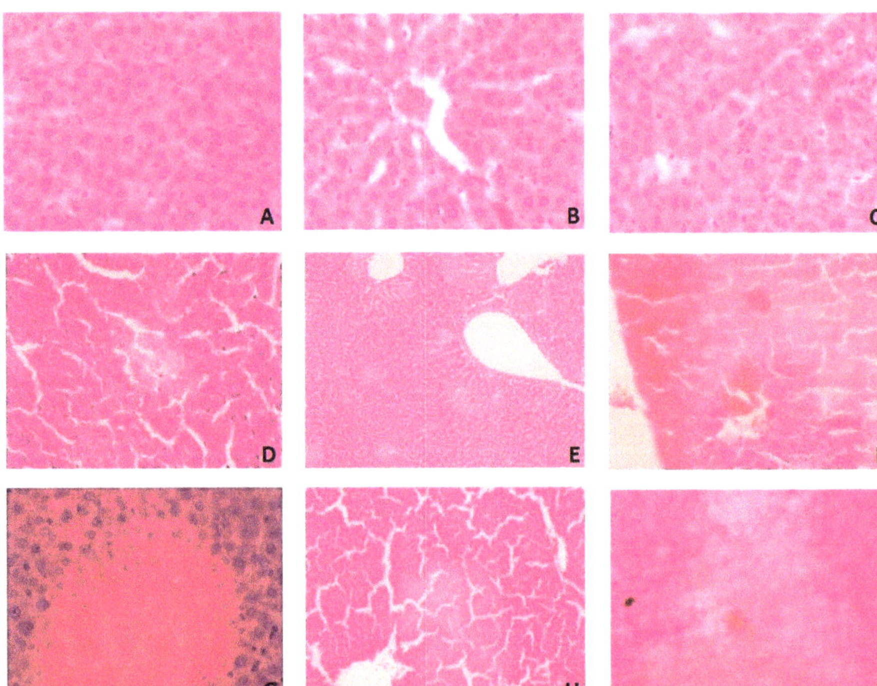

Figure 7. Liver histological examination of WPC-80-fed rats and the control group. **A** (C7), **B** (C14), **C** (C21), **D** (0.3 WPC 7), **E** (0.3 WPC 14), **F** (0.3 WPC 21), **G** (0.5 WPC 7), **H** (0.5 WPC 14), **I** (0.5 WPC 21).

4. Discussion

Our study is the first to indicate increased catabolism of liver glycoconjugates in the rats supplemented with whey protein concentrate WPC-80. We observed significantly higher activity of most lysosomal exoglycosidases as well as increased GSH concentration in the liver of rats receiving WPC-80. Despite increased glutathione biosynthesis, whey induces oxidative stress, which may lead to liver tissue damage.

Lysosomal exoglycosidases are responsible for the decomposition of sugar chains of glycoconjugates, that is, glycoproteins, glycolipids and proteoglycans in cell membranes and extracellular matrix [9,12]. Thus, changes in exoglycosidases activity may indicate catabolism and degree of remodelling of tissues/extracellular matrix [9]. Increased activity of exoglycosidases was recorded in the course of metabolic diseases [31], autoimmune diseases [32], cancer [33] and liver diseases [34–36]. The activity of exoglycosidases may be modified by environmental factors, diet and lifestyle [9]. Recently, a diet with high protein content (over 30% of the total energy intake) is becoming increasingly popular [37]. Excessive supply of dietary protein may affect the function of organs involved in protein metabolism (liver) and excretion of the products of its metabolism (kidneys) [7]. This condition leads to increased degradation of proteins due to the activity of, inter alia, hydrolytic lysosomal enzymes [7]. Therefore, changes in lysosomal exoglycosidases activity may reflect the intensity of metabolic changes occurring in liver tissue.

The liver is the main 'metabolic organ' of the human body. Its primary functions include decomposition of endogenous substances and xenobiotics (like toxins, alcohol and medicines), conversion of toxic ammonia into urea (in the so-called urea cycle) and participation in the metabolism of proteins, carbohydrates and lipids [7]. The results of our research indicate increased degradation of oligosaccharide chains of glycoconjugates in the liver of rats supplemented with WPC-80 concentrate. It is well known that hepatic glycoconjugates include structural, transport and secretory proteins, as well as tissue compatibility (histocompatibility) antigens encoded by MHC genes. The oligosaccharide chains of hepatic glycoproteins are also found on the outer surface of cell membrane, which participate in signal transduction and immune response pathways, while the glycoprotein transporters are involved in the transport of bile acids, glucose and growth factors [34–36,38]. It is suggested that increased catabolism of hepatic glycoconjugates may affect the cell structure and organisation of the liver tissue [39]. We found significant increase in the activity of most of the studied lysosomal hydrolases (↑HEX, ↑GLU, ↑MAN, ↑FUC) resulting from prolonged WPC-80 administration. However, the activity of GAL, GLU and partly HEX, FUC and MAN does not depend on the supplemented whey dose. Only the activity of HEX increased after two weeks of WPC-80 administration at a dose of 0.5 g/kg body weight compared to the dose of 0.3 g/kg body weight. It appears that raised activity of lysosomal hydrolases may indicate intensified liver metabolic processes and also impairment of liver function as a result of WPC-80 supplementation. Increased activity of exoglycosidases has been reported in numerous liver diseases, such as: primary biliary cirrhosis (PBC), autoimmune hepatitis (AIH), non-alcoholic fatty liver disease (NAFLD) and hepatic cholestasis [34–36,38]. It has been demonstrated that in inflammatory conditions lysosomal exoglycosidases are released from the liver into the blood, where they are caught by specific receptors located on the surface of macrophages [39]. In our study, the cytokines (IL-1β, TGF-β1) level was significantly higher in the liver of animals receiving WPC-80 at a dose of 0.5 g/kg body weight for 21 days (the highest dose and time of WPC-80 administration). It should be noted that TGF-β1 (transforming growth factor-β1) is one of the most important cytokines involved in the liver fibrosis [40]. It participates in the apoptosis of hepatocytes and activates inflammatory cells at the site of liver tissue damage. It is also the strongest factor stimulating the production of collagen and other extracellular matrix components [40]. Therefore, higher concentrations of TGF-β1 may predispose to the liver fibrosis in rats supplemented with high doses of WPC-80. Additionally, we observed a significant increase in GLU activity in the liver of WPC-80-supplemented rats compared to the controls. It is known that the activity of GLU increases in the course of numerous diseases of inflammatory aetiology [9]. This enzyme is released from the granular leukocytes and is one of the markers of the influx of neutrophils [41,42]. Numerous studies have described the relationship between GLU activity and concentration of proinflammatory cytokines and other inflammatory markers (e.g., IL-1, IL-6, TNF-α and CRP) [42,43]. Also in our experiment, the activity of GLU correlated with IL-1β level. Therefore, it may indicate intensified inflammatory processes in the liver parenchyma depending on the dose and time of administration of WPC-80. However, in the histopathological examination we did not observe any features of inflammation in the WPC-80-supplemented rats. Bearing in mind lysosomal exoglycosidases are an early marker of the inflammatory processes [42,43], an increase in their activity may suggest an initial stage of inflammation despite no changes were found in the histological studies. However, in WPC-80-fed rats we showed hepatocellular damage with the observed features of ischemic necrosis. Morphological changes of hepatocytes depended mainly on the duration of WPC-80 administration. Supplementation of WPC-80 at a dose of 0.5 g/kg body weight for 21 days resulted in a loss of nuclei as well as obliteration of cell membranes of the hepatocytes. Under such conditions, liver lysosomes may be damaged and proteolytic enzymes (including exoglycosidases) may be released. This may lead to further liver injury.

Oxidative stress may be one of the mechanisms responsible for the increase in the exoglycosidases activity in the liver. It is believed that a diet containing more than 33–45% protein may lead to increased production of ROS and initiate oxidative stress in various organs [18,20]. It is postulated that the increased production of free radicals is primarily a result of disorders of energy process in the mitochondrial respiratory chain [44]. In addition, it has been demonstrated that a long-term high-protein diet causes significant biochemical and ultrastructural changes in rat liver mitochondria and thus increase ROS production [45]. In our study, we found an increase of the MDA concentration in the liver of rats receiving WPC-80 at a dose of 0.5 g/kg of body weight compared to the control group. MDA is a marker of cell membrane lipid oxidation, which indicates oxidative stress in rats fed with WPC-80. MDA is also known to be a mutagenic and carcinogenic compound [46]. By forming adducts with proteins and nucleic acids, it promotes their accumulation in tissues and causes further oxidative damage [46,47]. MDA is also one of key oxidative stress mediators leading to liver damage through inflammation and fibrosis [48]. Lipid peroxidation may also cause necrosis of hepatocytes [46], which may partly explain the results of our histological studies. It is known that during hepatic ischemia, mitochondrial damage dramatically increases the ROS production, which intensifies further oxidative damage [49]. However, in our study we also observed an increase in the concentration of reduced glutathione—the most important liver antioxidant. This is not surprising as WPC-80 is a rich source of cysteine and methionine—precursors to GSH biosynthesis [3]. Yet, despite increased concentration of GSH in the group of rats receiving WPC-80, oxidative liver damage (↑MDA) occurs under these conditions. Therefore, the increased supply of WPC-80 does not effectively protect against excessive production of free oxygen radicals under the influence of increased protein supply. Moreover, it can be assumed that intensified GSH production is also an adaptive response of the body to increased ROS production, especially at high doses of WPC-80. Positive correlation between MDA and lysosomal exoglycosidases (HEX, GLU and MAN) in the liver of WPC-80-supplemented rats may prove the potential relationship between oxidative stress and catabolism of glycoconjugates, as it is suggested that oxidative stress increases permeability of lysosomal membranes and leakage of lysosomal exoglycosidases into the bloodstream.

In the literature, there are only a few studies evaluating the influence of a high-protein diet on the profile of lysosomal exoglycosidases in the liver. Witek et al. [50] analysed the activity of selected hydrolases (HEX, GLU, GAL, acid phosphatase, leucine and alanine aminopeptidase, cathepsins D and L) in the liver and kidneys of mice receiving a diet of varied (10% and 16%) protein content. A significant increase in lysosomal exoglycosidases activity as well as a considerable decrease in aminopeptidase and cathepsin activity was found in the liver of rats fed on a higher protein content diet. However, the reasons for the observed changes are still unknown. Colombo et al. [51] demonstrated significantly higher activity of AST, ALT and GGT in the liver of rats receiving a diet containing 32% and 51% protein versus the controls. Moreover, Mutlu et al. [52] reported increased activity of hepatic aminotransferases, as well as increased concentration of albumins with concomitant abdominal pain, which may suggest the need for caution in case of a high-protein diet. In our study, we showed increased aminotransferases activity in rats receiving WPC-80 at a dose of 0.5 g/kg body weight versus control group. Importantly, serum ALT and AST correlated with the activity of hepatic exoglycosidases (HEX, GLU), further confirming the usefulness of lysosomal hydrolases as markers of the liver function.

We did not observe any significant changes in the body weight, liver weight and liver index of rats receiving WPC-80 compared to controls. Although a high-protein diet is known to regulate the fat deposition in the liver [53], in our research, whey protein concentrate was not the primary source of food. It was administered as the intragastric supplementation, which may explain the observed lack of differences. However, in addition to the liver, also kidneys play a major role in the metabolism of proteins. Although this was not a direct goal of the present study, it may be presumed that high WPC-80 doses may interfere with kidney function as evidenced by the increase in serum creatinine and urea. However, this assumption requires further research especially because the remaining biochemical (albumin, uric acid) and morphological parameters did not differ significantly between individual groups of rats.

To sum up, WPC-80 is responsible for intensified reconstruction of liver tissue and induction of oxidative stress. We observed a significant increase in the activity of most lysosomal exoglycosidases and raised oxidative damage compared to the controls. In addition, whey protein concentrate leads to hepatocellular damage with the observed features of ischemic necrosis. High activity of exoglycosidases may result from their participation in liver tissue remodelling or involvement in an ongoing inflammatory process, particularly under the influence of high doses of WPC-80 (0.5 g/kg body weight). Since our experiment does not explain the reasons for the observed changes, we would like to highlight the need of conducting further studies to assess the effect of WPC-80 on liver damage parameters. We believe that it is particularly important to properly select the dose and time of WPC-80 administration.

Finally, it is also worth noting that our work had certain limitations. We evaluated only the selected lysosomal enzymes and biomarkers of oxidative stress and inflammation, so we cannot fully characterize the catabolism of liver glycoconjugates or changes caused by free radicals as a result of WPC-80 supplementation. What is more, our study assessed an animal model that can never fully replace tests on humans. However, despite relatively many reports on the antioxidant properties of whey, our study is the first to indicate the induction of liver oxidative stress under the influence of whey protein concentrate. We also point out that WPC-80 enhances catabolism of liver glycoconjugates and changes the morphology of hepatocytes. Therefore, whey should be cautiously used in liver diseases and disorders of the gastrointestinal tract. Our research is also a starting point for future basic and clinical research.

Supplementary Materials: The following are available online at http://www.mdpi.com/2072-6643/10/9/1178/s1, T Table S1: Protein and amino acids in analysed WPC-80., Table S2: Fatty acids in analysed WPC-80. Table S3: Vitamins and minerals in analysed WPC-80.

Author Contributions: M.Ż.-G. conceptualized and conducted the study, interpreted of results and wrote the manuscript; M.M. conceptualized and conducted the study, performed the statistical analysis, interpreted of results and wrote the manuscript; A.Z. conducted the study; K.G.-U. conducted the study; A.T. conducted the study; H.C. conceptualized and conducted the study, provided final approval of the version to be published.

Acknowledgments: The authors would like to thank Stanisław Jamiołkowski from the Dairy Cooperative in Mońki for the provision of WPC-80 and for financial support for the WPC-80 composition testing; Prof. Barbara Malinowska from Department of Experimental Physiology and Pathophysiology and Prof. Ewa Chabielska from Laboratory of Biopharmacy, Medical University of Bialystok for allowing animal studies as well as Anna Sadowska, Kamil Bienias and Sławomir Prokopiuk for their help in conducting the research on animals.

Conflicts of Interest: The authors declare no conflict of interest.

References

1. Kita, M.; Obara, K.; Kondo, S.; Umeda, S.; Ano, Y. Effect of supplementation of a whey peptide rich in tryptophan-tyrosine-related peptides on cognitive performance in healthy adults: A randomized, double-blind, placebo-controlled study. *Nutrients* **2018**, *10*, 887. [CrossRef] [PubMed]
2. Teba, C.D.; da Silva, E.M.M.; Chávez, D.W.H.; de Carvalho, C.W.P; Ascheri, J.L.R. Effects of whey protein concentrate, feed moisture and temperature on the physicochemical characteristics of a rice-based extruded flour. *Food Chem.* **2017**, *228*, 287–296. [CrossRef] [PubMed]

3. Falkowski, M.; Maciejczyk, M.; Koprowicz, T.; Mikołuć, B.; Milewska, A.; Zalewska, A.; Car, H. Whey protein concentrate wpc-80 improves antioxidant defense systems in the salivary glands of 14-month wistar rats. *Nutrients* **2018**, *10*, 782. [CrossRef] [PubMed]
4. Nabuco, H.C.G.; Tomeleri, C.M.; Sugihara Junior, P.; Fernandes, R.R.; Cavalcante, E.F.; Antunes, M.; Ribeiro, A.S.; Teixeira, D.C.; Silva, A.M.; Sardinha, L.B.; et al. Effects of whey protein supplementation pre- or post-resistance training on muscle mass, muscular strength and functional capacity in pre-conditioned older women: A randomized clinical trial. *Nutrients* **2018**, *10*, 563. [CrossRef] [PubMed]
5. Ignowski, E.; Winter, A.N.; Duval, N.; Fleming, H.; Wallace, T.; Manning, E.; Koza, L.; Huber, K.; Serkova, N.J.; Linseman, D.A. The cysteine-rich whey protein supplement, Immunocal®, preserves brain glutathione and improves cognitive, motor and histopathological indices of traumatic brain injury in a mouse model of controlled cortical impact. *Free Radic. Biol. Med.* **2018**, *124*, 328–341. [CrossRef] [PubMed]
6. Díaz-Rúa, R.; Keijer, J.; Palou, A.; van Schothorst, E.M.; Oliver, P. Long-term intake of a high-protein diet increases liver triacylglycerol deposition pathways and hepatic signs of injury in rats. *J. Nutr. Biochem.* **2017**, *46*, 39–48. [CrossRef] [PubMed]
7. Jean, C.; Rome, S.; Mathé, V.; Huneau, J.F.; Aattouri, N.; Fromentin, G.; Achagiotis, C.L.; Tomé, D. Metabolic evidence for adaptation to a high protein diet in rats. *J. Nutr.* **2001**, *131*, 91–98. [CrossRef] [PubMed]
8. Diez-Fernandez, C.; Häberle, J. Targeting CPS1 in the treatment of Carbamoyl phosphate synthetase 1 (CPS1) deficiency, a urea cycle disorder. *Expert Opin. Ther. Targets* **2017**, *21*, 391–399. [CrossRef] [PubMed]
9. Chojnowska, S.; Kępka, A.; Szajda, S.D.; Waszkiewicz, N.; Bierć, M.; Zwierz, K. Exoglycosidase markers of diseases. *Biochem. Soc. Trans.* **2011**, *39*, 406–409. [CrossRef] [PubMed]
10. Witek, B.; Rochon-Szmejchel, D.; Stanisławska, I.; Łyp, M.; Wróbel, K.; Zapała, A.; Kamińska, A.; Kołataj, A. Activities of lysosomal enzymes in alloxan-induced diabetes in the mouse. *Adv. Exp. Med. Biol.* **2018**, *1040*, 73–81. [CrossRef] [PubMed]
11. Lysek-Gladysinska, M.; Wieczorek, A.; Walaszczyk, A.; Jelonek, K.; Jozwik, A.; Pietrowska, M.; Dörr, W.; Gabrys, D.; Widlak, P. Long-term effects of low-dose mouse liver irradiation involve ultrastructural and biochemical changes in hepatocytes that depend on lipid metabolism. *Radiat. Environ. Biophys.* **2018**, *57*, 123–132. [CrossRef] [PubMed]
12. Maciejczyk, M.; Kossakowska, A.; Szulimowska, J.; Klimiuk, A.; Knaś, M.; Car, H.; Niklińska, W.; Ładny, J.R.; Chabowski, A.; Zalewska, A. lysosomal exoglycosidase profile and secretory function in the salivary glands of rats with streptozotocin-induced diabetes. *J. Diabetes Res.* **2017**, *2017*. [CrossRef] [PubMed]
13. Bee Ling, T.; Mohd Esa, N.; Winnie-Pui-Pui, L. Nutrients and oxidative stress: Friend or foe? *Oxid. Med. Cell. Longev.* **2018**, *2018*. [CrossRef]
14. Żukowski, P.; Maciejczyk, M.; Waszkiel, D. Sources of free radicals and oxidative stress in the oral cavity. *Arch. Oral Biol.* **2018**, *92*, 8–17. [CrossRef] [PubMed]
15. Pietrucha, B.; Heropolitanska-Pliszka, E.; Maciejczyk, M.; Car, H.; Sawicka-Powierza, J.; Motkowski, R.; Karpinska, J.; Hryniewicka, M.; Zalewska, A.; Pac, M.; et al. Comparison of selected parameters of redox homeostasis in patients with ataxia-telangiectasia and nijmegen breakage syndrome. *Oxid. Med. Cell. Longev.* **2017**, *2017*. [CrossRef] [PubMed]
16. Żukowski, P.; Maciejczyk, M.; Matczuk, J.; Kurek, K.; Waszkiel, D.; Zendzian-Piotrowska, M.; Zalewska, A. Effect of N-Acetylcysteine on antioxidant defense, oxidative modification and salivary gland function in a rat model of insulin resistance. *Oxid. Med. Cell. Longev.* **2018**, *2018*, 6581970. [CrossRef] [PubMed]
17. Fejfer, K.; Buczko, P.; Niczyporuk, M.; Ładny, J.R.; Hady, R.H.; Knaś, M.; Waszkiel, D.; Klimiuk, A.; Zalewska, A.; Maciejczyk, M. Oxidative modification of biomolecules in the nonstimulated and stimulated saliva of patients with morbid obesity treated with bariatric surgery. *Biomed. Res. Int.* **2017**, *2017*. [CrossRef] [PubMed]
18. Camiletti-Moirón, D.; Aparicio, V.A.; Nebot, E.; Medina, G.; Martínez, R.; Kapravelou, G.; Andrade, A.; Porres, J.M.; López-Jurado, M.; Aranda, P. High-protein diet induces oxidative stress in rat brain: Protective action of high-intensity exercise against lipid peroxidation. *Nutr. Hosp.* **2015**, *31*, 866–874. [CrossRef]
19. Gu, C.; Xu, H. Effect of oxidative damage due to excessive protein ingestion on pancreas function in mice. *Int. J. Mol. Sci.* **2010**, *11*, 4591–4600. [CrossRef] [PubMed]
20. Kołodziej, U.; Maciejczyk, M.; Niklińska, W.; Waszkiel, D.; Żendzian-Piotrowska, M.; Żukowski, P.; Zalewska, A. Chronic high-protein diet induces oxidative stress and alters the salivary gland function in rats. *Arch. Oral Biol.* **2017**, *84*, 6–12. [CrossRef] [PubMed]

21. Liu, Q.; Kong, B.; Han, J.; Sun, C.; Li, P. Structure and antioxidant activity of whey protein isolate conjugated with glucose via the Maillard reaction under dry-heating conditions. *Food Struct.* **2014**, *1*, 145–154. [CrossRef]
22. Hassan, A.M.; Abdel-Aziem, S.H.; Abdel-Wahhab, M.A. Modulation of DNA damage and alteration of gene expression during aflatoxicosis via dietary supplementation of Spirulina (Arthrospira) and whey protein concentrate. *Ecotoxicol. Environ. Saf.* **2012**, *79*, 294–300. [CrossRef] [PubMed]
23. Tokajuk, A.; Karpińska, O.; Zakrzeska, A.; Bienias, K.; Prokopiuk, S.; Kozłowska, H.; Kasacka, I.; Chabielska, E.; Car, H. Dysfunction of aorta is prevented by whey protein concentrate-80 in venous thrombosis-induced rats. *J. Funct. Foods* **2016**, *27*, 365–375. [CrossRef]
24. Zalewska, A.; Knaś, M.; Maciejczyk, M.; Waszkiewicz, N.; Klimiuk, A.; Choromańska, M.; Matczuk, J.; Waszkiel, D.; Car, H. Antioxidant profile, carbonyl and lipid oxidation markers in the parotid and submandibular glands of rats in different periods of streptozotocin induced diabetes. *Arch. Oral Biol.* **2015**, *60*, 1375–1386. [CrossRef] [PubMed]
25. Kolodziej, U.; Maciejczyk, M.; Miasko, A.; Matczuk, J.; Knas, M.; Zukowski, P.; Zendzian-Piotrowska, M.; Borys, J.; Zalewska, A. Oxidative modification in the salivary glands of high fat-diet induced insulin resistant rats. *Front. Physiol.* **2017**, *8*, 20. [CrossRef] [PubMed]
26. Borys, J.; Maciejczyk, M.; Antonowicz, B.; Krętowski, A.; Waszkiel, D.; Bortnik, P.; Czarniecka-Bargłowska, K.; Kocisz, M.; Szulimowska, J.; Czajkowski, M.; et al. Exposure to Ti4Al4V titanium alloy leads to redox abnormalities, oxidative stress and oxidative damage in patients treated for mandible fractures. *Oxid. Med. Cell. Longev.* **2018**, *2018*. [CrossRef] [PubMed]
27. Marciniak, J.; Zalewska, A.; Popko, J.; Zwierz, K. Optimization of an enzymatic method for the determination of lysosomal N-acetyl-β-D-hexosaminidase and β-glucuronidase in synovial fluid. *Clin. Chem. Lab. Med.* **2006**, *44*, 933–937. [CrossRef] [PubMed]
28. Chojnowska, S.; Minarowska, A.; Waszkiewicz, N.; Kępka, A.; Zalewska-Szajda, B.; Gościk, E.; Kowal, K.; Olszewska, E.; Konarzewska-Duchnowska, E.; Minarowski, Ł.; et al. The activity of N-acetyl-β-D-hexosaminidase A and B and β-glucuronidase in nasal polyps and hypertrophic nasal concha. *Otolaryngol. Pol.* **2014**, *68*, 20–24. [CrossRef] [PubMed]
29. Moron, M.; Depierre, J.; Mannervik, B. Levels of glutathione, glutathione reductase and glutathione S-transferase activities in rat lung and liver. *Biochim. Biophys. Acta-Gen. Subj.* **1979**, *582*, 67–78. [CrossRef]
30. Buege, J.A.; Aust, S.D. Microsomal lipid peroxidation. *Methods Enzymol.* **1978**, *52*, 302–310. [PubMed]
31. Sims-Robinson, C.; Bakeman, A.; Rosko, A.; Glasser, R.; Feldman, E.L. the role of oxidized cholesterol in diabetes-induced lysosomal dysfunction in the brain. *Mol. Neurobiol.* **2016**, *53*, 2287–2296. [CrossRef] [PubMed]
32. Pásztói, M.; Nagy, G.; Géher, P.; Lakatos, T.; Tóth, K.; Wellinger, K.; Pócza, P.; György, B.; Holub, M.C.; Kittel, Á.; et al. Gene expression and activity of cartilage degrading glycosidases in human rheumatoid arthritis and osteoarthritis synovial fibroblasts. *Arthritis Res. Ther.* **2009**, *11*, R68. [CrossRef] [PubMed]
33. Ramessur, K.T.; Greenwell, P.; Nash, R.; Dwek, M. V Breast cancer invasion is mediated by beta-N-acetylglucosaminidase (beta-NAG) and associated with a dysregulation in the secretory pathway of cancer cells. *Br. J. Biomed. Sci.* **2010**, *67*, 189–196. [CrossRef] [PubMed]
34. Hultberg, B.; Pålsson, B.; Isaksson, A.; Masson, P. Beta-hexosaminidase in bile and plasma from patients with cholestasis. *Liver* **1995**, *15*, 153–158. [CrossRef] [PubMed]
35. Humaloja, K.; Salaspuro, M.; Roine, R.P. Biliary excretion of dolichols and β-hexosaminidase—Effect of ethanol and glucagon. *Lipids* **1997**, *32*, 1169–1172. [CrossRef] [PubMed]
36. Maenhout, T.M.; Poll, A.; Wuyts, B.; Lecocq, E.; Van Vlierberghe, H.; De Buyzere, M.L.; Delanghe, J.R. Microheterogeneity of Serum β-Hexosaminidase in Chronic Alcohol Abusers in a Driver's License Regranting Program. *Alcohol. Clin. Exp. Res.* **2013**, *37*, 1264–1270. [CrossRef] [PubMed]
37. Pesta, D.H.; Samuel, V.T. A high-protein diet for reducing body fat: Mechanisms and possible caveats. *Nutr. Metab.* **2014**, *11*, 53. [CrossRef] [PubMed]
38. Fawzy Montaser, M.; Amin Sakr, M.; Omar Khalifa, M. Alpha-l-fucosidase as a tumour marker of hepatocellular carcinoma. *Arab. J. Gastroenterol.* **2012**, *13*, 9–13. [CrossRef] [PubMed]
39. Halvorson, M.R.; Campbell, J.L.; Sprague, G.; Slater, K.; Noffsinger, J.K.; Peterson, C.M. Comparative evaluation of the clinical utility of three markers of ethanol intake: The effect of gender. *Alcohol. Clin. Exp. Res.* **1993**, *17*, 225–229. [CrossRef] [PubMed]

40. Fabregat, I.; Moreno-Càceres, J.; Sánchez, A.; Dooley, S.; Dewidar, B.; Giannelli, G.; ten Dijke, P. TGF-β signalling and liver disease. *FEBS J.* **2016**, *283*, 2219–2232. [CrossRef] [PubMed]
41. Shimoi, K.; Nakayama, T. Glucuronidase deconjugation in inflammation. *Methods Enzymol.* **2005**, *400*, 263–272. [CrossRef] [PubMed]
42. Panagiotopoulou, E.C.; Fouzas, S.; Douros, K.; Triantaphyllidou, I.E.; Malavaki, C.; Priftis, K.N.; Karamanos, N.K.; Anthracopoulos, M.B. Increased β-glucuronidase activity in bronchoalveolar lavage fluid of children with bacterial lung infection: A case-control study. *Respirology* **2015**, *20*, 1248–1254. [CrossRef] [PubMed]
43. Jiang, H.; Zhang, Y.; Xiong, X.; Harville, E.W.; Karmin, O.; Qian, X. Salivary and serum inflammatory mediators among pre-conception women with periodontal disease. *BMC Oral Health* **2016**, *16*, 131. [CrossRef] [PubMed]
44. Choromańska, M.; Klimiuk, A.; Kostecka-Sochoń, P.; Wilczyńska, K.; Kwiatkowski, M.; Okuniewska, N.; Waszkiewicz, N.; Zalewska, A.; Maciejczyk, M. Antioxidant defence, oxidative stress and oxidative damage in saliva, plasma and erythrocytes of dementia patients. Can salivary AGE be a marker of dementia? *Int. J. Mol. Sci.* **2017**, *18*, e2205. [CrossRef] [PubMed]
45. Jordá, A.; Zaragozá, R.; Portolés, M.; Báguena-Cervellera, R.; Renau-Piqueras, J. Long-term high-protein diet induces biochemical and ultrastructural changes in rat liver mitochondria. *Arch. Biochem. Biophys.* **1988**, *265*, 241–248. [CrossRef]
46. Ayala, A.; Muñoz, M.F.; Argüelles, S. Lipid peroxidation: Production, metabolism and signaling mechanisms of malondialdehyde and 4-hydroxy-2-nonenal. *Oxid. Med. Cell Longev.* **2014**, *2014*. [CrossRef] [PubMed]
47. Maciejczyk, M.; Szulimowska, J.; Skutnik, A.; Taranta-Janusz, K.; Wasilewska, A.; Wiśniewska, N.; Zalewska, A. Salivary Biomarkers of Oxidative Stress in Children with Chronic Kidney Disease. *J. Clin. Med.* **2018**, *7*, e209. [CrossRef] [PubMed]
48. Kim, S.; Park, S.; Kim, B.; Kwon, J. Toll-like receptor 7 affects the pathogenesis of non-alcoholic fatty liver disease. *Sci. Rep.* **2016**, *6*, 27849.02. [CrossRef] [PubMed]
49. Elias-Miró, M.; Jiménez-Castro, M.B.; Rodés, J.; Peralta, C. Current knowledge on oxidative stress in hepatic ischemia/reperfusion. *Free Radic. Res.* **2013**, *47*, 555–568. [CrossRef] [PubMed]
50. Witek, B.; Ochwanowska, E.; Stanisławska, I.; Wróbel, A.; Mierzwa, W.; Kołątaj, A.; Bagnicka, E. Effect of testosterone on the activity of lysosomal enzymes in the mouse liver and kidney maintained on the different protein level in diet. *Vet. Med.-Sci. Pract.* **2007**, *63*, 1084–1089.
51. Colombo, J.-P.; Cervantes, H.; Kokorovic, M.; Pfister, U.; Perritaz, R. Effect of different protein diets on the distribution of amino acids in plasma, liver and brain in the rat. *Ann. Nutr. Metab.* **1992**, *36*, 23–33. [CrossRef] [PubMed]
52. Mutlu, E.; Keshavarzian, A.; Mutlu, G. Hyperalbuminemia and elevated transaminases associated with high-protein diet. *Scand. J. Gastroenterol.* **2006**, *41*, 759–760. [CrossRef] [PubMed]
53. French, W.W.; Dridi, S.; Shouse, S.A.; Wu, H.; Hawley, A.; Lee, S.O.; Gu, X.; Baum, J.I. A high-protein diet reduces weight gain, decreases food intake, decreases liver fat deposition and improves markers of muscle metabolism in obese Zucker rats. *Nutrients* **2017**, *9*, e587. [CrossRef] [PubMed]

nutrients MDPI

Review

ACEI-Inhibitory Peptides Naturally Generated in Meat and Meat Products and Their Health Relevance

Leticia Mora, Marta Gallego and Fidel Toldrá *

Instituto de Agroquímica y Tecnología de Alimentos (CSIC), Avenue Agustín Escardino 7, 46980 Paterna, Valencia, Spain; lemoso@iata.csic.es (L.M.); mgallego@iata.csic.es (M.G.)
* Correspondence: ftoldra@iata.csic.es; Tel.: +34-963-900-022 (ext. 2112); Fax: +34-963-636-301

Received: 31 July 2018; Accepted: 3 September 2018; Published: 7 September 2018

Abstract: Meat and meat products have been described as a very good source of angiotensin I converting enzyme (ACEI)-inhibitory peptides. The generation of bioactive peptides can occur through the action of endogenous muscular enzymes during processing, gastrointestinal digestion, or by using commercial enzymes in laboratory or industry under controlled conditions. Studies of bioavailability are necessary in order to prove the positive health effect of bioactive peptides in the body as they should resist gastrointestinal digestion, cross the intestinal barrier, and reach blood stream and target organs. However, in order to better understand their effect, interactions, and bioavailability, it is necessary to consider food matrix interactions and continue the development of quantitative methodologies in order to obtain more data that will enable advances in the field of bioactive peptides and the determination of their influence on health.

Keywords: meat; peptides; antihypertensive; peptidomics

1. Introduction

Bioactive peptides derived from food proteins can exert different effects after their absorption in the human body, such as prevention of diseases or physiological modulation. Physiological properties such as antihypertensive, antioxidant, antithrombotic, or hypocholesterolemic activity in the cardiovascular system [1,2]; mineral binding, antidiabetic, antimicrobial, or anti-inflammatory effects in the gastrointestinal system [3,4]; cytomodulatory or immunomodulatory actions in the immune system [5]; and opioid agonist or antagonist activity in the nervous system [6] have been recently described to be exerted by different food-derived peptides [7].

The activity of angiotensin I-converting enzyme (ACEI) inhibitors has been extensively studied over the last decade. The main reason for this interest is the relevance of hypertension in the development of cardiovascular diseases, which is the most important public health problem of this century. In this respect, different synthetic drugs are available on the market for the treatment of hypertension but their numerous side effects have focused researchers' interest on the search of alternative non-toxic and naturally generated peptides for controlling blood pressure [8].

ACEI is a dipeptidyl carboxypeptidase enzyme that participates in the renin–angiotensin system (RAS) and converts angiotensin-I into the vasoconstrictor angiotensin-II by cleaving two amino acids at the same time, thus inactivating the vasodilator bradykinin. The role of ACEI inhibitors is to maintain the balance between the vasoconstrictive and salt-retentive effects of angiotensin-II and vasodilator effects of bradykinin (Figure 1). Thus, the main interest for studying ACEI-inhibitory natural peptides is due to their capacity to inhibit ACEI, which lead to a decrease in blood pressure by inactivating the formation of angiotensin-II [9].

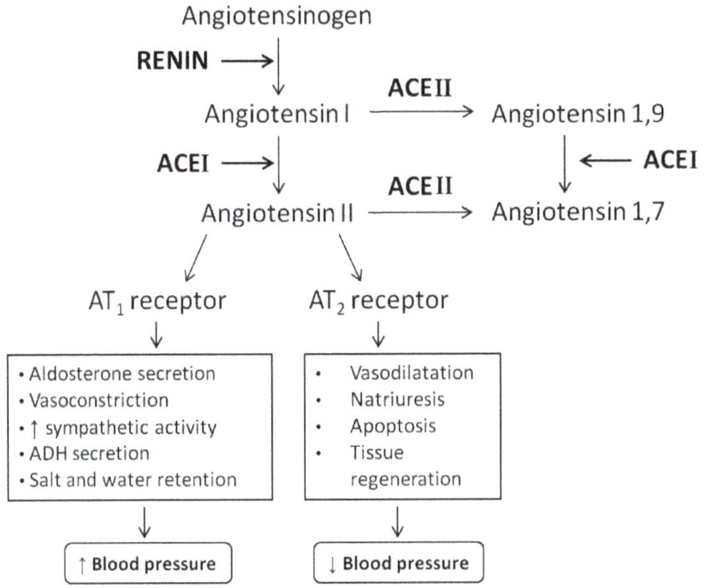

Figure 1. The renin-angiotensin system (RAS). ACEI: angiotensin I-converting enzyme; ACEII: angiotensin II-converting enzyme.

In this article, the generation of ACEI-inhibitory peptides from meat and meat products and their identification by empirical and in silico approaches have been reviewed, as well as the latest studies on bioavailability from the point of view of their health relevance. A discussion about current limitations and challenges to be overcome in order to advance in the state-of-the-art of this field is also included.

2. Generation of Meat-Derived ACEI-Inhibitory Peptides

ACEI-inhibitory peptides are usually small peptides with sizes comprising between 2 and 20 amino acids. Their function depends on the protein source, hydrolysis conditions, degree of hydrolysis, molecular mass, and amino acid composition as well as the position of amino acids in the peptide sequences. In this respect, ACEI-inhibitory peptides have been described that have hydrophobic and branched-chain amino acids in their structure. According to the literature, the type of amino acids located in the three positions close to the C-terminal end of the ACEI-inhibitory peptide is important for activity. The presence of aromatic, positively-charged, and basic amino acids in these positions is important for competitive binding to the ACEI active site. In fact, milk-derived tripeptides containing prolines might have different *cis/trans* configurations of bonds which could influence their access/binding to the ACEI complex [10–14]. Milk proteins have been described as a very good source of antihypertensive peptides, released during gastrointestinal digestion or food processing. The tripeptides Ile-Pro-Pro and Val-Pro-Pro, that are released from casein during the fermentation of milk, have been described as antihypertensive in several animal models as well as in clinical studies [15].

ACEI-inhibitory peptides obtained from food sources are inactive within the intact parent protein but can exert their activity once they are released by hydrolysis. Different ways of generating ACEI-inhibitory peptides have been utilised, as shown in Figure 2.

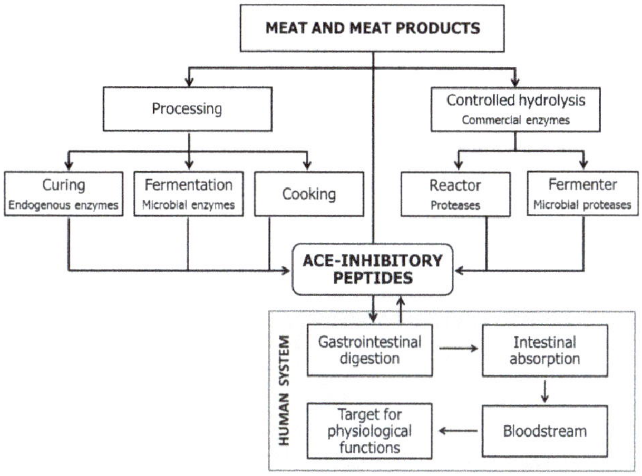

Figure 2. Different ways to generate ACEI-inhibitory peptides.

2.1. Bioactive Peptides Generated during Gastrointestinal Digestion

Gastrointestinal digestion (GI) is the last step for the generation of bioactive peptides from foods. After food ingestion, gastrointestinal peptidases such as pepsin, trypsin, or chymotrypsin are the main proteases responsible for the generation of multiple peptides, including bioactive sequences. In the laboratory, gastrointestinal digestion can be simulated using specific commercial enzymes and controlled conditions of pH and temperature. Thus, a simulated gastrointestinal digestion of raw pork meat using pepsin and pancreatin indicated that the physiological digestion of pork proteins could generate peptides with biological activity [16]. These results were later confirmed in vitro with the ACEI-inhibitory peptides KAPVA (Lys-Ala-Pro-Val-Ala) and PTPVP (Pro-Thr-Pro-Val-Pro), showing half maximal inhibitory concentration (IC_{50}) values of 46.56 and 256.41 μM, respectively [17], using the ACEI-inhibitory method described by Sentandreu and Toldrá (2006) [18]. Later, it was confirmed that these peptides also produced in vivo a decrease in the systolic blood pressure (SBP) of spontaneously hypertensive rats (SHRs) of 33.72 ± 8.01 mmHg and 25.66 ± 6.84 mmHg, respectively, after single oral administration of the synthesised peptides dissolved in distilled water at a concentration of 2 mg/mL and adjusted to 1 mg of peptide/kg of body weight administered by gastric intubation. The SBP was measured by the tail cuff method with a programmed electro-sphygmomanometer, and the effect lasted up to 6 h after single administration [19]. A recent study evaluated the digestion of beef proteins by studying the kinetics of peptide release in vivo by regularly sampling the gastric contents using a cannula. The obtained results were evaluated with bioinformatics tools in order to identify potentially bioactive peptides [20].

On the other hand, GI simulation has also been used in studies of bioavailability of certain peptide sequences in order to demonstrate whether they could exert a positive health effect in the body, as they should resist further GI digestion, cross the intestinal barrier, and reach the blood stream and target organs.

Finally, necessary treatments of meat before consumption such as cooking could facilitate the later generation of bioactive peptides due to denatured proteins being more susceptible to be hydrolysed by the enzymes of the intestinal tract.

2.2. Hydrolysis Treatments with Commercial Enzymes

The most used methodology for the generation of bioactive peptides is the hydrolysis of proteins with commercial enzymes. Proteases from different sources such as of microbial, plant, or animal origin, have been used for the hydrolysis of food proteins. In meat and meat products, Flavourzyme from *Aspergillus oryzae*, and Neutrase and Alcalase from *Bacillus subtilis* and *Bacillus lincheniformis*, respectively, have been the most used in the generation of bioactive peptides. In addition, proteases from plant origin such as bromelain and papain have been described as interesting enzymes for the hydrolysis of meat proteins by their contribution to meat tenderisation. These enzymes show a wider specificity in comparison with other enzymes such as trypsin or pepsin, cleaving peptide bonds from a wide variety of regions and frequently acting as either endopeptidases, or as exopeptidases hydrolysing amino acids from N- and C-terminal sites. In fact, the activity and hydrolytic specificity of many commercial peptidases is not clearly defined by manufacturers and thus, the degree of hydrolysis and final content of peptides is difficult to predict [8].

Several studies have reported the generation and identification of ACEI-inhibitory peptides resulting from hydrolysates of pork [17,21,22], chicken [23,24], and beef [25]. However, proteins obtained from by-products constitute good substrates that can be used to obtain bioactive peptides through this methodology [26,27], giving an extra added value to these products as well as reducing their environmental impact. In fact, this is the most commonly used procedure when the objective is to obtain high amounts of bioactive peptides for commercialisation, because its efficiency is optimised in a laboratory and later scaled up for pilot plant and industrial production.

2.3. *Bioactive Peptide Generation during Ageing and the Processing of Meat*

Bioactive peptides can be generated through the action of endogenous enzymes in ageing and curing processes as well as in combination with microbial peptidases such as in fermentation processes. Proteolysis by endogenous proteases is the most important phenomena occurring in the ageing of meat that influences its final characteristics with endogenous peptidases as main figures. Broadly speaking, endopeptidases such as calpains and cathepsins are first responsible for the hydrolysis of proteins into large fragments and oligopeptides, which affect the texture of meat during ageing and the initial steps of curing processes. Later, the activity of exopeptidases such as aminopeptidases and carboxypeptidases will generate small peptides and free amino acids, responsible for the characteristic flavour of dry-cured products. Some of the generated small peptides have also been described as bioactive peptides, exerting activities such as ACEI-inhibitory activity and antihypertensive, antioxidant, antilisteria, dipeptidyl peptidase IV (DPP-IV) inhibitory, and anti-inflammatory activity.

Dry-fermented sausages are elaborated using shorter processes with microorganisms such as lactic acid bacteria (LAB) (as a starter), yeasts, or moulds that are responsible for fermentation followed by ripening/drying. Lactic acid bacteria such as *Lactobacillus sakei*, *Lactobacillus curvatus*, *Lactobacillus plantarum* and *Lactobacillus casei* alone or in combination with staphylococci, *Kocuria*, yeast, or moulds, exert proteolysis through the action of endo- and exopeptidases. In general, these fermentation processes are involved in the liberation of small peptides and free amino acids that not only affect flavour development but also contribute to the generation of bioactive peptides [28].

The presence of ACEI-inhibitory peptides naturally generated during the processing of meat products such as dry-cured hams or dry-fermented sausages has also been described [29–33].

3. Identification of ACEI-Inhibitory Peptides

Traditionally, empirical approaches have been the method of choice for the identification of bioactive peptides from food matrices. However, it is very challenging when the objective is to generate specific peptide sequences that are able to exert certain activity. Then, the experimental design can be simplified by using bioinformatics for computer simulation in silico.

Empirical approaches used for the identification of bioactive peptides including ACEI-inhibitory peptides in complex sample matrices such as meat and meat products involve: (1) the release of the bioactive sequences from the parent protein; (2) preliminary in vitro assays to screen for bioactivity; (3) purification and separation through the use of high-resolution techniques, such as chromatography; (4) additional in vitro assays to determine the most active fractions; (5) identification of peptides by mass spectrometry (MS) techniques; (6) selection and synthesis of potential bioactive peptides; and (7) in vitro and in vivo confirmation of the bioactivity [34]. A scheme of the traditional empirical procedure for the identification and confirmation of bioactive peptides from food matrices is shown in Figure 3.

In vitro ACEI-inhibitory activity is typically measured by monitoring the conversion of a specific substrate by ACEI in the presence and absence of inhibitors. Spectrophotometric and chromatographic methods have been commonly used to measure the hydrolysis of substrates such as Hippuryl-His-Leu (HHL) or the fluorogenic *o*-aminobenzoylglycyl-*p*-nitrophenylalanylproline. However, the inhibitory activities of these peptides on ACEI activity do not always correlate with antihypertensive effects. In this regard, SHRs are the animal model most frequently used to verify the in vivo efficacy of ACEI-inhibitory peptides. Some studies have evaluated the effects on SBP of SHRs after oral administration of meat hydrolysates or peptide extracts showing ACEI-inhibitory activity [19,35–37]. Table 1 shows the antihypertensive effects of meat-derived peptides after single oral administration to SHR [38–44]. As a last step, human clinical trials are the most accurate method to assess the efficacy and physiological functions of meat-derived antihypertensive peptides, although few studies have been done in this respect due to the complexity and expensive costs. Hodgson et al. (2006) suggested that a partial substitution of carbohydrate intake with protein-rich foods such as lean red meat may lower SBP in hypertensive persons [45], whereas a clinical study done by Saiga-Egusa et al. (2009) using chicken collagen hydrolysate observed a SBP reduction in mildly hypertensive subjects by inhibiting ACEI and plasma renin activity [46]. Additionally, it has been reported that the regular consumption of dry-cured ham would not increase blood pressure despite its high salt content, and even could exert other beneficial effects on cardiovascular health related to glucose and lipid metabolism, and inflammatory processes [47–49].

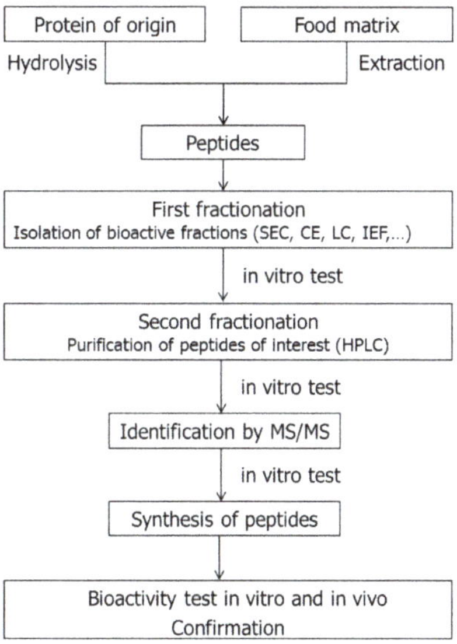

Figure 3. Scheme of the traditional empirical procedure for the identification and confirmation of bioactive peptides from food matrices. SEC: size-exclusion chromatography; CE: capillary electrophoresis; LC: liquid chromatography; IEF: isolectric focusing; HPLC: high performance liquid chromatography; MS/MS: mass spectrometry in tandem.

Table 1. Angiotensin I-converting enzyme (ACEI)-inhibitory peptides identified in meat and meat products with antihypertensive effects in spontaneously hypertensive rats.

Source	Peptide Sequence	Parent Protein	Hydrolysis Treatment	IC_{50} (μM) [a]	Dose (mg/kg BW) [b]	SBP (mmHg) [c]	Time (h) [d]	Reference
Chicken muscle	IKW	—	Thermolysin	0.21	60	−0.17	4	[23]
Chicken muscle	LKP	Aldolase	Thermolysin	0.32	60	−0.18	4	[23]
Chicken muscle	FKGRYYP	Creatine kinase	Thermolysin	0.55	60	0	—	[23]
Chicken muscle	GA(Hyp)GL(Hyp)GP	Collagen	Proteases	29.4	4.5	−0.18	6	[39]
Chicken bone	YYRA	Inmunoglobin heavy chain	Pepsin	57.2	10	−0.20	6	[40]
Porcine muscle	MNPPK	Myosin	Thermolysin	945.5	1	−0.23	6	[35]
Porcine muscle	ITTNP	Myosin	Thermolysin	549	1	−0.21	6	[35]
Porcine muscle	VKKVLGNP	Myosin light chain	Pepsin	29	10	−0.24	3	[41]
Porcine muscle	KRQKYDI	Troponin	Pepsin	26.2	10	−0.9	6	[42]
Porcine muscle	KRVITY	Myosin heavy chain	Pepsin	6.1	10	−0.23	6	[43]
Porcine muscle	VKAGF	Actin	Pepsin	20.3	10	−0.17	6	[43]
Porcine muscle	RPR	Nebulin	Pepsin + pancreatin	382	1	−0.33	6	[19]
Porcine muscle	KAPVA	Titin	Pepsin + pancreatin	46.56	1	−0.33	6	[19]
Porcine muscle	PTPVP	Titin	Pepsin + pancreatin	256.41	1	−0.25	6	[19]
Porcine skin	GF(Hyp)GP	Collagen	*Aspergillus* protease	91	10	−0.20	8	[44]
Goat muscle	FQPS	—	Protamex® + Flavourzyme®	27.0	2.39	−0.10	8	[45]
Spanish dry-cured ham	AAATP	Allantoicase	No treatment	100	1	−0.26	8	[19]

[a] IC_{50} value is the peptide concentration that inhibits 50% of ACE activity; [b] Oral administration of the peptide expressed as mg/kg body weight of rat; [c] Maximum decrease in systolic blood pressure (SBP) after administration of the peptide to spontaneously hypertensive rats; [d] Time after peptide administration to exert the maximum decrease in systolic blood pressure.

In addition to empirical approaches, the use of in silico analyses that combine bioinformatics tools and peptide databases has been increasingly used as a cost- and time-effective alternative. This predictive strategy enables to obtain biological and chemometric information on peptide sequences to be obtained through a series of steps: (1) selection of proteins of interest with known amino acid sequences by predicting their potential as precursors of novel bioactive peptides; (2) in silico protein digestion by selected proteolytic enzymes; (3) in silico identification and characterisation of peptides; (4) bioactivity prediction using a combination of sequence biochemical properties and databases of known bioactive peptides; (5) peptide synthesis; and (6) in vitro or in vivo confirmation of the bioactivity [50]. Figure 4 shows the main steps of in silico approaches and suggests open access databases and bioinformatics tools for the selection of the protein, hydrolysis simulation and bioactivity prediction. In this regard, BIOPEP is a widely used database for the study and identification of food-derived bioactive peptides as well as for in silico digestion and prediction of their bioactivities. In addition, computational models such as quantitative structure-activity relationships (QSAR), quantitative structure-property relationships (QSPR), and molecular docking simulations allow the discovery and characterisation of structural and physical-chemical properties such as hydrophilicity-hydrophobicity, molecular size, and electronic and steric characteristics, and results in very useful information to evaluate the potential affinity between the biopeptide sequence of interest and the target [50,51].

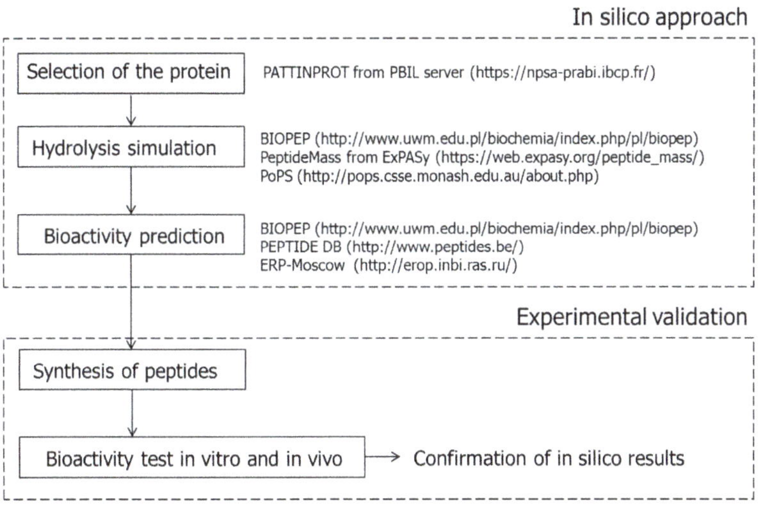

Figure 4. Main steps of in silico approaches and open access databases for the selection of the protein, hydrolysis simulation and bioactivity prediction.

In silico approaches have shown that some bovine, porcine and chicken proteins such as collagen, connectin, and myosin are good sources of ACEI-inhibitory peptides, which could be released from the parent protein through the action of determined enzymes [52–54]. Moreover, computer simulations are fundamental for understanding molecular mechanisms and ACEI-peptide interactions such as the fact that the C-terminal tripeptide sequence, hydrophobicity, and positive charge of the amino acid residues in this region of the peptide have a major influence on ACEI inhibition [55].

At the end, empirical and in silico approaches converge in the need for the confirmation of both the identity of the generated/predicted peptide sequences and their activity in the complexity of the matrix (see Figure 4).

4. Bioavailability of ACEI-Inhibitory Peptides

Bioavailability studies are necessary to assess whether the bioactive peptide can reach its target site in active form and sufficient quantity to exert health effects in the organism. The action of gastrointestinal enzymes, intestinal absorption, cellular uptake, and action of blood plasma peptidases can modify the structure of ACEI-inhibitory peptides or hydrolyse them leading to a loss, maintenance, or gain of bioactivity [11,56].

The use of digestion models and LC-MS techniques combined with in silico and in vitro/in vivo approaches have enabled evaluation of the stability of ACEI-inhibitory peptides from beef, chicken and pork meat in gastrointestinal digestion as well as the identification and quantification of the resulting products [17,20,30,57–59]. On the other hand, cell models such as heterogeneous human epithelial colorectal adenocarcinoma cells (Caco-2 cell) monolayers have been useful to study the transepithelial transport of ACEI-inhibitory peptides derived from meat proteins, being able to determine structural changes and amount of peptides transported or the involved transport pathway [60–62]. The ability of peptides to resist enzymatic degradation and be transported across intestinal membranes into blood circulation depends on their characteristics, length, and amino acid composition. In this regard, proline-rich peptides are more resistant to be attacked by gastrointestinal enzymes, and di- and tri-peptides could be absorbed intact by peptide transporter systems and hydrolysed later [63]. The low transport ability of oligopeptides compared to di- and tri-peptides is probably due to their length and involve paracellular route, while the hydrophobicity of peptides does not seem to influence absorption [64]. Additionally, the absorption of peptides could be affected by co-existing peptides and food components, which can share the transport pathway or participate in its regulation [64].

The bioavailability and bioaccessibility of bioactive peptides can also be affected by processing/storage conditions and food matrix-peptide interactions that can lead to peptide modifications with changes in its native structure and activity [65]. Several studies have evaluated the stability of ACEI-inhibitory peptides after household cooking preparations of pork and beef meat [66], different temperatures and pH used when processing meat products [30,67], and the effect of ageing under industrial conditions (vacuum-packed and chilled-storage) and cooking of beef meat [68].

5. Challenges and Limitations

Currently, with the basis of knowledge for the identification of bioactive peptides already clear, it is necessary to continue the research in bioactive peptides to achieve a better understanding of their effect, interactions, and bioavailability. In this sense, several authors have established the need for serious consideration of food matrix interactions, especially when the objective is to use the bioactive peptides as a functional ingredient [65]. Increasingly, once the peptide has been identified in a food matrix, it is synthesised and characterised as an individual molecule. However, the expected in vitro and/or in vivo activity may differ when the peptide interacts with the complex mixture of compounds that are taking part of any food.

On the other hand, increased effort on the development of quantitative methodologies for a better understanding of hydrolysis, bioactivity, and/or bioavailability is necessary. Data such as the quantity of specific naturally generated peptides in the original food and the dose of a bioactive peptide needed to exert an effect in vivo, as well as the final sequences and amount present in bloodstream and target organ after GI digestion are key data for advancing in the field of bioactive peptides and their health influence. In fact, determining the quantity of ACEI-inhibitory peptides in the meat sample that are able to reach the target site in the human system is of fundamental importance in bioavailability studies to better understand the effects and mechanisms of action of these peptides. The main limitation for quantitation is the nature of sample: small peptides often comprise fewer than four amino acids at low abundance, and there is high complexity of the matrix [69]. Current advances in mass spectrometry instrumentation, bioinformatics tools, and updated protein databases are contributing to progress in quantitative peptidomics [68].

6. Conclusions

Meat and meat products have been described as a very good source of ACEI-inhibitory peptides. With proteins being a major constituent of meats, the generation of bioactive peptides from meat proteins has been described as occurring either through the action of endogenous muscular enzymes during processing, during GI digestion, or by using commercial enzymes in the laboratory or in industrial processes under controlled conditions. The identification of ACEI-inhibitory peptides has been traditionally done using empirical approaches, although currently there is an increasing interest in in silico approaches based on bioinformatics as they are less time-consuming and cheaper methodologies. However, despite the identification of bioactive peptides being clear, there is an increasing need to study food matrix interactions, especially when the objective is to use the bioactive peptides as a functional ingredient. The quantitation of these peptides for a better understanding of their health influence and bioavailability is necessary to advance in this field.

Author Contributions: Writing—Original Draft Preparation, L.M. and M.G.; Writing—Review and Editing, L.M., M.G. and F.T.; Supervision, F.T.; Project Administration, F.T. and L.M.; Funding Acquisition, F.T. and L.M.

Funding: This research was funded by grant AGL2017-89381-R and FEDER funds from the Spanish Ministry of Science, Innovation, and Universities.

Acknowledgments: Ramón y Cajal postdoctoral contract to L.M. is also acknowledged.

Conflicts of Interest: The authors declare no conflict of interest.

References

1. Gallego, M.; Mora, L.; Toldrá, F. Health relevance of antihypertensive peptides in foods. *Curr. Opin. Food Sci.* **2018**, *19*, 8–14. [CrossRef]
2. Lorenzo, J.M.; Munekata, P.E.S.; Gómez, B.; Barba, F.J.; Mora, L.; Pérez-Santaescolástica, C.; Toldrá, F. Bioactive peptides as natural antioxidants in food products—A review. *Trends Food Sci. Technol.* **2018**, *79*, 136–147. [CrossRef]
3. Santos, J.C.P.; Sousa, R.C.S.; Otoni, C.G.; Moraes, A.R.F.; Souza, V.G.L.; Medeiros, E.A.A.; Espitia, P.J.P.; Pires, A.C.S.; Coimbra, J.S.R.; Soares, N.F.F. Nisin and other antimicrobial peptides: Production, mechanisms of action, and application in active food packaging. *Innov. Food Sci. Emerg. Technol.* **2018**, *48*, 179–194. [CrossRef]
4. Moughan, P.J.; Rutherfurd-Markwick, K. Food bioactive proteins and peptides: antimicrobial, immunomodulatory and anti-inflammatory effects. In *Diet, Immunity and Inflammation*; Calder, P.C., Parveen, Y., Eds.; Woodhead Publishing Series in Food Science, Technology and Nutrition; Woodhead Publishing: Sawston, UK, 2013; pp. 313–340. ISBN 9780857090379.
5. Chalamaiah, M.; Yu, W.; Wu, J. Immunomodulatory and anticancer protein hydrolysates (peptides) from food proteins: A review. *Food Chem.* **2018**, *245*, 205–222. [CrossRef] [PubMed]
6. Arısoy, S.; Üstün-Aytekin, Ö. Hydrolysis of food-derived opioids by dipeptidyl peptidase IV from *Lactococcus lactis* spp. *Lactis*. *Food Res. Int.* **2018**, *111*, 574–581. [CrossRef] [PubMed]
7. Mora, L.; Aristoy, M.C.; Toldrá, F. Chapter Bioactive peptides. In *Encyclopedia of Food Chemistry*, 1st ed.; Varelis, P., Melton, L., Shahidi, F., Eds.; Elsevier: New York, NY, USA, 2018; ISBN 9780128140260.
8. Toldrá, F.; Reig, M.; Aristoy, M.C.; Mora, L. Generation of bioactive peptides during processing. *Food Chem.* **2018**, *267*, 395–404. [CrossRef] [PubMed]
9. Wu, J.; Liao, W.; Udenigwe, C.C. Revisiting the mechanisms of ACE inhibitory peptides from food proteins. *Trends Food Sci. Technol.* **2017**, *69*, 214–219. [CrossRef]
10. Girgih, A.T.; He, R.; Malomo, S.; Offengenden, M.; Wu, J.; Aluko, R.E. Structural and functional characterization of hemp seed (*Cannabis sativa* L.) protein derived antioxidant and antihypertensive peptides. *J. Funct. Foods* **2014**, *6*, 384–394. [CrossRef]
11. Hernández-Ledesma, B.; del Mar Contreras, M.; Recio, I. Antihypertensive peptides: Production, bioavailability and incorporation into foods. *Adv. Colloid Interface Sci.* **2011**, *165*, 23–35. [CrossRef] [PubMed]
12. Lassoued, I.; Mora, L.; Nasri, R.; Jridi, M.; Toldrá, F.; Aristoy, M.-C.; Nasri, M. Characterization and comparative assessment of antioxidant and ACE inhibitory activities of thornback ray gelatin hydrolysates. *J. Funct. Foods* **2015**, *13*, 225–238. [CrossRef]

13. Shahidi, F.; Zhong, Y. Bioactive peptides. *J. AOAC Int.* **2008**, *91*, 914–931. [PubMed]
14. Zheng, Y.; Li, Y.; Zhang, Y.; Ruan, X.; Zhang, R. Purification, characterization, synthesis, in vitro ACE inhibition and in vivo antihypertensive activity of bioactive peptides derived from oil palm kernel glutelin-2 hydrolysates. *J. Funct. Foods* **2017**, *28*, 48–58. [CrossRef]
15. Jäkälä, P.; Vapaatalo, H. Antihypertensive peptides from milk proteins. *Pharmaceuticals* **2010**, *3*, 251–272. [CrossRef] [PubMed]
16. Escudero, E.; Sentandreu, M.A.; Toldrá, F. Characterization of peptides released by in vitro digestion of pork meat. *J. Agric. Food Chem.* **2010**, *58*, 5160–5165. [CrossRef] [PubMed]
17. Escudero, E.; Sentandreu, M.A.; Arihara, K.; Toldrá, F. Angiotensin I converting enzyme inhibitory peptides generated from in vitro gastrointestinal digestion of pork meat. *J. Agric. Food Chem.* **2010**, *58*, 2895–2901. [CrossRef] [PubMed]
18. Sentandreu, M.A.; Toldrá, F. A rapid, simple and sensitive fluorescence method for the assay of angiotensin-I converting enzyme. *Food Chem.* **2006**, *97*, 546–554. [CrossRef]
19. Escudero, E.; Toldrá, F.; Sentandreu, M.A.; Nishimura, H.; Arihara, K. Antihypertensive activity of peptides identified in the in vitro gastrointestinal digest of pork meat. *Meat Sci.* **2012**, *91*, 382–384. [CrossRef] [PubMed]
20. Sayd, T.; Dufour, C.; Chambon, C.; Buffière, C.; Remond, D.; Santé-Lhoutellier, V. Combined in vivo and in silico approaches for predicting the release of bioactive peptides from meat digestion. *Food Chem.* **2018**, *249*, 111–118. [CrossRef] [PubMed]
21. Arihara, K.; Nakashima, Y.; Mukai, T.; Ishikawa, S.; Itoh, M. Peptide inhibitors for angiotensin I-converting enzyme from enzymatic hydrolysates of porcine skeletal muscle proteins. *Meat Sci.* **2001**, *57*, 319–324. [CrossRef]
22. Katayama, K.; Tomatsu, M.; Fuchu, H.; Sugiyama, M.; Kawahara, S.; Yamauchi, K.; Kawamura, Y.; Muguruma, M. Purification and characterization of an angiotensin I-converting enzyme inhibitory peptide derived from porcine troponin C. *Anim. Sci. J.* **2003**, *74*, 53–58. [CrossRef]
23. Fujita, H.; Yokoyama, K.; Yoshikawa, M. Classification and antihypertensive activity of angiotensin I-converting enzyme inhibitory peptides derived from food proteins. *J. Food Sci.* **2000**, *65*, 564–569.
24. Terashima, M.; Baba, T.; Ikemoto, N.; Katayama, M.; Morimoto, T.; Matsumura, S. Novel angiotensin-converting enzyme (ACE) inhibitory peptides derived from boneless chicken leg meat. *J. Agric. Food Chem.* **2010**, *58*, 7432–7436. [CrossRef] [PubMed]
25. Jang, A.; Lee, M. Purification and identification of angiotensin converting enzyme inhibitory peptides from beef hydrolysates. *Meat Sci.* **2005**, *69*, 653–661. [CrossRef] [PubMed]
26. Adje, E.Y.; Balti, R.; Guillochon, D.; Nedjar-Arroume, N. α 67–106 of bovine hemoglobin: A new family of antimicrobial and angiotensin I-converting enzyme inhibitory peptides. *Eur. Food Res. Technol.* **2011**, *232*, 637–646. [CrossRef]
27. Banerjee, P.; Shanthi, C. Isolation of novel bioactive regions from bovine Achilles tendon collagen having angiotensin I-converting enzyme-inhibitory properties. *Process Biochem.* **2012**, *47*, 2335–2346. [CrossRef]
28. Mora, L.; Gallego, M.; Escudero, E.; Reig, M.; Aristoy, M.C.; Toldrá, F. Small peptides hydrolysis in dry-cured meats. *Int. J. Food Microbiol.* **2015**, *212*, 9–15. [CrossRef] [PubMed]
29. Escudero, E.; Mora, L.; Fraser, P.D.; Aristoy, M.C.; Arihara, K.; Toldrá, F. Purification and identification of antihypertensive peptides in Spanish dry-cured ham. *J. Proteomics* **2013**, *78*, 499–507. [CrossRef] [PubMed]
30. Escudero, E.; Mora, L.; Toldrá, F. Stability of ACE inhibitory ham peptides against heat treatment and in vitro digestion. *Food Chem.* **2014**, *161*, 305–311. [CrossRef] [PubMed]
31. Mora, L.; Escudero, E.; Toldrá, F. Characterization of the peptide profile in Spanish Teruel, Italian Parma and Belgian dry-cured hams and its potential bioactivity. *Food Res. Int.* **2016**, *89*, 638–646. [CrossRef] [PubMed]
32. Mejri, L.; Vásquez-Villanueva, R.; Hassouna, M.; Marina, M.L.; García, M.C. Identification of peptides with antioxidant and antihypertensive capacities by RP-HPLC-Q-TOF-MS in dry fermented camel sausages inoculated with different starter cultures and ripening times. *Food Res. Int.* **2017**, *100*, 708–716. [CrossRef] [PubMed]
33. Gallego, M.; Mora, L.; Escudero, E.; Toldrá, F. Bioactive peptides and free amino acids profiles in different types of European dry-fermented sausages. *Int. J. Food Microbiol.* **2018**, *276*, 71–78. [CrossRef] [PubMed]
34. Sánchez-Rivera, L.; Martínez-Maqueda, D.; Cruz-Huerta, E.; Miralles, B.; Recio, I. Peptidomics for discovery, bioavailability and monitoring of dairy bioactive peptides. *Food Res. Int.* **2014**, *63*, 170–181. [CrossRef]

35. Nakashima, Y.; Arihara, K.; Sasaki, A.; Mio, H.; Ishikawa, S.; Itoh, M. Antihypertensive activities of peptides derived from porcine skeletal muscle myosin in spontaneously hypertensive rats. *J. Food Sci.* **2002**, *67*, 434–437. [CrossRef]
36. Saiga, A.I.; Iwai, K.; Hayakawa, T.; Takahata, Y.; Kitamura, S.; Nishimura, T.; Morimatsu, F. Angiotensin I-converting enzyme-inhibitory peptides obtained from chicken collagen hydrolysate. *J. Agric. Food Chem.* **2008**, *56*, 9586–9591. [CrossRef] [PubMed]
37. Mora, L.; Escudero, E.; Arihara, K.; Toldrá, F. Antihypertensive effect of peptides naturally generated during Iberian dry-cured ham processing. *Food Res. Int.* **2015**, *78*, 71–78. [CrossRef] [PubMed]
38. Iwai, K.; Saiga-Egusa, A.; Hayakawa, T.; Shimizu, M.; Takahata, Y.; Morimatsu, F. An angiotensin I-converting enzyme (ACE)-inhibitory peptide derived from chicken collagen hydrolysate lowers blood pressure in spontaneously hypertensive rats. *J. Jpn. Soc. Food Sci.* **2008**, *55*, 602–605. [CrossRef]
39. Nakade, K.; Kamishima, R.; Inoue, Y.; Ahhmed, A.; Kawahara, S.; Nakayama, T.; Maruyama, M.; Numata, M.; Ohta, K.; Aoki, T.; et al. Identification of an antihypertensive peptide derived from chicken bone extract. *Anim. Sci. J.* **2008**, *79*, 710–715. [CrossRef]
40. Katayama, K.; Mori, T.; Kawahara, S.; Miake, K.; Kodama, Y.; Sugiyama, M.; Kawamura, Y.; Nakayama, T.; Maruyama, M.; Muguruma, M. Angiotensin-I converting enzyme inhibitory peptide derived from porcine skeletal muscle myosin and its antihypertensive activity in spontaneously hypertensive rats. *J. Food Sci.* **2007**, *72*, S702–S706. [CrossRef] [PubMed]
41. Katayama, K.; Anggraeni, H.E.; Mori, T.; Ahhmed, A.M.; Kawahara, S.; Sugiyama, M.; Nakayama, T.; Maruyama, M.; Muguruma, M. Porcine skeletal muscle troponin is a good source of peptides with angiotensin-I converting enzyme inhibitory activity and antihypertensive effects in spontaneously hypertensive rats. *J. Agric. Food Chem.* **2008**, *56*, 355–360. [CrossRef] [PubMed]
42. Muguruma, M.; Ahhmed, A.M.; Katayama, K.; Kawahara, S.; Maruyama, M.; Nakamura, T. Identification of pro-drug type ACE inhibitory peptide sourced from porcine myosin B: Evaluation of its antihypertensive effects in vivo. *Food Chem.* **2009**, *114*, 516–522. [CrossRef]
43. Ichimura, T.; Yamanaka, A.; Otsuka, T.; Yamashita, E.; Maruyama, S. Antihypertensive effect of enzymatic hydrolysate of collagen and Gly-Pro in spontaneously hypertensive rats. *Biosci. Biotechnol. Biochem.* **2009**, *73*, 2317–2319. [CrossRef] [PubMed]
44. Mirdhayati, I.; Hermanianto, J.; Wijaya, C.H.; Sajuthi, D.; Arihara, K. Angiotensin converting enzyme (ACE) inhibitory and antihypertensive activities of protein hydrolysate from meat of Kacang goat (*Capra aegagrus hircus*). *J. Sci. Food Agric.* **2016**, *96*, 3536–3542. [CrossRef] [PubMed]
45. Hodgson, J.M.; Burke, V.; Beilin, L.J.; Puddey, I.B. Partial substitution of carbohydrate intake with protein intake from lean red meat lowers blood pressure in hypertensive persons. *Am. J. Clin. Nutr.* **2006**, *83*, 780–787. [CrossRef] [PubMed]
46. Saiga-Egusa, A.; Iwai, K.; Hayakawa, T.; Takahata, Y.; Morimatsu, F. Antihypertensive effects and endothelial progenitor cell activation by intake of chicken collagen hydrolysate in pre- and mild-hypertension. *Biosci. Biotechnol. Biochem.* **2009**, *73*, 422–424. [CrossRef] [PubMed]
47. López, M.R.C.; Bes-Rastrollo, M.; Zazpe, I.; Martínez, J.A.; Cuervo, M.; Martínez-González, M.A. Consumo de jamón curado e incidencia de episodios cardiovasculares, hipertensión arterial o ganancia de peso. *Med. Clin.* **2009**, *133*, 574–580. [CrossRef] [PubMed]
48. Montoro-García, S.; Zafrilla-Rentero, M.P.; Celdrán-de Haro, F.M.; Piñero-de Armas, J.J.; Toldrá, F.; Tejada-Portero, L.; Abellán-Alemán, J. Effects of dry-cured ham rich in bioactive peptides on cardiovascular health: A randomized controlled trial. *J. Funct. Foods* **2017**, *38*, 160–167. [CrossRef]
49. Martínez-Sánchez, S.M.; Minguela, A.; Prieto-Merino, D.; Zafrilla-Rentero, M.P.; Abellán-Alemán, J.; Montoro-García, S. The effect of regular intake of dry-cured ham rich in bioactive peptides on inflammation, platelet and monocyte activation markers in humans. *Nutrients* **2017**, *9*, 321. [CrossRef] [PubMed]
50. Agyei, D.; Ongkudon, C.M.; Wei, C.Y.; Chan, A.S.; Danquah, M.K. Bioprocess challenges to the isolation and purification of bioactive peptides. *Food Bioprod. Process.* **2016**, *98*, 244–256. [CrossRef]
51. Carrasco-Castilla, J.; Hernández-Álvarez, A.J.; Jiménez-Martínez, C.; Gutiérrez-López, G.F.; Dávila-Ortiz, G. Use of proteomics and peptidomics methods in food bioactive peptide science and engineering. *Food Eng. Rev.* **2012**, *4*, 224–243. [CrossRef]
52. Gu, Y.; Majumder, K.; Wu, J. QSAR-aided in silico approach in evaluation of food proteins as precursors of ACE inhibitory peptides. *Food Res. Int.* **2011**, *44*, 2465–2474. [CrossRef]

53. Minkiewicz, P.; Dziuba, J.; Michalska, J. Bovine meat proteins as potential precursors of biologically active peptides-a computational study based on the BIOPEP database. *Food Sci. Technol. Int.* **2011**, *17*, 39–45. [CrossRef] [PubMed]
54. Lafarga, T.; O'Connor, P.; Hayes, M. Identification of novel dipeptidyl peptidase-IV and angiotensin-I-converting enzyme inhibitory peptides from meat proteins using in silico analysis. *Peptides* **2014**, *59*, 53–62. [CrossRef] [PubMed]
55. Pripp, A.H.; Isaksson, T.; Stepaniak, L.; Sørhaug, T. Quantitative structure-activity relationship modelling of ACE-inhibitory peptides derived from milk proteins. *Eur. Food Res. Technol.* **2004**, *219*, 579–583. [CrossRef]
56. Vermeirssen, V.; Van Camp, J.; Verstraete, W. Bioavailability of angiotensin I converting enzyme inhibitory peptides. *Br. J. Nutr.* **2004**, *92*, 357–366. [CrossRef] [PubMed]
57. Mora, L.; Bolumar, T.; Heres, A.; Toldrá, F. Effect of cooking and simulated gastrointestinal digestion on the activity of generated bioactive peptides in aged beef meat. *Food Funct.* **2017**, *8*, 4347–4355. [CrossRef] [PubMed]
58. Sangsawad, P.; Roytrakul, S.; Yongsawatdigul, J. Angiotensin converting enzyme (ACE) inhibitory peptides derived from the simulated in vitro gastrointestinal digestion of cooked chicken breast. *J. Funct. Foods* **2017**, *29*, 77–83. [CrossRef]
59. Dellafiora, L.; Paolella, S.; Dall'Asta, C.; Dossena, A.; Cozzini, P.; Galaverna, G. Hybrid in silico/in vitro approach for the identification of angiotensin I converting enzyme inhibitory peptides from Parma dry-cured ham. *J. Agric. Food Chem.* **2015**, *63*, 6366–6375. [CrossRef] [PubMed]
60. Fu, Y.; Young, J.F.; Rasmussen, M.K.; Dalsgaard, T.K.; Lametsch, R.; Aluko, R.E.; Therkildsen, M. Angiotensin I–converting enzyme–inhibitory peptides from bovine collagen: Insights into inhibitory mechanism and transepithelial transport. *Food Res. Int.* **2016**, *89*, 373–381. [CrossRef] [PubMed]
61. Gallego, M.; Grootaert, C.; Mora, L.; Aristoy, M.C.; Van Camp, J.; Toldrá, F. Transepithelial transport of dry-cured ham peptides with ACE inhibitory activity through a Caco-2 cell monolayer. *J. Funct. Foods* **2016**, *21*, 388–395. [CrossRef]
62. Sangsawad, P.; Choowongkomon, K.; Kitts, D.D.; Chen, X.M.; Li-Chan, E.C.; Yongsawatdigul, J. Transepithelial transport and structural changes of chicken angiotensin I-converting enzyme (ACE) inhibitory peptides through Caco-2 cell monolayers. *J. Funct. Foods* **2018**, *45*, 401–408. [CrossRef]
63. Segura-Campos, M.; Chel-Guerrero, L.; Betancur-Ancona, D.; Hernandez-Escalante, V.M. Bioavailability of bioactive peptides. *Food Rev. Int.* **2011**, *27*, 213–226. [CrossRef]
64. Shen, W.; Matsui, T. Current knowledge of intestinal absorption of bioactive peptides. *Food Funct.* **2017**, *8*, 4306–4314. [CrossRef] [PubMed]
65. Udenigwe, C.C.; Fogliano, V. Food matrix interaction and bioavailability of bioactive peptides: Two faces of the same coin? *J. Funct. Foods* **2017**, *35*, 9–12. [CrossRef]
66. Jensen, I.J.; Dort, J.; Eilertsen, K.E. Proximate composition, antihypertensive and antioxidative properties of the semimembranosus muscle from pork and beef after cooking and in vitro digestion. *Meat Sci.* **2014**, *96*, 916–921. [CrossRef] [PubMed]
67. Fu, Y.; Young, J.F.; Dalsgaard, T.K.; Therkildsen, M. Separation of angiotensin I-converting enzyme inhibitory peptides from bovine connective tissue and their stability towards temperature, pH and digestive enzymes. *Int. J. Food Sci. Technol.* **2015**, *50*, 1234–1243. [CrossRef]
68. Mora, L.; Gallego, M.; Reig, M.; Toldrá, F. Challenges in the quantitation of naturally generated bioactive peptides in processed meats. *Trends Food Sci. Technol.* **2017**, *69*, 306–314. [CrossRef]
69. Arroume, N.; Froidevaux, R.; Kapel, R.; Cudennec, B.; Ravallec, R.; Flahaut, C.; Bazinet, L.; Jacques, P.; Dhulster, P. Food peptides: Purification, identification and role in the metabolism. *Curr. Opin. Food Sci.* **2016**, *7*, 101–107. [CrossRef]

nutrients

MDPI

Article

Dose-Related Antihypertensive Properties and the Corresponding Mechanisms of a Chicken Foot Hydrolysate in Hypertensive Rats

Anna Mas-Capdevila [1], Zara Pons [1], Amaya Aleixandre [2], Francisca I. Bravo [1,*] and Begoña Muguerza [1,3]

[1] Nutrigenomics Research Group, Department of Biochemistry and Biotechnology, Universitat Rovira i Virgili, 43007 Tarragona, Spain; anna.mas@urv.cat (A.M.-C.); zara.pons@urv.cat (Z.P.); begona.muguerza@urv.cat (B.M.)

[2] Department of Pharmacology, School of Medicine, Universidad Complutense de Madrid, 28040 Madrid, Spain; amaya@med.ucm.es

[3] Technological Unit of Nutrition and Health, EURECAT-Technology Centre of Catalonia, 43204 Reus, Spain

* Correspondence: franciscaisabel.bravo@urv.cat; Tel.: +977-55-88-37

Received: 9 August 2018; Accepted: 10 September 2018; Published: 12 September 2018

Abstract: The antihypertensive properties of different doses of a chicken foot hydrolysate, Hpp11 and the mechanisms involved in this effect were investigated. Spontaneously hypertensive rats (SHR) were administered water, Captopril (50 mg/kg) or Hpp11 at different doses (25, 55 and 85 mg/kg), and the systolic blood pressure (SBP) was recorded. The SBP of normotensive Wistar-Kyoto (WKY) rats administered water or Hpp11 was also recorded. Additionally, plasmatic angiotensin-converting enzyme (ACE) activity was determined in the SHR administered Hpp11. Moreover, the relaxation caused by Hpp11 in isolated aortic rings from Sprague-Dawley rats was evaluated. Hpp11 exhibited antihypertensive activity at doses of 55 and 85 mg/kg, with maximum activity 6 h post-administration. At this time, no differences were found between these doses and Captopril. Initial SBP values of 55 and 85 mg/kg were recovered 24 or 8 h post-administration, respectively, 55 mg/kg being the most effective dose. At this dose, a reduction in the plasmatic ACE activity in the SHR was found. However, Hpp11 did not relax the aortic ring preparations. Therefore, ACE inhibition could be the mechanism underlying Hpp11 antihypertensive effect. Remarkably, Hpp11 did not modify SBP in WKY rats, showing that the decreased SBP effect is specific to the hypertensive state.

Keywords: hypertension; protein hydrolysate; angiotensin-converting enzyme; ACE-inhibitory activity; endothelial dysfunction; bioactive peptides

1. Introduction

Cardiovascular diseases (CVD) are the leading cause of mortality in Europe, and hypertension (HTN) is one of the main CVD risk factors [1]. In this sense, the lowering of blood pressure (BP) through behavioural and pharmacological interventions has been showed to remarkably improve CVD [2]. Currently, one of the most popular pharmacologic therapies to treat HTN is based on the use of angiotensin-converting enzyme (ACE) inhibitors such as Captopril or Enalapril [3]. ACE is the key enzyme of the renin-angiotensin-aldosterone system (RAAS), which is one of the most important systems in the regulation of blood volume and systemic vascular resistance. ACE hydrolyses the decapeptide angiotensin I (Ang I) to the octapeptide angiotensin II (Ang II), which is a potent vasoconstrictor but also breaks down bradykinin, a vasodilator [4]. Although pharmacological ACE inhibitors are widely used to decrease BP, some undesirable side effects have been described for these drugs, such as angioedema, dry cough, disturbance in taste, and skin reactions, among others [5].

In consequence, the study of natural bioactive compounds has received great attention, and their use has been considered a good strategy to decrease the risk of HTN [6].

Specifically, the hydrolysis of food proteins is considered a potential source of peptides with ACE inhibitory activities and/or antihypertensive effects [7–10]. Different protein sources have been reported to release ACE inhibitor peptides, such as milk and egg [11], fish [12,13] or meat [14], among others. Considering this, the interest in proteins derived from food by-products as sources of ACE inhibitor peptides has increased. The use of food by-products allows the reuse of waste materials, making the food and agricultural industries more environmentally friendly [15–17]. In this regard, our group has used chicken feet, a poultry industry by-product, to obtain hydrolysates that present ACE inhibitory (ACEI) activity [18]. Chicken feet is considered a by-product in Spain and in most countries in Europe, and since a few years ago, the conversion of animal by-products to feed and certain legislations in some countries disallows indiscriminate dumping or landfilling of animal wastes [19]. Thus, this chicken by-product represents environmental and economic problems for meat processors if they are not correctly treated. Considering this, the chicken industry considered that it is no longer practical to discard by-products and wastes, especially when a significant amount of valuable raw materials have a strong economic potential like the production of new products and functional ingredients with a significant added-value [20]. It is known that chicken proteins, especially chicken collagen, has been demonstrated to be a source of bioactive peptides, able to inhibit ACE and exhibit antihypertensive activity [21–23]. Nevertheless, the in vitro ACEI activity and in vivo antihypertensive effects of protein hydrolysates are not always correlated, since the physiological transformations during digestion determine the bioavailability of these peptides and, as a result, their bioactivity. Moreover, it has also been demonstrated that the in vivo ACEI activity is not the only mechanism underlying the antihypertensive effects of some bioactive peptides. In this sense, certain food bioactive peptides have shown direct effects on relaxation in vascular smooth muscle [24].

In a previous study, we observed that the administration of 5 mL/kg bw (body weight) of a chicken foot hydrolysate, Hpp11, exhibited an antihypertensive effect in spontaneously hypertensive rats (SHR), which is considered to be a model for human essential HTN [25]. Thus, considering that 100 mg/kg bw dose of other protein hydrolysates showed substantial antihypertensive effects [26–28], doses lower than the antihypertensive demonstrated dose of 100 mg/kg bw; 85, 55 and 25 mg/kg bw of Hpp11, were administered to SHR. Therefore, the aims of the present study were to evaluate the most effective Hpp11 dose to obtain a significant antihypertensive effect in SHR and to investigate the mechanisms underlying the Hpp11 antihypertensive effect. Moreover, the effect of Hpp11 on the arterial SBP of Wistar-Kyoto (WKY) rats, the normotensive control for SHR, was also studied to rule out a potential hypotensive effect of this hydrolysate.

2. Materials and Methods

2.1. Chemicals and Reagents

Chicken feet from *Gallus gallus domesticus* were provided by a local farm (Granja Gaià, La Riera de Gaià, Spain). Protamex® (Novozymes, Bagsværd, Denmark) (EC 3.4.21.62 and 3.4.24.28, 1.5 AU/g from *Bacillus licheniformis* and *Bacillus amyloliquefaciens*), was kindly provided by Novozymes (Bagsværd, Denmark). ACE (angiotensin-converting enzyme, EC 3.4.15.1), *N*-Hippuryl-His-Leu (Hip-His-Leu), Captopril (PubChem CID: 44093) were purchased from Santa Cruz Biotechnology (Dallas, TX, USA) and o-aminobenzoylglicil-p-nitrofenilalanilprolina (o-Abz-Gly-p-Phe(NO_2)-Pro-OH, PubChem CID: 128860) was provided by Bachem Feinchemikalien (Bubendorf, Switzerland). Acetylcholine (PubChem CID: 187), methoxamine hydrochloride (PubChem CID: 6081) and heparin heparin (PubChem CID: 772) were purchased from Sigma-Aldrich (Madrid, Spain). All other chemical solvents used were of analytical grade.

2.2. Chicken Foot Hydrolysate Hpp11: Obtainment and Characterisation

Chicken feet were mechanically disrupted, and sieves were utilized to obtain the protein hydrolysate, Hpp11 [18]. Protein powder with a size ≤2 mm was suspended in distilled water (20 mg/mL, *w*/*v*) and incubated for 1.5 h in a water bath set at 100 °C at 100 rpm. Subsequently, an enzymatic solution, Protamex®, was added at a final concentration of 2.67 µg/mL (enzyme/substrate ratio, 0.4 AU/g protein). Hydrolysis was carried out at 50 °C for 2 h at pH 7.0 in a MaxQ Orbital Shaker Thermo Scientific (Thermo Fisher Scientific, Waltham, MA, USA). At the end of the reaction, the enzyme was heat inactivated (80 °C, 10 min) in a water bath. Then, hydrolysate was centrifuged at 10,000× *g* for 20 min at 4 °C, and the supernatant was filtered through a 0.45 µm membrane, collected and lyophilized. Hpp11 was reconstituted in water to carry out the following experiments.

Hpp11 was characterized before its administration to SHR. Hpp11 protein content was estimated by the determination of total nitrogen compounds content of Hpp11 by the Kjeldahl method, multiplying the determined nitrogen content by 6.25 and the humidity determination was carried out following the AOAC official methods [29]. The degree of hydrolysis was determined by the TNBS method according to Adler-Nissen (1979) [30], in which free α-amino groups were determined. The Hpp11 ACEI activity was determined according to Quirós et al. [31]. The fluorescence measurements were performed after 30 min in a multi-scan microplate fluorimeter (FLUOstar optima, BMG Labtech, Offeuburg, Germany). The excitation and emission wavelengths were 360 and 400 nm, respectively. The software used to process the data was FLUOstar control (version 1.32 R2, BMG Labtech, Offeuburg, Germany).

The inhibition pattern of Hpp11 on the ACE substrate o-Abz-Gly-p-Phe(NO_2)-Pro-OH was assayed at the following concentrations: 7.2, 3.6, 1.8, 0.9, 0.45, 0.23 and 0 mM. The inhibition kinetics of ACE in the presence of Hpp11 was determined by Lineweaver–Burk plots [30].

All the analyses were performed in triplicate.

2.3. Experimental Procedure in the SHR and WKY Rats

Male SHR and WKY rats (17–20-week-old, weighing 300–350 g) were obtained from Charles River Laboratories España S.A. (Barcelona, Spain). The animals were housed at a temperature of 23 °C with 12 h light/dark cycles and consumed tap water and a standard diet (A04 Panlab, Barcelona, Spain) ad libitum during the experiments.

Different doses of the hydrolysate (25, 55 and 85 mg/kg bw) or a single dose of Hpp11 (55 mg/kg bw) were administered by gastric intubation to SHR or WKY rats, respectively, between 9 and 10 am. Tap water was used as a negative control for the SHR and WKY rats, and 50 mg/kg Captopril dissolved in tap water was given as a positive control to the SHR. The total volume of water, Captopril or Hpp11 orally administered to the rats was between 1.5 and 2 mL.

The systolic blood pressure (SBP) was recorded in the rats by the tail-cuff method [32] before and 2, 4, 6, 8, 24 and 48 h post-administration. Before the measurement, the animals were kept at 38 °C for 10 min in order to detect the pulsations of the tail artery. Changes in the SBP were expressed as the differences between the mean values of these variables before and after the administration of the treatment. To minimize stress-induced variations in BP, all measurements were taken by the same person, in the same peaceful environment. Moreover, before starting the experiments, we established a 2-week training period for the rats to become accustomed to the procedure. Data are expressed as the mean values ± standard error of the means (SEM) for a minimum of six experiments.

Additionally, twelve 20–23-week-old SHR weighing 350–380 g were administered Hpp11 at 55 mg/kg bw or water to determine the plasmatic ACE activity. The Hpp11 and water were orally administered by gastric intubation between 9 and 10 am. Blood samples were collected at 6 h post-administration via the saphenous vein using heparin vials. The samples were centrifuged at 2000× *g* for 15 min at 4 °C to obtain plasma. The procedure that was used to determine the plasmatic ACE activity is described below.

2.4. Determination of the Plasmatic ACE Activity

The plasmatic ACE activity was performed by a fluorometric method reported by Miguel et al. [28]. The measurements were performed in a multi-scan microplate fluorimeter (FLUOstar optima, BMG Labtech) at 37 °C and 350 nm excitation with 520 nm emission filters. ACE at different concentrations was added to each plate to obtain a calibration curve. ACE activity was expressed as the mean ± SEM mU ACE/mL of plasma for at least three replicates.

2.5. Experiments in Aorta Rings

Male 17–22-week-old, non-treated Sprague-Dawley (SD) rats weighing 250–300 g were sacrificed by decapitation. The thoracic aorta was excised from the animal's thorax, and excess fat and connective tissue were removed. To obtain the aorta preparations, the tissue was placed in a dissecting dish containing Krebs-Henseleit solution (NaCl, 118 mM: KCl, 4.7 mM; $CaCl_2$, 2.5 mM; KH_2PO_4, 1.2 mM; $MgSO_4$, 1.2 mM; $NaHCO_3$, 25 mM; and glucose, 10.0 mM) and cut into 3–4 mm rings. The aorta rings were mounted between two steel hooks in organ baths containing Krebs-Henseleit solution at 37 °C and continuously bubbled with a 95% O_2 and 5% CO_2 mixture, which gave a pH of 7.4. An optimal tension of 2 g was applied to all the aortic rings and adjusted every 15 min during the 60–90 min equilibration period, before adding the assayed compounds. The isometric tension was recorded by using an isometric force displacement transducer connected to an acquisition system (Protos 5, Panlab, Barcelona, Spain). After the equilibration period, 80 mM KCl was added to verify their functionality, and when the contraction had reached the steady state (approximately 15 min after the administration), the preparations were washed until the basal tension was recovered. The rings were then exposed to 10^{-5} M methoxamine, and when the contraction had reached the steady state, 10 μL Hpp11 was added to the organ bath at cumulative doses to reach concentrations between 0.01 mg/mL and 5 mg/mL. Water (10 μL) was used as negative control. The relaxant responses were expressed as a percentage of the pre-contraction induced by methoxamine, which was considered 100 percent. Results are expressed as the means ± SEM for at least eight experiments using aorta rings extracted from different animals. Concentration–response curves were fitted to the logistic equation, and statistical analysis was performed to compare concentration–response curves.

All the animal protocols followed in this study were approved by the Bioethical Committee of the Universitat Rovira i Virgili (European Comission Directive 86/609) and the Spanish Royal Decree 223/1988.

2.6. Statistical Analysis

The results are expressed as the mean ± SEM. Differences between the Hpp11 doses in the SHR were analysed by a two-way analysis of variance (ANOVA), and the Hpp11 effect on the WKY rats was analysed by a one-way analysis of variance (one-way ANOVA). To analyse differences between multiple independent groups, one-way analysis of variance followed by Tukey's or Dunnet's T3 post hoc test were used when required. The plasmatic ACE results were analysed by Student's *t*-test. Differences between concentration–response curves were analysed by two-way analysis of variance (two-way ANOVA). All the analyses were performed using IBM SPSS Statistics (SPSS, Chicago, IL, USA). Outliers were determined by using Grubbs' test. Differences between groups were considered significant when $p < 0.05$.

3. Results

3.1. Chicken Foot Hydrolysate Hpp11

Chicken foot hydrolysate, Hpp11, was characterized before the in vivo experiments. According to ACE inhibition, it was observed that the IC_{50} value (concentration of the hydrolysate needed to inhibit 50% of the original ACE activity) of Hpp11 was 0.027 mg/mL. Table 1 shows the results of the Hpp11 determination of protein content, expressed as the total nitrogen compounds content, the humidity, the ash content, the degree of hydrolysis and the ACE inhibition as percentage.

Table 1. Protein content, humidity, ash content and degree of hydrolysis of the chicken foot hydrolysate Hpp11.

Determinations	(%)
Total protein content [a]	0.67
Humidity	98.93
Ash content [b]	0.17
Degree of hydrolysis [c]	18.85
ACE inhibition [d]	95.11

[a] Protein content was estimated by the measure of total nitrogen compounds content measured by the Kjeldahl method, expressed as *w/v*; [b] Ash content is expressed as g ash/100 g of product; [c] Degree of hydrolysis was measured by the TNBS method in which free α-amino groups were determined. The data shown are mean values of each parameter for at least two different hydrolysates assayed under the same conditions. [d] Angiotensin-converting enzyme (ACE) inhibitory activity (%).

3.2. *Hpp11 In Vitro Inhibition Pattern on ACE*

Figure 1 shows the Lineweaver-Burk plot of ACE activity in presence of Hpp11. Considering that the Lineweaver-Burk plot obtained by changing the substrate concentration intersects with the *y*-axis, the inhibition of ACE by Hpp11 corresponds to competitive inhibition.

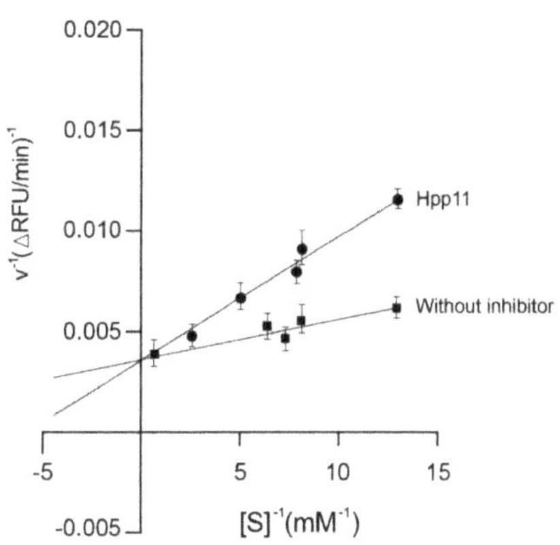

Figure 1. Lineweaver-Burk plot of angiotensin-converting enzyme (ACE) inhibition by chicken foot hydolysate Hpp11 and the control (without inhibitor). The Hpp11 effects at varying concentrations of ACE substrate (0–7.2 mM).

3.3. *Effect of Different Doses of Hpp11 on Blood Pressure in Hypertensive and Normotensive Rats*

Figure 2 shows the effect of three different doses of Hpp11 in SHR. Initial values of the SBP in the SHR were 195.9 ± 3.15 mmHg. As expected, the rats that only received water did not change their SBP values. In contrast, administration of Captopril (50 mg/kg bw) caused a clear decrease in the SBP, reaching the maximum decrease at 6 h post-administration. Regarding the hydrolysate, oral administration of 25 mg/kg bw did not produce an antihypertensive effect in the SHR. However, Hpp11 at 55 or 85 mg/kg bw resulted in a significant decrease in the SBP, reaching the maximum decrease at 6 h post-administration (−26.33 ± 2.1 and −30.45 ± 1.65 mmHg, respectively). At this time, the SBP decreases produced by both doses were similar to the decreases caused by Captopril. In fact, no significant differences between the decrease in BP produced by both Hpp11 doses was observed; however, the 55 mg/kg bw dose produced a more sustained antihypertensive effect than

85 mg/kg bw, showing a similar behaviour when compared to Captopril. In this sense, the SBP initial values were recovered 24 or 8 h post-administration at 55 and 85 mg/kg bw, respectively.

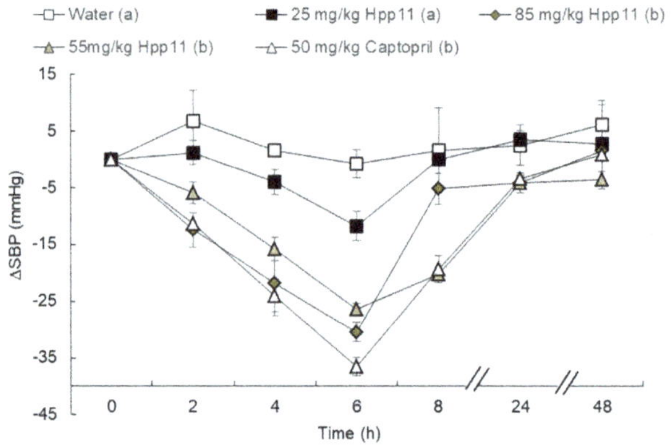

Figure 2. Decrease in the systolic blood pressure (SBP) in spontaneously hypertensive rats after the administration of water, Captopril (50 mg/kg bw) or different doses of chicken foot hydrolysate Hpp11: 25 mg/kg bw, 55 mg/kg bw and 85 mg/kg bw. Data are expressed as the mean ± SEM. All of the experimental groups include a minimum of six animals. Different letters represent significant differences ($p < 0.05$). p was estimated by two-way ANOVA.

In addition, oral administration of Hpp11 at a single dose of 55 mg/kg bw did not modify the arterial SBP in the normotensive WKY rats during the experiment (Figure 3). In fact, the SBP from the treated group showed similar values as the group administered with water.

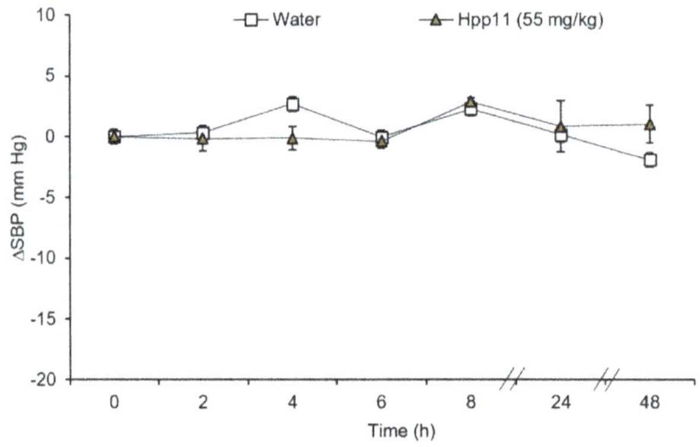

Figure 3. Decrease in the systolic blood pressure (SBP) in Wistar–Kyoto rats after administration of water or 55 mg/kg bw of chicken foot hydrolysate Hpp11. Data are expressed as the mean ± SEM. Both experimental groups have a minimum of six animals. No significant differences were observed.

3.4. Mechanisms Involved in the Antihypertensive Effect of Hpp11

The plasmatic ACE activity was measured in the rats administered 55 mg/kg bw of Hpp11 or water, 6 h post-administration. A reduction of 21% in the plasmatic ACE activity was found in the group administered Hpp11, being significantly lower than plasmatic ACE activity presented by the group administered water (Figure 4).

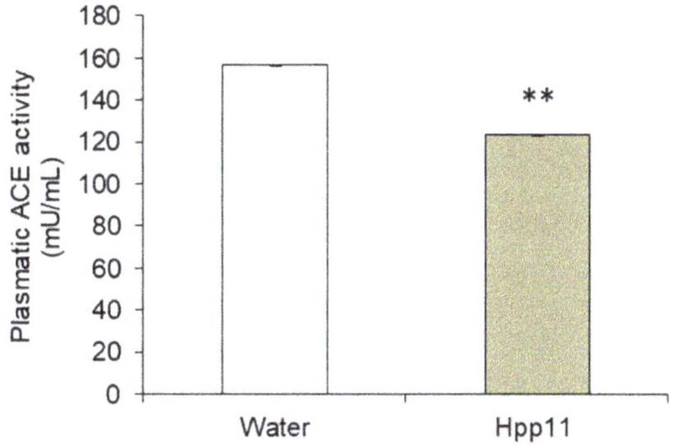

Figure 4. The plasmatic angiotensin-converting enzyme activity (ACE) in spontaneously hypertensive rats, 6 h after administration of 55 mg/kg chicken foot hydrolysate Hpp11 or water. Data are expressed as the mean ± SEM. The experimental groups include a minimum of six animals. The asterisks indicate differences between groups at $p < 0.01$ (**). p was calculated by Student's t-test.

In addition, to evaluate the existence of other mechanisms of antihypertensive activity in addition to ACE inhibition, the vascular effects of Hpp11 in aorta of SD rats was investigated. As demonstrated in Figure 5, Hpp11 did not produce relaxation in the aortic segments pre-contracted by methoxamine showing a similar effect to the control group.

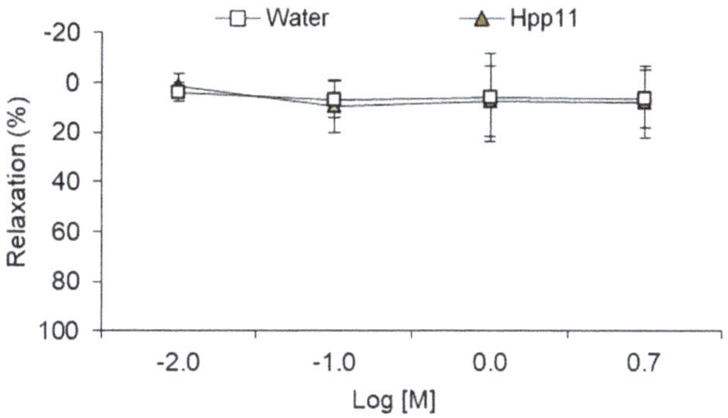

Figure 5. Cumulative concentration–response curves of chicken foot hydrolysate Hpp11 (0.01–5 M) in methoxamine pre-constricted aortic rings from Sprague-Dawley rats. Water was employed as a control, adding the same volume used to carry out the concentration-response curves of Hpp11. Data are mean values ± SEM. Both experimental groups have a minimum of six animals. No significant differences were observed between control group and Hpp11 group.

4. Discussion

The beneficial effects of bioactive peptides derived from hydrolyzed dietary proteins have been reported in many studies [33,34]. Some of these peptides demonstrate antihypertensive effects among other activities. Considering that commonly used antihypertensive drugs could present undesirable side effects, the interest in the use of protein hydrolysates to alleviate HTN has increased in recent years [35]. It is well known that chicken proteins are a good source of antihypertensive peptides. Onuh et al. demonstrated that peptides included in chicken skin protein hydrolysates were able to produce an antihypertensive effect after their administration to SHR [22]. Similar results were obtained from Saiga et al., postulating that chicken is a great source of bioactive peptides in part due to its high content of collagen [36], previously demonstrated to be a precursor of bioactive peptides [37]. Considering this, in a previous study our group it was demonstrated that chicken foot proteins are a potential source of antihypertensive peptides [18]. In this previous study, chicken foot hydrolysates were obtained and one of the hydrolysates (Hpp11) exhibited a clear antihypertensive effect when administered at a dose of 5 mL/kg bw to the SHR as well as in vitro ACEI activity [18]. In this sense, protein hydrolysates administered at 100 mg/kg bw have been demonstrated to exert substantial antihypertensive effects [22,28]. Thus, in this study, three different lower doses 85, 55 and 25 mg/kg bw were administered to SHR to identify the dose with the maximum antihypertensive effect. Only the doses of 55 and 85 mg/kg bw exhibited the antihypertensive effect, reaching, in both cases, the maximum decrease at 6 h post-administration. Importantly, no differences between Hpp11 at 55 and 85 mg/kg bw and Captopril 50 mg/kg bw were found, suggesting the potential antihypertensive effect of this hydrolysate. In this sense, many studies reported the beneficial effects of protein hydrolysates in treating HTN conditions [21,22,38,39]; however, it is important to note that the doses used in this study are significantly lower than the doses reported for different protein-derived hydrolysates. Accordingly, the blood pressure-lowering effect exhibited by Hpp11 at 55 and 85 mg/kg bw (-26.33 ± 2.1 and -30.45 ± 1.65 mmHg, respectively) was similar to those reported by Miguel et al. for the antihypertensive hydrolysate from egg white. However, in this study, 100 mg/kg bw dose was required to observe this antihypertensive effect [28]. Interestingly, chicken-leg bone protein hydrolysate showed similar antihypertensive results (−26 mmgHg) being administered at a dose of 50 mg/kg bw [39], demonstrating the antihypertensive potential effect of chicken by-products. Nevertheless, the dose used to obtain this reduction in BP was 600 mg/kg bw [40], significantly higher than the dose of Hpp11 used in the present study. As mentioned before, both doses (55 and 85 mg/kg bw) presented similar antihypertensive effects, but it was only the 55 mg/kg bw dose that maintained the antihypertensive effect 8 h post-administration. The SBP from the Hpp11 treated groups at 55 and 85 mg/kg bw were completely restored 24 h post-administration. It is known that ACE inhibitory activity in vitro does not always correspond to an antihypertensive effect in vivo. This is mainly due to the bioavailability of the ACE inhibitory peptides after oral administration and the fact that peptides may influence blood pressure by mechanisms other than ACE inhibition. In vivo protein digestion could produce peptide modifications that could inactivate or activate antihypertensive peptides [41,42]. Considering this, in vivo assays are always required to demonstrate in vivo bioactivity of these protein hydrolysates able to inhibit ACE in vitro. These observations indicate that the ACE-inhibiting peptides in the 55 and 85 mg/kg bw Hpp11 were bioavailable either intact or in modified forms to exert short-term antihypertensive effects. Then, these peptides were rapidly metabolized into inactive products leading to the subsequent reduction in activity, especially for 85 mg/kg bw Hpp11, with no apparent antihypertensive by 8 h post-administration. A similar antihypertensive pattern was recently described by Udenigwe et al. using by-product hen meat protein hydrolysates [43]. These results showed that at relatively low doses, Hpp11 was able to reduce the SBP in the same manner as Captopril, demonstrating its potential applicability in HTN treatment. Moreover, the fact that relatively low doses are enough to obtain a potent antihypertensive effect increases its industrial value.

It is also important to point out that the administration of Hpp11 to normotensive WKY rats did not modify the BP of these animals. This indicates that the effect of Hpp11 is specific to the hypertensive condition. Therefore, these products could be used as functional foods without any risk in normotensive subjects.

One of the most common mechanisms likely involved in the BP-lowering effect of food peptides is ACE inhibition. Therefore, hydrolysate selection by their ACEI activity in vitro is a potential strategy for the selection of antihypertensive hydrolysates and peptides [6]. In fact, Hpp11 was selected by its great ability to inhibit ACE in vitro. However, in vitro ACEI activity does not always correspond to the same bioactivity in vivo because of the physiological transformations during protein digestion. Thus, plasmatic ACE activity in the SHR treated with 55 mg/kg bw was evaluated 6 h post-administration. ACE activity was significantly reduced in the Hpp11 treated group compared to the water treated group. Similar results were reported after the administration of the ACE-inhibitory peptides contained in egg yolk [44] and soya protein [45].

Moreover, the inhibitory pattern of Hpp11 on in vitro ACE was studied. It was demonstrated that the peptides contained in the hydrolysate bind competitively at the active site of ACE to produce its inhibition. Quirós et al. [46] reported the same inhibition pattern for β-casein-peptides with antihypertensive properties. In this sense, it is well known that the most common mechanism of action of peptides in ACE inhibition is different from that of synthetic drugs. Generally, drugs indiscriminately block ACE and interfere with its activity, while ACE inhibitory peptides competitively block the binding of Ang I to ACE, thereby inhibiting the formation of Ang II [14,47]. Considering our results, Hpp11 produced its in vivo antihypertensive action by inhibiting the ACE activity, which suggests a possible reduction in Ang II release. However, many other systems different from RAAS can contribute to the control of BP. In this context, hydrolysates are complex mixtures of different peptides, and mechanisms of action other than ACE inhibition could be involved in their antihypertensive effect. In fact, it has been reported that antihypertensive food peptides can also have antioxidant, vasodilator, and/or opioid activities. In this sense, Sipola et al. [48] reported on the vasodilator-mediated antihypertensive effect of milk-derived peptides. Similar results were reported by Fujita et al., who reported that the antihypertensive effect of human casein-derived peptides was mediated by inducing relaxation in arteries [49]. To evaluate the potential Hpp11 vasodilator effect, aortic rings from SD rats were pre-contracted with methoxamine and then Hpp11 at increasing doses was administered. To evaluate the potential effects of different compounds on the vasculature, normotensive animals are used. SD rats are normotensive animals, such as WKY. However, SD rats are widely used to perform this type of study, considering that they offer higher response to contractile and relaxing agents than WKY, allowing it to demonstrate more clearly the effect of the tested compound [50].

Nevertheless, Hpp11 did not induce any relaxation in these preparations, showing similar behaviour to the control (water). However, it should be highlighted that SD rats are normotensive animals and Hpp11 may have different effects in the arteries of hypertensive animals. Future studies evaluating the Hpp11 effect on aortic rings from SHR could be performed to analyse the possible differences in their arterial responses to Hpp11. Moreover, the aorta is a conduit artery, and the resistance arteries determine the arterial BP more so than large vessels [51]. Therefore, we also suggest the use of resistance arteries for future studies to evaluate the Hpp11 vasodilator effect.

5. Conclusions

In this study, we demonstrated that the most effective antihypertensive dose of the chicken foot hydrolysate Hpp11 was 55 mg/kg after an acute administration. Our results indicate that Hpp11 produces its antihypertensive effect through the inhibition of ACE. Therefore, Hpp11 at low doses could be used as a functional food ingredient with potential therapeutic benefits in the prevention and treatment of HTN. Nevertheless, considering that HTN is a chronic pathology that requires chronic treatment, the evaluation of long-term administration of Hpp11 is necessary in animals and humans before the use of Hpp11 as an antihypertensive functional ingredient. Moreover, further studies are needed to determine the amino acid sequences present in Hpp11, responsible for the observed antihypertensive effect.

6. Patents

Patent application "Hydrolysates of chicken leg, their peptides and their uses": application number P201731065.

Author Contributions: Conceptualization, B.M. and F.I.B.; Formal analysis, A.M.-C., Z.P. and F.I.B.; Funding acquisition, B.M. and F.I.B.; Investigation, A.M.-C., Z.P. and F.I.B.; Methodology, A.M.-C., Z.P. and F.I.B.; Supervision, B.M., F.I.B. and A.A.; Writing—Original Draft, A.M.-C.; Writing—Review & Editing, B.M., F.I.B. and A.A.

Funding: This work has been supported by Grant Numbers AGL-2013-40707-R and AGL-2016-77105-R from the Spanish Government.

Acknowledgments: A.M.-C. and F.I.B. are recipients of a predoctoral fellowship from Universitat Rovira i Virgili—Martí i Franquès (Grant number: 2015PMF-428 PIPF-51) and postdoctoral mobility grant from the Fundación Triptolemos and Spanish Government (Ministerio de Educación, Cultura y Deportes), respectively. We would like to thank Niurka Llopiz, Rosa Pastor and Manuel Bas for technical assistance.

Conflicts of Interest: The authors declare no conflict of interest.

References

1. Messerli, F.H.; Williams, B.; Ritz, E. Essential hypertension. *Lancet* **2007**, *370*, 591–603. [CrossRef]
2. Hedayati, S.; Elsayed, E.; Reilly, R. Non-pharmacological aspects of blood pressure management: What are the data? *Kidney Int.* **2011**, *79*, 1061–1070. [CrossRef] [PubMed]
3. Zhuang, Y.; Sun, L.; Zhang, Y.; Liu, G. Antihypertensive effect of long-term oral administration of jellyfish (*Rhopilema esculentum*) collagen peptides on renovascular hypertension. *Mar. Drugs* **2012**, *10*, 417–426. [CrossRef] [PubMed]
4. Cheng, F.Y.; Wan, T.C.; Liu, Y.T.; Chen, C.M.; Lin, L.C.; Sakata, R. Determination of angiotensin-I converting enzyme inhibitory peptides in chicken leg bone protein hydrolysate with alcalase. *Anim. Sci. J.* **2009**, *80*, 91–97. [CrossRef] [PubMed]
5. Sica, D.A. Angiotensin-converting enzyme inhibitors side effects—Physiologic and non-physiologic considerations. *J. Clin. Hypertens.* **2004**, *6*, 410–416. [CrossRef]
6. Margalef, M.; Bravo, F.I.; Arola-Arnal, A.; Muguerza, B. Natural angiotensin converting enzyme (ACE) inhibitors with antihypetensive properties. In *Natural Products Targeting Clinically Relevant Enzymes*; Andrade, P., Valentao, P., Pereira, D.M., Eds.; Wiley-VCH Verlag GmbH & Co.: Weinheim, Germany, 2017; pp. 45–67.
7. Iwaniak, A.; Minkiewicz, P.; Darewicz, M. Food-originating ACE inhibitors, including antihypertensive peptides, as preventive food components in blood pressure reduction. *Compr. Rev. Food Sci. Food Saf.* **2014**, *13*, 114–134. [CrossRef]
8. Chakrabarti, S.; Wu, J. Bioactive peptides on endothelial function. *Food Sci. Hum. Wellness* **2016**, *5*, 1–7. [CrossRef]
9. Fang, H.; Luo, M.; Sheng, Y.; Li, Z.; Wu, Y.; Liu, C. The antihypertensive effect of peptides: A novel alternative to drugs? *Peptides* **2008**, *29*, 1062–1071.
10. Martínez-Maqueda, D.; Miralles, B.; Recio, I.; Hernández-Ledesma, B. Antihypertensive peptides from food proteins: A review. *Food Funct.* **2012**, *3*, 350. [CrossRef] [PubMed]
11. Aleixandre, A.; Miguel, M.; Muguerza, B. Péptidos antihipertensivos derivados de proteínas de leche y huevo. *Nutr. Hosp.* **2008**, *23*, 313–318. [PubMed]
12. Huang, J.; Liu, Q.; Xue, B.; Chen, L.; Wang, Y.; Ou, S.; Peng, X. Angiotensin-I-converting enzyme inhibitory activities and in vivo Antihypertensive Effects of Sardine Protein Hydrolysate. *J. Food Sci.* **2016**, *81*, H2831–H2840. [CrossRef] [PubMed]
13. Slizyte, R.; Rommi, K.; Mozuraityte, R.; Eck, P.; Five, K.; Rustad, T. Bioactivities of fish protein hydrolysates from defatted salmon backbones. *Biotechnol. Rep.* **2016**, *11*, 99–109. [CrossRef] [PubMed]
14. Ahhmed, A.M.; Muguruma, M. A review of meat protein hydrolysates and hypertension. *Meat Sci.* **2010**, *86*, 110–118. [CrossRef] [PubMed]
15. Ketnawa, S.; Rawdkuen, S. Angiotensin converting enzyme inhibitory peptides from aquatic and their processing by-Products: A review. *Int. J. Sci. Innov. Discov.* **2013**, *2*, 185–199.
16. Karamaæ, M.; Flaczyk, E.; Wanasundara, P.K.J.P.D.; Amarowicz, R. Angiotensin I-converting enzyme (ACE) inhibitory activity of hydrolysates obtained from muscle food industry by-products—A short report. *Pol. J. Food Nutr. Sci.* **2005**, *14*, 133–137.
17. Mora, L.; Reig, M.; Toldrá, F. Bioactive peptides generated from meat industry by-products. *Food Res. Int.* **2014**, *65*, 344–349. [CrossRef]
18. Bravo, F.I.; Arola, L.; Muguerza, B. Procedure for obtaining a hydrolysate claw chicken leg with antihypertensive activity, and peptides obtained hydrolysate containing. Patent No. ES2606954B1, 11 December 2017.

19. Lasekan, A.; Abu Bakar, F.; Hashim, D. Potential of chicken by-products as sources of useful biological resources. *Waste Manag.* **2013**, *33*, 552–565. [CrossRef] [PubMed]
20. Toldrá, F.; Aristoy, M.C.; Mora, L.; Reig, M. Innovations in value-addition of edible meat by-products. *Meat Sci.* **2012**, *92*, 290–296. [CrossRef] [PubMed]
21. Onuh, J.O.; Girgih, A.T.; Aluko, R.E.; Aliani, M. Inhibitions of renin and angiotensin converting enzyme activities by enzymatic chicken skin protein hydrolysates. *Food Res. Int.* **2013**, *53*, 260–267. [CrossRef]
22. Onuh, J.O.; Girgih, A.T.; Malomo, S.A.; Aluko, R.E.; Aliani, M. Kinetics of in vitro renin and angiotensin converting enzyme inhibition by chicken skin protein hydrolysates and their blood pressure lowering effects in spontaneously hypertensive rats. *J. Funct. Foods* **2015**, *14*, 133–143. [CrossRef]
23. Onuh, J.O.; Girgih, A.T.; Nwachukwu, I.; Ievari-Shariati, S.; Raj, P.; Netticadan, T.; Aluko, R.E.; Aliani, M. A metabolomics approach for investigating urinary and plasma changes in spontaneously hypertensive rats (SHR) fed with chicken skin protein hydrolysates diets. *J. Funct. Foods* **2016**, *22*, 20–33. [CrossRef]
24. Majumder, K.; Wu, J. Molecular Targets of Antihypertensive Peptides: Understanding the mechanisms of action based on the pathophysiology of hypertension. *Int. J. Mol. Sci.* **2015**, *16*, 256–283. [CrossRef] [PubMed]
25. Miguel, M.; Manso, M.; Aleixandre, A.; Alonso, M.J.; Salaices, M.; Lopez-Fandino, R. Vascular effects, angiotensin I-converting enzyme (ACE)-inhibitory activity, and antihypertensive properties of peptides derived from egg white. *J. Agric. Food Chem.* **2007**, *55*, 10615–10621. [CrossRef] [PubMed]
26. Girgih, A.T.; Nwachukwu, I.D.; Onuh, J.O.; Malomo, S.A.; Aluko, R.E. Antihypertensive properties of a pea protein hydrolysate during short- and long-term oral administration to spontaneously hypertensive rats. *J. Food Sci.* **2016**, *81*, H1281–H1287. [CrossRef] [PubMed]
27. Lin, H.-C.; Alashi, A.M.; Aluko, R.E.; Sun Pan, B.; Chang, Y.-W. Antihypertensive properties of tilapia (*Oreochromis* spp.) frame and skin enzymatic protein hydrolysates. *Food Nutr. Res.* **2017**, *61*, 1391666. [CrossRef] [PubMed]
28. Miguel, M.; Alonso, M.J.; Salaices, M.; Aleixandre, A.; López-Fandiño, R. Antihypertensive, ACE-inhibitory and vasodilator properties of an egg white hydrolysate: Effect of a simulated intestinal digestion. *Food Chem.* **2007**, *104*, 163–168. [CrossRef]
29. Association of Official Analytical Chemists (AOAC) (Ed.) *Official Methods of Analysis*, 16th ed.; Association of Official Analytical Chemists: Arlington, VA, USA, 1995.
30. Adler-Nissen, J. Determination of the degree of hydrolysis of food protein hydrolysates by trinitrobenzenesulfonic acid. *J. Agric. Food Chem.* **1979**, *27*, 1256–1262. [CrossRef] [PubMed]
31. Quirós, A.; del Contreras, M.M.; Ramos, M.; Amigo, L.; Recio, I. Stability to gastrointestinal enzymes and structure–activity relationship of β-casein-peptides with antihypertensive properties. *Peptides* **2009**, *30*, 1848–1853. [CrossRef] [PubMed]
32. Buñag, R.D. Validation in awake rats of a tail-cuff method for measuring systolic pressure. *J. Appl. Physiol.* **1973**, *34*, 279–282. [CrossRef] [PubMed]
33. Yamamoto, N. Antihypertensive peptides derived from food proteins. *Biopolym. Pept. Sci. Sect.* **1997**, *43*, 129–134. [CrossRef]
34. Udenigwe, C.C.; Mohan, A. Mechanisms of food protein-derived antihypertensive peptides other than ACE inhibition. *J. Funct. Foods* **2014**, *8*, 45–52. [CrossRef]
35. Hou, Y.; Wu, Z.; Dai, Z.; Wang, G.; Wu, G. Protein hydrolysates in animal nutrition: Industrial production, bioactive peptides, and functional significance. *J. Anim. Sci. Biotechnol.* **2017**, *8*, 1–13. [CrossRef] [PubMed]
36. Saiga, A.; Iwai, K.; Hayakawa, T.; Takahata, Y.; Kitamura, S.; Nishimura, T.; Morimatsu, F. Angiotensin I-converting enzyme-inhibitory peptides obtained from chicken collagen hydrolysate. *J. Agric. Food Chem.* **2008**, *56*, 9586–9591. [CrossRef] [PubMed]
37. Fu, Y.; Therkildsen, M.; Aluko, R.E.; Lametsch, R. Exploration of collagen recovered from animal by-products as a precursor of bioactive peptides: Successes and challenges. *Crit. Rev. Food Sci. Nutr.* **2018**, *8398*, 1–17. [CrossRef] [PubMed]
38. Balti, R.; Bougatef, A.; Ali, N.E.H.; Zekri, D.; Barkia, A.; Nasri, M. Influence of degree of hydrolysis on functional properties and angiotensin I-converting enzyme-inhibitory activity of protein hydrolysates from cuttlefish (*Sepia officinalis*) by-products. *J. Sci. Food Agric.* **2010**, *90*, 2006–2014. [CrossRef] [PubMed]
39. Cheng, F.Y.; Wan, T.C.; Liu, Y.T.; Lai, K.M.; Lin, L.C.; Sakata, R. A study of in vivo antihypertensive properties of enzymatic hydrolysate from chicken leg bone protein. *Anim. Sci. J.* **2008**, *79*, 614–619. [CrossRef]

40. Li, G.-H.; Qu, M.-R.; Wan, J.-Z.; You, J.-M. Antihypertensive effect of rice protein hydrolysate with in vitro angiotensin I-converting enzyme inhibitory activity in spontaneously hypertensive rats. *Asia Pac. J. Clin. Nutr.* **2007**, *16* (Suppl. 1), 275–280.
41. Vermeirssen, V.; Van Camp, J.; Verstraete, W. Bioavailability of angiotensin I converting enzyme inhibitory peptides. *Br. J. Nutr.* **2004**, *92*, 357. [CrossRef] [PubMed]
42. Jao, C.-L.; Huang, S.-L.; Hsu, K.-C. Angiotensin I-converting enzyme inhibitory peptides: Inhibition mode, bioavailability, and antihypertensive effects. *BioMedicine* **2012**, *2*, 130–136. [CrossRef]
43. Udenigwe, C.C.; Girgih, A.T.; Mohan, A.; Gong, M.; Malomo, S.A.; Aluko, R.E. Antihypertensive and bovine plasma oxidation-inhibitory activities of spent hen meat protein hydrolysates. *J. Food Biochem.* **2017**, *41*, 1–8. [CrossRef]
44. Yoshii, H.; Tachi, N.; Ohba, R.; Sakamura, O.; Takeyama, H.; Itani, T. Antihypertensive effect of ACE inhibitory oligopeptides from chicken egg yolks. *Comp. Biochem. Physiol. C* **2001**, *128*, 27–33. [CrossRef]
45. Yang, H.-Y.; Yang, S.-C.; Chen, J.-R.; Tzeng, Y.-H.; Han, B.-C. Soyabean protein hydrolysate prevents the development of hypertension in spontaneously hypertensive rats. *Br. J. Nutr.* **2004**, *92*, 507. [CrossRef] [PubMed]
46. Quirós, A.; Ramos, M.; Muguerza, B.; Delgado, M.A.; Miguel, M.; Aleixandre, A.; Recio, I. Identification of novel antihypertensive peptides in milk fermented with *Enterococcus faecalis*. *Int. Dairy J.* **2007**, *17*, 33–41. [CrossRef]
47. Alderman, C.P. Adverse effects of the angiotensin-converting enzyme inhibitors. *Ann Pharmacoter.* **1996**, *30*, 55–61. [CrossRef] [PubMed]
48. Sipola, M.; Finckenberg, P.; Vapaatalo, H.; Pihlanto-Leppälä, A.; Korhonen, H.; Korpela, R.; Nurminen, M.-L. Alpha-lactorphin and beta-lactorphin improve arterial function in spontaneously hypertensive rats. *Life Sci.* **2002**, *71*, 1245–1253. [CrossRef]
49. Fujita, H.; Suganuma, H.; Usui, H.; Kurahashi, K.; Nakagiri, R.; Sasaki, R.; Yoshikawa, M. Vasorelaxation by casomokinin L, a derivative of β-casomorphin and casoxin D, is mediated by NK1receptor. *Peptides* **1996**, *17*, 635–639. [CrossRef]
50. Rahmani, M.A.; DeGray, G.; David, V.; Ampy, F.R.; Jones, L. Comparison of calcium import as a function of contraction in the aortic smooth muscle of Sprague-Dawley, Wistar Kyoto and spontaneously hypertensive rats. *Front. Biosci.* **1999**, *4*, D408–D415. [PubMed]
51. Pons, Z.; Arola, L. Involvement of nitric oxide and prostacyclin in the antihypertensive effect of low-molecular-weight procyanidin rich grape seed extract in male spontaneously hypertensive rats. *J. Funct. Foods* **2014**, *6*, 419–427.

nutrients

MDPI

Review

Hairless Canaryseed: A Novel Cereal with Health Promoting Potential

Emily Mason [1,2], Lamia L'Hocine [1,*], Allaoua Achouri [1] and Salwa Karboune [2]

1 Saint-Hyacinthe Research and Development Centre, Agriculture and Agri-Food Canada, 3600 Casavant Boulevard West, St-Hyacinthe, QC J2S 8E3, Canada; emily.mason2@mail.mcgill.ca (E.M.); allaoua.achouri@Canada.ca (A.A.)

2 Department of Food Science and Agricultural Chemistry, Macdonald Campus, McGill University 21, 111 Lakeshore, Ste Anne de Bellevue, QC H9X 3V9, Canada; salwa.karboune@mcgill.ca

* Correspondence: lamia.lhocine@Canada.ca; Tel.: +1-450-768-7944

Received: 30 August 2018; Accepted: 16 September 2018; Published: 19 September 2018

Abstract: Glabrous canaryseeds were recently approved for human consumption as a novel cereal grain in Canada and the United States. Previously, canaryseeds were exclusively used as birdseed due to the presence of carcinogenic silica fibers; therefore the nutritional value of the seeds has been seriously overlooked. Two cultivars of glabrous canaryseeds (yellow and brown) were created from the hairy varieties. They are high in protein compared to other cereal grains, and contain high amounts of tryptophan, an amino acid normally lacking in cereals, and are gluten-free. Bioactive peptides of canaryseeds produced by in vitro gastrointestinal digestion have shown antioxidant, antidiabetic, and antihypertensive activity. The seeds contain other constituents with health promoting effects, including unsaturated fatty acids, minerals, and phytochemicals. Anti-nutritional components in the seeds are comparable to other cereal grains. Because of their beneficial health effects, canaryseeds should be regarded as a healthy food and have immense potential as a functional food and ingredient. Further research is required to determine additional bioactive peptide activity and capacity, as well as differences between the yellow and brown cultivars.

Keywords: canaryseed; cereal protein; bioactive peptide; antioxidant; ACE inhibitor; DPP-IV inhibitor; gluten-free; functional food

1. Introduction

Due to the growing global demand for protein, there will be increased need for good sources of high quality plant protein for food uses. Discovering new sources of plant food proteins, besides the conventional ones (ex. wheat, soybean, pulses) provide promising opportunities in terms of environmental sustainability, economic profitability, and nutritional advantages. The consumption of different plant proteins can ensure an adequate supply of essential amino acids for meeting human physiological requirements. Opportunities are endless for using plant proteins as a functional ingredient in formulated food products to increase nutritional quality, as well as to provide desirable health promoting effects.

In 2015, Health Canada and the Food and Drug Administration (FDA) gave GRAS (Generally Regarded as Safe) status to glabrous canaryseeds (*Phalaris canariensis* L.) and approved them as a novel food product. Previously, the seeds had limited use as birdseed, because they were lined with fine, hair-like silica fibers, that were deemed hazardous to human health [1]. The Crop Development Center at the University of Saskatchewan in Canada developed a new 'hairless' or 'glabrous' canaryseed from the hairy variety, which is safe for human consumption. Caged and wild birds have consumed hairy canaryseeds for centuries, alone or mixed with other grains, such as millet, sunflower seeds, and flaxseeds [2]. Nonetheless, very little research has been conducted on the seeds, since they had no nutritional value for humans. The new glabrous canaryseed, regarded as a true cereal grain, has tremendous potential in the food industry, due to its unique properties and characteristics. Canaryseed groats contain approximately 61% starch, 20% protein, 8% crude fat and 7% total dietary fiber [3,4]. Compared to other cereal grains in the same family, such as oats, barley, wheat, and rye, they are extremely high in protein. Some studies have shown the potential of hairy canaryseed proteins to produce bioactive peptides with beneficial health effects, such as antioxidant, antihypertensive, and antidiabetic activity [5,6]. Furthermore, unlike wheat, canaryseeds are gluten-free. This review aims to overview the research conducted on canaryseeds to date, particularly the examination of canaryseed proteins and their exceptional health benefits, to ascertain their uniqueness compared to other cereal grains and potential applications in the food industry.

2. Canaryseed Development and Production

Hairy canaryseeds, like most grass species, have seeds lined with hair-like silica fibers that were found to be causing lung damage and even esophageal cancer [1]. Hucl, et al. [7], from the University of Saskatchewan's Crop Development Center (CDC), developed a hairless canaryseed containing no fine hair to decrease skin irritations and potential cancer development by farmers involved in harvesting the crop. The new silica-free or glabrous species was not only safe for individuals manipulating the seeds, but could also be safely consumed and utilized by the food industry as a new cereal grain. Using mutagenesis and breeding techniques, four hairless brown varieties have been created from the original seeds: CDC Maria, CDC Togo, CDC Bastia, and CDC Calvi [8]. In addition, yellow colored cultivars of the glabrous seeds were developed, which are thought to be more aesthetically pleasing for food use as compared to the brown colored cultivar [9] (Figure 1).

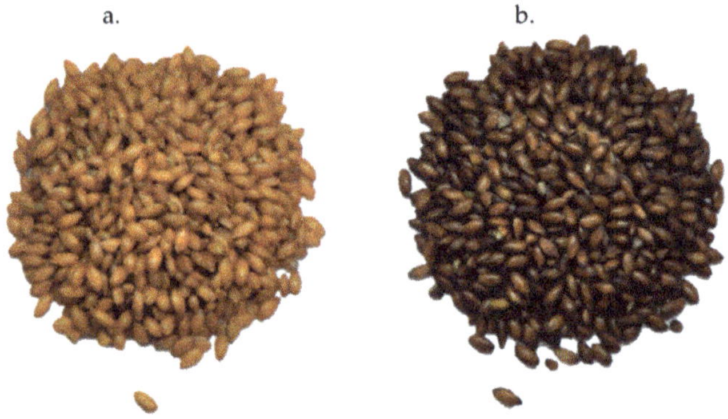

Figure 1. (**a**) Yellow (C09052) and (**b**) brown (CDC Calvi) cultivars of glabrous canaryseeds (*Phalaris canariensis* L.) produced by Hucl, et al. [7], at the Crop Development Center at the University of Saskatchewan.

Glabrous or hairless canaryseeds are members of the family *Poaceae*, along with other prevalent cereal grains, such as wheat, oat, barley, and rye [10]. The groats (hulled kernels of the grain) have an elliptical shape and measure approximately 4 mm in length and 2 mm in width, comparable to flaxseeds and sesame seeds [4]. The seeds are harvested from canarygrass; a grassy, herbaceous plant that grows optimally in any regions where wheat is cultivated, with growth and production cycles comparable to other winter cereals, such as spring wheat and oat. In addition, very few weeds, diseases, and insects have been reported in canarygrass, which would decrease canaryseed yields [2]. The Western provinces of Canada (Saskatchewan, Manitoba, and Alberta) cultivate the majority of canaryseeds in Canada, which produces over 80% of canaryseed exports worldwide, followed by Argentina and Hungary, mainly to countries with high proportions of caged birds [8]. On average, about 300,000 acres of canaryseed are grown in the province of Saskatchewan every year with yields ranging between 800 to 1400 pounds per acre, representing more than 95 percent of Canadian acreage and production [8], and which is still comprised of only the hairy varieties. The higher yield of the older hairy varieties has limited the uptake by producers of the glabrous varieties. The variety CDC Calvi has the highest yield of the developed glabrous varieties [8]. The approval of glabrous canaryseed varieties for human consumption opens up new opportunities in food applications instead of the sole use as birdseed, which is expected to create more demand for the production of canaryseed.

3. Canaryseed Proteins: A Novel Source of Plant Proteins

3.1. Protein Characteristics

Canaryseeds have been compared extensively with wheat and other cereals in the same family, and one of their distinguishing factors is their higher protein content (Table 1), which ranges between 20–23%, in comparison to 13% for wheat. Canaryseed proteins, along with other cereal proteins, can be separated into four fractions based on their solubility: prolamins, glutelins, globulins and albumins [11]. The prolamin and glutelin fractions, which are principally storage proteins, are more abundant in canaryseeds than wheat, however, the globulin and albumin fractions represent the lowest amount of overall protein [3,4], which is possibly indicative of a reduced amount of anti-nutritional factors, such as enzyme inhibitors [4]. Regardless of the variations in protein fraction proportions, wheat remains unique because of its ability to make dough, due to the exceptional viscoelastic properties of its proteins [11]. Nonetheless, to date, no published data is available on the breadmaking potential of 100% canary flour, although Abdel-Aal, et al. [12] reported that replacement of up to 25% of wheat flour with canaryseed flour in bread had no significant effects on bread quality and loaf volume, except for crumb color.

Table 1. Protein comparison between canaryseed and other cereals.

Cereal Variety	% Protein (Dry Basis)	Reference
Canaryseed	20–23%	[4,12]
Wheat	13%	[13]
Oat	10–13%	[14]
Barley	13–16%	[15]
Rye	11–16%	[16]
Millet	8.5–15%	[17]

A key trait of canaryseeds is their possible lack of gluten-like proteins, which elicit an allergic reaction known as coeliac disease in some sensitive individuals when they consume gluten-containing cereals, such as wheat, barley, and rye [18,19]. Gluten is a complex mixture of proteins called prolamins, which play key roles in conveying dough viscosity/elasticity. Wheat prolamins are termed gliadins and glutenins, barley prolamins are hordeins, and those from rye secalin. A common characteristic of these proteins is the presence of multiple proline and glutamine residues, making them resistant to gastrointestinal digestion and more exposed to deamination by tissue transglutaminase [20]. In a recent study conducted by Boye, et al. [21] to establish the safety of canaryseeds for human consumption from a food allergy perspective, glabrous canaryseeds were analyzed using three separate techniques (enzyme-linked immunosorbent assay (ELISA), mass spectroscopy, and Western blotting) which all yielded negative results for gluten, indicating the cereal is an excellent alternative for individuals with coeliac disease. Although canaryseeds do not contain gluten and may be represented as gluten-free, canaryseeds do however contain a newly reported allergen named granule-bound starch synthase (GBSS), which is present in rice and maize [22], and which cross-reacted with sera from wheat sensitive/allergic individuals [21]. GBSS was simultaneously identified through mass spectroscopy analysis in several cereals (wheat, oat, sorghum, millet, teff, quinoa, buckwheat) [21]. As such, Health Canada has deemed it inappropriate for canaryseed, or food containing canaryseed, to be labelled as "wheat-free". Health Canada also requires canaryseed and foods containing canaryseed to be labelled with a statement to the effect that the product "may not be suitable for people with wheat allergy", provided the food does not also contain wheat as an ingredient [10].

The amino acid profile of canaryseeds (Table 2) remains unique, due to its high content of tryptophan, an essential amino acid, which is usually lacking in most cereal grains. Abdel-Aal, et al. [4] reported a higher tryptophan content in the Keet cultivar of hairy canaryseed proteins (2.8 g/100 g of protein) as compared to wheat (1.2 g/100 g) and casein (1.0 g/100 g) protein, as well as higher amounts of essential amino acids phenylalanine, leucine, and isoleucine as compared to wheat. Similarly to other cereals, canaryseeds are deficient in essential amino acids lysine, threonine, and methionine, but possess comparable levels to wheat [4]. Glabrous canaryseeds would make an excellent addition to other cereal grain and legume products to ensure consumers meet the recommended dietary intake of essential amino acids. In addition, canaryseeds contain high amounts of glutamic acid. Glutamic acid is the most abundant amino acid in the brain, which plays significant roles in synaptic activity, memory, and learning, also, it was reported that changes in glutamic acid metabolism and regulation in the brain leads to the development of Alzheimer's disease [23]. Moreover, high content of glutamic acid in the seeds could indicate the presence of high gamma-aminobutyric acid (GABA), a functional compound produced in plants primarily by the decarboxylation of L-glutamic acid, which has several health promoting properties, including reducing blood pressure and blood cholesterol, anticancer, and anti-obesity activity [24]. GABA concentration, however, has not been directly determined in canaryseeds.

Table 2. Amino acid comparison between canaryseeds and other cereals.

Amino Acid	Canaryseed (g/100 g Protein)	Wheat (g/100 g Protein)	Oat (g/16 g N or g/100 g Protein)	Barley (g/100 g Protein)	Millet (g/100 g Protein)
Histidine	1.6	2.1	1.74	2.4	2.4
Isoleucine	3.9	2.8	2.32	3.5	4.4
leucine	7.6	5.3	5.26	7.7	11.5
lysine	2.6	1.9	2.73	3.9	2.8
Methionine	1.9	1.4	2.5	2.1	2.3
Phenylalanine	6.5	5.4	5.3	5.7	5.6
Threonine	2.7	2.8	2.46	3.9	4.2
Tryptophan	2.8	1.2	1.15	N/A	N/A
Valine	4.8	3.8	3.2	5.4	6.0
Alanine	4.5	3	3.59	4.4	8.8
Arginine	6.4	5.1	5.79	4.6	3.9
Aspartic acid	4.4	4.4	7.37	6.3	8.7
Cystine	2.5	2.3	2.74	1.4	1.2
Glutamic acid	26	33	19.12	28.1	22
Glycine	3.1	3.8	3.81	4.7	3.2
Proline	6.2	8.6	4.54	12.7	6.8
Serine	4.5	4.3	3.86	4.9	5.3
Tyrosine	3.6	3.5	1.82	2.8	2.4
Reference	[8]	[4]	[14,25]	[26]	[26]

N/A = not available.

3.2. *Health Promoting Properties of Canaryseed Proteins*

Chronic disease is of major global concern today and includes diseases such as cardiovascular disease, cancer, and diabetes, which are leading causes of death worldwide [27]. A balance between an active lifestyle and good eating habits are critical in the long term to prevent and combat chronic diseases. Beyond their physiological and metabolic effects, dietary proteins are intrinsically associated with health improvement and prevention of nutrition related chronic diseases (ex. cardiovascular diseases, hypertension, cancer, oxidative damage, etc.), and which need to be also considered when assessing protein quality [28]. This is particularly relevant as consumers are increasingly looking to natural food sources to help prevent specific diseases or illnesses. Some parts of world, such as Mexico, have utilized hairy canaryseeds as a traditional folk medicine for treatment of diabetes and hypertension for centuries [5]. However, because of the presence of toxic hairs, the seeds were not consumed directly but soaked in water, drained, dried and then processed to make canaryseed "milk", which can be safely consumed.

The health benefits associated with drinking canaryseed "milk" were found to be largely related to the bioactive peptides produced during digestion. Bioactive peptides are small, specific and active protein fragments released from food proteins by proteolytic enzymes during protein digestion, which positively affect an individual's overall health [29,30]. Bioactive peptides have been reported from many food sources, such as fish and crustaceans, dairy products (milk, cheese, yoghurt), eggs, meat, and vegetal sources (grains, legumes, seeds) [31]. Depending on the amino acid composition and sequence, bioactive peptides possess different types of activity, including antioxidant, antimicrobial, antihypertensive, radical scavenging, anti-inflammatory, opioid, immunomodulatory, anticancer, chelation activity, and antidiabetic activity among others [31,32]. In recent years, a lot of research has been focused on the ability of plant proteins from cereals, nuts, and pulses to generate bioactive peptides with measurable health benefits. Thus far, very little research has been conducted on the bioactivity of glabrous canaryseeds. Research on canaryseed proteins and peptide bioactivity has been tested exclusively in vitro to date, with no animal or human subjects, and predominantly using the hairy varieties. Although the nutrient profile between hairless and hairy canaryseeds are very similar, further investigation into hairless canaryseed bioactivity is required and ongoing.

3.2.1. Antidiabetic Activity

Dipeptidyl peptidase IV (DPP-IV) enzyme plays a major role in the development of hyperglycemia in individuals with type II diabetes, because it inactivates incretin hormones, thereby increasing blood glucose levels [29]. Incretin-based therapy is a common treatment for type II diabetes, but it remains less effective, because the half-life of the hormone is very short, due to inactivation by DPP-IV enzymes [30]. DPP-IV inhibitors improve the efficiency of incretin-based therapy by inactivating the enzyme and increasing the activity of the incretin hormones. Estrada-Salas, et al. [5] found that peptides produced by in vitro gastrointestinal digestion of canaryseed milk using pepsin, trypsin, and pancreatin, displayed inhibitory activity in a dose dependent manner against DPP-IV enzyme from porcine kidney. In addition, an in vivo and in vitro study have demonstrated an anti-obesity effect of a lipid extract (produced by hexane extraction) of hairless canaryseed [33,34]. The anti-obesity effect of canaryseeds in addition to the inhibitory action of DPP-IV by canaryseed peptides would make this grain an excellent nutritional approach to improve the efficiency of synthetic drugs, since food derived DPP-IV inhibitors lack the potency of synthetic drugs inhibitors [35]. Further characterization of the DPP-IV inhibitor peptides in canaryseeds remains necessary to establish their antidiabetic effects and capacity.

3.2.2. Antihypertensive Activity

The angiotensin-I converting enzyme (ACE) increases blood pressure and causes hypertension in inclined individuals. ACE converts the inactive angiotensin-I into angiotensin-II (a very powerful vasoconstrictor) and inactivates bradykinin (a vasodilator), which both lead to the direct increase in blood pressure [5,36]. Synthetic ACE inhibitors are produced as a treatment for hypertension, and although effective, the synthetic inhibitors cause side effects, including coughing, food taste alterations, rashes and reduced efficiency when used in the long term [36]. Food sources of ACE inhibitors are of great interest, since individuals with hypertension can consume them as part of a healthy diet to reduce their high blood pressure [37].

Recent research studies revealed that canaryseed bioactive peptides have great potential to lower blood pressure through the inhibition of the ACE enzyme. Estrada-Salas, et al. [5] showed that canaryseed flour proteins digested in vitro using pepsin, trypsin, and pancreatin, exhibited a maximum percent inhibition against the ACE enzyme of 73.5% and an IC_{50} value of 322 μg/mL, which was similar to the IC_{50} value of other peptides from chickpea, pea, soybean, wheat gliadin, and sardine muscle. Undigested canaryseed proteins had significantly lower inhibition activity, meaning the antihypertensive bioactive peptides are produced upon protein digestion [5]. Similarly, Valverde, et al. [6] found that canaryseed flour proteins from the prolamin fraction had the highest inhibition activity against the ACE enzyme, with an IC_{50} value of 217.4 μg/mL, after in vitro digestion with pepsin and pancreatin. They further identified five peptides by mass spectroscopy (LSLGT, TDQPAG, QQLQT, FEPLQLA, and KPQLYQPF) in the digested prolamin fraction that had both ACE and DPP-IV inhibition activity. Additionally, Passos, et al. [38] administered to rats an aqueous extract of canaryseeds (obtained by soaking the seeds in water), which successfully reduced systolic blood pressure in the animals while having no renal or toxicological effects. All these studies demonstrated the potential positive effect of canaryseeds on cardiovascular disease control.

3.2.3. Antioxidant Activity

The antioxidant potential of plants has received a great deal of attention, because increased oxidative stress has been identified as a major causative factor in the development and progression of several life threatening diseases, including neurodegenerative and cardiovascular diseases. Free radical species that are generated in the body by various endogenous systems cause extensive damage to body tissues by destroying cell membrane structure, modifying enzyme activity, and changing DNA leading to cancer development [39]. In this regard, bioactive peptides of canaryseeds demonstrated antioxidant activity by reacting with free radical species, thereby preventing tissue damage and decay. Valverde, et al. [6] used two in vitro radical scavenging assays on digested canaryseed protein fractions and found that the prolamins had the overall highest antioxidant activity. Mass spectroscopy analysis of the digested prolamin fraction identified five peptides, of which only one had antioxidant activity (KPQLYQPF). Protein fractions from digested canaryseeds had higher antioxidant activity in general as compared to raw flour, because the seed proteins undergo hydrolysis, increasing their antioxidant activity [6].

3.2.4. Other Bioactivities

Only very limited studies have been conducted on other bioactive properties of hairy canaryseed proteins. As an example, acetylcholinesterase inhibitors are currently employed as a form of treatment for individuals with Alzheimer's disease, because they help maintain levels of acetylcholine in the brain, which is essential for nerve impulses and transmission [40]. Kchaou, et al. [41] found that a methanol extract of a hairy Tunisian canaryseed variety had a percent inhibition against acetylcholinesterase enzyme of 65% at a concentration of 1 mg/mL, which was attributed predominantly to polyphenols and flavonoids in the extract. An antibacterial activity of hairy Tunisian canaryseed extracts, especially against gram-positive bacteria, was also reported by Kchaou, et al. [41]. These bioactivities could possibly be the result of canaryseed peptides, as it was previously demonstrated for hemp seed protein hydrolysates, which exhibited acetylcholinesterase inhibition [40], or for other cereal proteins, such as wheat and barley, for which antibacterial activity was reported [42]. Proteins and peptides from cereal grains and legumes (wheat, barley, amaranth, oat, rye, soybean etc.) are known to have antithrombotic, immunomodulatory, and anticancer activity [42–52]. Bioactivities of Canadian glabrous canaryseed peptides remain largely unknown, but because of the diverse bioactivity reported in similar cereal grains from the same family, it remains highly likely that canaryseed peptides possess additional health promoting properties, which still need to be confirmed.

3.3. *Protein Digestibility*

Protein digestibility is an important parameter to consider when assessing protein quality [53]. The health advantages of glabrous canaryseeds depends on their digestibility and bioavailability. Several in vivo studies indicated excellent protein digestibility of canaryseed in animals. Broiler chickens fed hairless canaryseed groats and hulled seeds exhibited similar ileal protein digestibility as other feed components, including corn, wheat, sorghum, and peas [54]. The same study showed high apparent ileal digestibility of amino acids cysteine (86%), phenylalanine (88%), and tryptophan (93%). Furthermore, weight gain between broiler chickens fed with wheat and chickens fed with canaryseeds were similar.

Later, Classen et al. [55] fed broiler chickens yellow glabrous canaryseeds and glabrous brown seeds and determined the seeds were equivalent in terms of feeding value. Magnuson, et al. [56] found no evidence of toxicity in rats when fed glabrous canaryseeds for a 90 day study and, furthermore, rat diets supplemented with 50% hulled and dehulled glabrous canaryseeds were comparable in terms of growth, hematology, and clinical parameters as rats with diets supplemented with 50% wheat. Thacker [57] showed that crude protein digestibility in pigs increased linearly with increasing proportions of canaryseeds in their diets. Moreover, he found that a pig's diet containing 25% canaryseeds promoted the highest growth rates in the pigs with a crude protein digestibility of approximately 78%. All these studies indicate that hairless canaryseeds make an excellent addition or supplement to conventional animal feed, as it promotes growth, but also enhances protein digestibility.

For human digestibility of canaryseed proteins, no in vivo study has been reported in the literature despite several in vitro studies that have been carried out to mimic human protein digestibility of canaryseeds under gastrointestinal conditions. Abdel-Aal, et al. [4] used a multienzyme approach with trypsin, chymotrypsin, and peptidase and established an in vitro protein digestibility of 84% in hairy canaryseeds. Interestingly, Rajamohamed, et al. [58] compared the effects of thermal treatment on canaryseed protein digestibility. The in vitro protein digestibility of raw, roasted, and boiled glabrous canaryseed flours was determined by gastric, duodenal, and sequential gastric-duodenal methods. The sequential gastric-duodenal method was most effective at digesting the proteins and, overall, thermal processing enhanced protein digestion. As a cereal, canaryseeds can be used in various forms, such as a whole groat, whole meal, or whole grain flour in several applications, such as a cereal, in pasta, and in baking to make products, such as bread, muffins, and cereal grain bars [10]. Since thermal processing increased protein digestibility, the heating and thermal processing of canaryseeds in the development and production of baked goods will contribute to its improved nutritive value.

4. Other Health Promoting Canaryseed Components

4.1. Starch

Canaryseeds are comprised of 61% starch, which serves as the main energy store in the plants [59]. Canaryseed starch granules are small and polygonal in shape with reported sizes ranging from 0.5 to 7.5 μm [60–62]. X-ray diffraction patterns of the starch exhibit the traits of an A-type starch, characteristic of most cereal grains [61,62]. Starch is comprised of two glucose polymers; linear amylose and branched amylopectin. Abdel-Aal, et al. [62] reported a range of amylose content in hairy canaryseeds of 16.2–19.5% of total starch and Irani, et al. [61] determined an average of 23.6% and 22.5% for a brown and yellow hairless cultivar, respectively, which is typical of most starches [63]. The amylose to amylopectin ratio is indicative of its digestibility because, in general, high amylose starches are harder to digest whereas waxy starches are more readily digested [64].

Starches of the yellow and brown cultivars of glabrous canaryseeds have been extensively compared. Overall, their properties appear similar, but some researchers report differences among the two colored cultivars. Irani, et al. [65] observed differences in starch granule shape between a yellow and brown hairless canaryseed variety (CO5041 and CDC Maria, respectively) in dilute solution. The yellow cultivar starch showed both spherical and ellipsoidal structure, whereas the brown cultivar and wheat starch showed only ellipsoidal structure. An investigation of the rheological properties of canaryseed starches revealed C05041 starch was less sensitive to temperature and with increasing concentration, displayed higher thixotrophy and pseudoplastic behavior as compared to CDC Maria starch [66].

Retrogradation, the process of heating starch in the presence of water followed by cooling, results in a critical change in the ordered amylose/amylopectin structure, and hence, in changes to its physiochemical and functional properties. Although starch retrogradation is mostly considered an undesirable phenomenon, such as its involvement in the staling of bread and sensory and quality loss in high starch foods over time, it also plays a nutritionally important role [67]. The retrogradation process can produce resistant starch (also known as resistant starch 3 (RS3)), because the amylose and amylopectin structures become more compact and therefore resistant to enzymatic hydrolysis. Resistant starch is characterized as starch that remains mostly undigested by enzymes in the small intestine, thereby passing into the large intestine where it undergoes fermentation by the colons microflora [68]. There is no rapid release of glucose into the bloodstream and the starch acts like a prebiotic for the gut microflora. Canaryseed starch demonstrated greater rates of hydrolysis in the presence of pancreatic α-amylase as compared to wheat starch, which could be due to its small granule size and relatively low amylose composition [62]. Nonetheless, canaryseed starch also had a higher tendency for retrogradation, potentially forming RS3, a nutritionally valuable starch. Resistant starches promote probiotic bacteria, lower the glycemic index of foods, have hypocholesterolemic effects, reduce gallstone formation, improve mineral absorption, have high satiety, and aid in weight management [69].

Overall, canaryseed starch does possess unique characteristics as compared to wheat starch. Its properties in dilute solution are similar to that of wheat and demonstrate a potential use as a thickener or stabilizer in food products [61]. Canaryseed starches, although easily digestible, have a higher tendency to retrograde into RS3, which could make them more available for digestion by the colons microflora [61,62]. This functionality, however, would need to be further investigated.

4.2. Fiber

Besides starch and protein, fiber represents a minor component of the total composition of canaryseeds. Canaryseeds consist of approximately 7% dietary fiber, considerably lower compared to other cereal grains, especially wheat, which contains double the amounts on average [4,12,70]. The bran portion of the grain contains more dietary fiber than the whole grain and white flour portions in both canaryseeds and wheat [12]. Several purification steps are usually required to obtain a high purity fiber, due to high contamination with starch and protein. The extraction order also plays a role on fiber extraction purity, since the removal of starch and protein prior to fiber in an ethanol, alkaline, and water wet milling extraction technique results in a higher fiber purity [3]. Overall, canaryseeds still remain a poor source of dietary fiber compared to other grains from the same cereal family.

4.3. Lipids

Similarly to fiber, lipids are minor components of the seeds as compared to starch and protein. To extract oil from canaryseeds, ethanol has proved a very suitable solvent. Abdel-Aal, et al. [3] reported a crude oil content of 8.3% with an extraction efficiency of 75% when the ethanol extraction step was repeated three times. Oil from canaryseed would be produced primarily as a byproduct, since its removal is necessary to obtain purified starch and protein fractions from the seeds.

The crude fat content in glabrous canaryseed is high as compared to other cereal grains and the fatty acids are largely unsaturated (Table 3). Canaryseeds lipids consist of 54% linoleic, 29% oleic, 11% palmitic, 2.4% linolenic, and 1% stearic acids [8]. In comparison, wheat grain lipids consist of 62% linoleic, 16% oleic, 17% palmitic, 4% linolenic, and 1% stearic acids [4]. Diets high in saturated fatty acids have been correlated with increased incidence of chronic heart disease, whereas diets higher in monounsaturated fatty acids (oleic acid) and especially polyunsaturated fatty acids (linoleic acid, linolenic acid) promote cardiovascular health, neurological function, and improved immune response [71]. Canaryseeds contain high amounts of unsaturated fatty acids, which is advantageous for a healthy diet, but could make them prone to oxidation and rancidity. However, the presence of certain antioxidants in canaryseed oil, such as caffeic acid esters, could potentially reduce these detrimental effects [72]. Furthermore, Ben Salah, et al. [73] reported health promoting activity in canaryseed oil, produced from a hairy Tunisian canaryseed variety, which demonstrated antioxidant, antibacterial, and antiacetylcholinesterase activity, which was largely attributed to the high total polyphenol content in the oil.

Table 3. Crude fat and lipid composition of canaryseed and other cereal grains.

	Canaryseed	Wheat	Oat	Barley	Millet
Crude Fat (% dry basis)	6.7	4.4	4.79	3.4	4.7
Reference	[8]	[4]	[14]	[74]	[74]
FA (% total lipids)					
Palmitic (C16)	11.38	16.6	19.2	23.0	7.42
Stearic (C18)	1.22	0.8	1.46	1.12	6.84
Oleic (C18:1)	29.1	16.2	30.8	11.4	16.11
Linoleic (C18:2)	53.39	62.1	46.4	58.8	66.68
Linolenic (C18:3)	2.42	4.0	2.13	7.78	2.48
Reference	[8]	[4]	[75]	[75]	[76]

4.4. Minerals

In terms of nutrients, glabrous canaryseeds contain several essential minerals and are higher in phosphorous, magnesium, and manganese compared to wheat, oat, barley, and millet, nonetheless, although comparable to levels present in wheat, canaryseeds contain less iron and calcium as other cereal grains (Table 4). Canaryseeds contain higher amounts of vitamin B1 (thiamine) as compared to wheat and an equivalent amount of vitamin B2 (riboflavin), but are poor in niacin [12].

Table 4. Nutrient comparison between glabrous canaryseeds and other cereal grains.

Mineral	Canaryseed (mg/100 g)	Wheat Grain (mg/100 g)	Oat Grain (mg/100 g)	Barley (mg/100 g)	Millet (mg/100 g)
Phosphorous	640	430	340	457	288
Magnesium	200	155	140	197	149
Manganese	6.3	5.9	5.1	0.92	0.81
Iron	6.5	4.2	4.5	12.8	20
Zinc	3.9	2.5	3.5	7.4	6.6
Calcium	40	20	62	73.6	51
Potassium	385	355	420	457	280
Reference	[12]	[12]	[77]	[78]	[78]

4.5. Phytochemicals

Phytochemicals, including polyphenols, terpenoids, and alkaloids, are naturally occurring chemicals produced by plants and, when consumed, promote positive overall health. Research indicates that glabrous canaryseeds are a good source of different types of phytochemicals. Ferulic acid is the most abundant phenolic acid in canaryseeds [79–81]. Ferulic acid displays a broad range of health promoting effects, including anti-inflammatory, antidiabetic, antiaging, neuroprotective, radioprotective, and hepatoprotective activity, mainly due to its strong antioxidant activity [82]. Li et al. [81] compared the total phenolic and flavonoid content in nineteen different samples of brown and yellow varieties of canaryseed groats. They found the yellow and brown colored seeds had the same flavonoid profiles and that ferulic acid was the dominating phenolic acid, followed by caffeic and coumaric acid, but unlike their flavonoid profiles, brown cultivars had higher amounts of ferulic and caffeic acid relative to the yellow cultivars [81]. *O*-pentosyl isovitexin, identified as the major flavonoid in canaryseeds, displays diversified activity including anti-hypotensive, anti-inflammatory, antimicrobial, antiplatelet, and antioxidant [81].

Carotenoids are another class of phytochemicals that, when ingested, perform a number of beneficial biological functions, including antioxidant activity, immune response improvement, suppression of reactive oxygen species, and lowering the risk of cardiovascular disease [83]. Cereals in general possess only small amounts of carotenoids as compared to fruits and vegetables, nonetheless, the pigment remains present and concentrated mostly in the bran fraction. The major carotenoids present in cereals are xanthophylls like lutein, zeaxanthin, and β-cryptoxanthin with only small amounts of carotenes [83]. Li and Beta [84] evaluated the total carotenoid content in brown and yellow glabrous canaryseed cultivars and determined lutein, zeaxanthin, and β-carotene were the three major carotenoids present. Surprisingly, β-carotene was present in the largest quantities in all canaryseed varieties and far outweighed the β-carotene content of other crops, including wheat, rice, barley, and corn [84]. The carotenoid content of the brown and yellow canaryseed cultivars were relatively similar, in contrast, canaryseed flour was significantly higher in total carotenoid content (11.28 mg/kg) compared to the whole meal (9.27 mg/kg), and bran (8.32 mg/kg) fractions [84]. The results indicate canaryseed flour is a good source of carotenoids. However, carotenoids are highly sensitive molecules and changes in carotenoid stability during storage and processing still need to be addressed.

4.6. Anti-Nutritional Components

Like all cereal grains, canaryseeds contain certain anti-nutritional factors, including enzyme inhibitors, amylase inhibitors, phytate, and heavy metals. Enzyme inhibitors play important roles in living plants by preventing proteins and carbohydrates from degradation during growth and protection against threats by animals, insects and some microorganisms [11]. Trypsin inhibitor is a type of enzyme inhibitor present in raw cereals and legumes and, upon consumption, could lead to reduced protein and nutrient digestibility and even cause growth inhibition [79]. Likewise, amylase inhibitors form aggregates with amylase, resulting in a reduction of starch digestion when consumed [85].

Phytate can also be considered as both nutritional and anti-nutritional component in cereals. Phytate has chelating properties and could reduce the availability of some essential minerals, like calcium, iron, and zinc, thereby decreasing their absorption in the small intestine, but on the other hand, exhibits antioxidant activity showing positive effects in cancer treatment, hypercholesterolemia, hypercalcuria, and kidney stones [79]. Similarly, heavy metals present in raw cereals are essential to human health and provide beneficial effects (acting as cofactors to essential enzymes and aiding in the production of amines and amino acids).

Abdel-Aal, et al. [79] evaluated the trypsin inhibitor, amylase inhibitor, phytate and heavy metal content in the bran, wholegrain flour, and white flour of hairy canaryseeds, hairless canaryseeds, and wheat. All hairless canaryseed fractions contained significantly more phytate than wheat (28–41%), but no significant difference in trypsin inhibitor content compared to wheat. Canaryseed amylase inhibitor content was higher in the white flour fraction, but lower in the bran fraction as compared to wheat.

With regards to heavy metals, the hairless canaryseed variety CDC Maria contained higher amounts of the essential heavy metals zinc (44.8 mg/kg), nickel (2.27 mg/kg), and copper (38.0 mg/kg) as compared to the wheat control (32.24 mg/kg, 0.34 mg/kg, and 24.4 mg/kg for zinc, nickel, and copper respectively), however, the molybdenum content was higher in wheat (0.64 mg/kg) as compared to CDC Maria (0.51 mg/kg) [79]. There was no significant difference in neutral metal content (antimony, cobalt, selenium, tellurium, tungsten), and toxic metal content (arsenic, cadmium, lead, mercury), between CDC Maria and the wheat control, and all toxic metals were present in acceptable levels to human health for both grains.

In summary, the anti-nutritional components of wheat and glabrous canaryseeds are very similar and the anti-nutrients are present in low enough quantities that they do not outweigh their positive health benefits. To date, no studies compare the anti-nutritional components of multiple varieties of glabrous yellow and brown seeds. Li, et al. [81] reported a difference in phenolic acid content between brown and yellow canaryseed cultivars and a similar trend could exist in terms of their anti-nutritional content.

5. Potential as a Functional Food and Alternative to Major Allergens

Functional foods are a growing trend among consumers today, because consumers not only eat food to satisfy their hunger, but they eat specific foods to maintain or improve their overall health [86]. Although there is no official definition of a functional food, the general idea is their consumption provides exceptional nutritional health benefits above and beyond basic nutrition. Some food products, designated as "superfoods", offer more than one health promoting property and recent superfood trends among consumers include oats, hemp seeds, almonds, kale, acai berries, blueberries, and green tea among others [87–89]. Oats contain large proportions of beta-glucan, a type of water soluble fiber present in the grain that possess several health promoting effects, such as reducing cholesterol and lowering postprandial glucose and insulin levels in the blood, which is especially beneficial for individuals with type II diabetes [90]. Likewise, canaryseeds demonstrate exceptional nutritional qualities, including their antioxidant, antidiabetic, antihypertensive, and even anti-obesity activity. Furthermore, their phytochemical content (phenolic acids, carotenoids, and flavonoids) and relatively low abundance of anti-nutritional factors contribute to their nutritional qualities. The grains themselves could be used as a functional ingredient in food products (such as granola bars, bread, pasta, and cereals) to improve their nutritional value. In addition, canaryseeds are gluten-free. Using canaryseed to replace wheat or gluten-containing cereals will create more options for gluten-sensitive individuals and also produces new opportunities to develop gluten-free products. Moreover, because of their size and shape, canaryseeds offer the possibility to replace sesame seeds in products, such as baked goods, snack foods, and toppings, creating new products for individuals with allergies to sesame seeds.

6. Conclusions

Glabrous canaryseed, technically an ancient grain, is an excellent new source of plant based protein. Confirmation of the broad spectra of its potential bioactivities and health benefits would make this cereal an excellent nutritional and therapeutic aid to help combat non-communicable diseases, including cancer, diabetes, and heart disease. Due to a lack of knowledge, and because the seed is "new", this unique cereal is currently underutilized by consumers and the industry. However, growing trends among consumers, including the consumption of functional foods and gluten-free products, have created high demands in the food industry that can be supported with the use of glabrous canaryseeds.

Author Contributions: E.M., L.L. and A.A. contributed to the process of writing, revising, and editing of the manuscript. S.K contributed to critically revising the manuscript. All authors approved the final version.

Funding: This study has been supported by the Agriculture and Agri-Food Canada's Science and Innovation Strategic Action Plan (Project J-001308).

Conflicts of Interest: The authors declare no conflict of interest.

References

1. Bhatt, T.; Coombs, M.; O'Neill, C. Biogenic silica fibre promotes carcinogenesis in mouse skin. *Int. J. Cancer* **1984**, *34*, 519–528. [CrossRef] [PubMed]
2. Cogliatti, M. Canaryseed crop. *Sci. Agropecu.* **2012**, *3*, 75–88. [CrossRef]
3. Abdel-Aal, E.-S.M.; Hucl, P.; Patterson, C.A.; Gray, D. Fractionation of hairless canary seed (*phalaris canariensis*) into starch, protein, and oil. *J. Agric. Food Chem.* **2010**, *58*, 7046–7050. [CrossRef] [PubMed]
4. Abdel-Aal, E.-S.M.; Hucl, P.J.; Sosulski, F.W. Structural and compositional characteristics of canaryseed (*Phalaris canariensis* L.). *J. Agric. Food Chem.* **1997**, *45*, 3049–3055. [CrossRef]
5. Estrada-Salas, P.A.; Montero-Moran, G.M.; Martinez-Cuevas, P.P.; Gonzalez, C.; Barba de la Rosa, A.P. Characterization of antidiabetic and antihypertensive properties of canary seed (*Phalaris canariensis* L.) peptides. *J. Agric. Food Chem.* **2014**, *62*, 427–433. [CrossRef] [PubMed]

6. Valverde, M.E.; Orona-Tamayo, D.; Nieto-Rendón, B.; Paredes-López, O. Antioxidant and antihypertensive potential of protein fractions from flour and milk substitutes from canary seeds (*Phalaris canariensis* L.). *Plant Foods Hum. Nutr.* **2017**, *72*, 20–25. [CrossRef] [PubMed]
7. Hucl, P.; Matus-Cadiz, M.; Vandenberg, A.; Sosulski, F.W.; Abdel-Aal, E.S.M.; Hughes, G.R.; Slinkard, A.E. Cdc maria annual canarygrass. *Can. J. Plant Sci.* **2001**, *81*, 115–116. [CrossRef]
8. Canaryseed Development Commission of Saskatchewan. about Canaryseed. Available online: https://www.canaryseed.ca/about.html (accessed on 15 March 2017).
9. Matus-Cádiz, M.A.; Hucl, P.; Vandenberg, A. Inheritance of hull pubescence and seed color in annual canarygrass. *Can. J. Plant Sci.* **2003**, *83*, 471–474. [CrossRef]
10. Health Canada. Novel food information—Glabrous canary seed (*Phalaris canariensis* L.). Available online: http://www.hc-sc.gc.ca/fn-an/gmf-agm/appro/canary-seed-lang-graine-alpiste-decision-eng.php#share (accessed on 15 March 2017).
11. Koehler, P.; Wieser, H. Chemistry of cereal grains. In *Handbook on Sourdough Biotechnology*; Gobbetti, M., Gänzle, M., Eds.; Springer: Boston, MA, USA, 2013; pp. 11–45. [CrossRef]
12. Abdel-Aal, E.-S.M.; Hucl, P.; Shea Miller, S.; Patterson, C.A.; Gray, D. Microstructure and nutrient composition of hairless canary seed and its potential as a blending flour for food use. *Food Chem.* **2011**, *125*, 410–416. [CrossRef]
13. Belderok, B.; Mesdag, J.; Donner, D.A. The wheat grain. In *Bread-Making Quality of Wheat: A Century of Breeding in Europe*; Donner, D.A., Ed.; Springer: Dordrecht, The Netherlands, 2000; pp. 15–20.
14. Biel, W.; Bobko, K.; Maciorowski, R. Chemical composition and nutritive value of husked and naked oats grain. *J. Cereal Sci.* **2009**, *49*, 413–418. [CrossRef]
15. Asare, E.K.; Jaiswal, S.; Maley, J.; Båga, M.; Sammynaiken, R.; Rossnagel, B.G.; Chibbar, R.N. Barley grain constituents, starch composition, and structure affect starch in vitro enzymatic hydrolysis. *J. Agric. Food Chem.* **2011**, *59*, 4743–4754. [CrossRef] [PubMed]
16. Nyström, L.; Lampi, A.-M.; Andersson, A.A.M.; Kamal-Eldin, A.; Gebruers, K.; Courtin, C.M.; Delcour, J.A.; Li, L.; Ward, J.L.; Fra, A.; et al. Phytochemicals and dietary fiber components in rye varieties in the healthgrain diversity screen. *J. Agric. Food Chem.* **2008**, *56*, 9758. [CrossRef] [PubMed]
17. Abdalla, A.A.; El Tinay, A.H.; Mohamed, B.E.; Abdalla, A.H. Proximate composition, starch, phytate and mineral contents of 10 pearl millet genotypes. *Food Chem.* **1998**, *63*, 243–246. [CrossRef]
18. Arendt, E.K.; Zannini, E. Wheat and other triticum grains. In *Cereal Grains for the Food and Beverage Industries*; Woodhead Publishing: Cambridge, UK, 2013; pp. 1–67.
19. Tatham, A.S.; Shewry, P.R. Allergens to wheat and related cereals. *Clin. Exp. Allergy* **2008**, *38*, 1712–1726. [CrossRef] [PubMed]
20. Comino, I.; Moreno Mde, L.; Real, A.; Rodríguez-Herrera, A.; Barro, F.; Sousa, C. The gluten-free diet: Testing alternative cereals tolerated by celiac patients. *Nutrients* **2013**, *5*, 4250–4268. [CrossRef] [PubMed]
21. Boye, J.I.; Achouri, A.; Raymond, N.; Cleroux, C.; Weber, D.; Koerner, T.B.; Hucl, P.; Patterson, C.A. Analysis of glabrous canary seeds by elisa, mass spectrometry, and western blotting for the absence of cross-reactivity with major plant food allergens. *J. Agric. Food Chem.* **2013**, *61*, 6102–6112. [CrossRef] [PubMed]
22. Krishnan, H.B.; Chen, M.-H. Identification of an abundant 56 kda protein implicated in food allergy as granule-bound starch synthase. *J. Agric. Food Chem.* **2013**, *61*, 5404–5409. [CrossRef] [PubMed]
23. Esposito, Z.; Belli, L.; Toniolo, S.; Sancesario, G.; Bianconi, C.; Martorana, A. Amyloid β, glutamate, excitotoxicity in alzheimer's disease: Are we on the right track? *CNS Neurosci. Ther.* **2013**, *19*, 549–555. [CrossRef] [PubMed]
24. Zhang, Q.; Xiang, J.; Zhang, L.; Zhu, X.; Evers, J.; van der Werf, W.; Duan, L. Optimizing soaking and germination conditions to improve gamma-aminobutyric acid content in japonica and indica germinated brown rice. *J. Funct. Foods* **2014**, *10*, 283–291. [CrossRef]
25. Pomeranz, Y.; Robbins, G.S.; Briggle, L.W. Amino acid composition of oat groats. *J. Agric. Food Chem.* **1971**, *19*, 536–539. [CrossRef]
26. Ejeta, G.; Hassen, M.M.; Mertz, E.T. In vitro digestibility and amino acid composition of pearl millet (pennisetum typhoides) and other cereals. *Proc. Natl. Acad. Sci. USA* **1987**, *84*, 6016–6019. [CrossRef] [PubMed]

27. World Health Organization (WHO). *Global Status Report on Noncommunicable Diseases*; WHO: Geneva, Switzerland, 2014. Available online: http://www.who.int/nmh/publications/ncd-status-report-2014/en/ (accessed on 15 March 2017).
28. Food and Agriculture Organization (FAO). *Dietary Protein Quality Evaluation in Human Nutrition: Report of an FAO Expert Consultation*; FAO: Rome, Italy, 2013; p. 51. Available online: http://www.fao.org/ag/humannutrition/35978-02317b979a686a57aa4593304ffc17f06.pdf (accessed on 15 March 2017).
29. Patil, P.; Mandal, S.; Tomar, S.K.; Anand, S. Food protein-derived bioactive peptides in management of type 2 diabetes. *Eur. J. Nutr.* **2015**, *54*, 863–880. [CrossRef] [PubMed]
30. Velarde-Salcedo, A.J.; Barrera-Pacheco, A.; Lara-González, S.; Montero-Morán, G.M.; Díaz-Gois, A.; González de Mejia, E.; Barba de la Rosa, A.P. In vitro inhibition of dipeptidyl peptidase iv by peptides derived from the hydrolysis of amaranth (*amaranthus hypochondriacus* L.) proteins. *Food Chem.* **2013**, *136*, 758–764. [CrossRef] [PubMed]
31. Sánchez, A.; Vázquez, A. Bioactive peptides: A review. *Food Qual. Saf.* **2017**, *1*, 29–46. [CrossRef]
32. David, D.K.; Katie, W. Bioactive proteins and peptides from food sources. Applications of bioprocesses used in isolation and recovery. *Curr. Pharm. Des.* **2003**, *9*, 1309–1323. [CrossRef]
33. Perez Gutierrez, R.M.; Madrigales Ahuatzi, D.; Cruz Victoria, T. Inhibition by seeds of *Phalaris canariensis* extracts of key enzymes linked to obesity. *Altern. Ther. Health Med.* **2016**, *22*, 8–14. [PubMed]
34. Perez Gutierrez, R.M.; Mota-Flores, J.M.; Madrigales Ahuatzi, D.; Cruz Victoria, T.; Horcacitas, M.D.C.; Garcia Baez, E. Ameliorative effect of hexane extract of *Phalaris canariensis* on high fat diet-induced obese and streptozotocin-induced diabetic mice. *Evid.-Based Complement. Altern. Med.* **2014**. [CrossRef] [PubMed]
35. Power, O.; Nongonierma, A.B.; Jakeman, P.; FitzGerald, R.J. Food protein hydrolysates as a source of dipeptidyl peptidase iv inhibitory peptides for the management of type 2 diabetes. *Proc. Nutr. Soc.* **2014**, *73*, 34–46. [CrossRef] [PubMed]
36. Chen, J.; Wang, Y.; Zhong, Q.; Wu, Y.; Xia, W. Purification and characterization of a novel angiotensin-i converting enzyme (ace) inhibitory peptide derived from enzymatic hydrolysate of grass carp protein. *Peptides* **2012**, *33*, 52–58. [CrossRef] [PubMed]
37. Iwaniak, A.; Minkiewicz, P.; Darewicz, M. Food-originating ace inhibitors, including antihypertensive peptides, as preventive food components in blood pressure reduction. *Compr. Rev. Food Sci. Food Saf.* **2014**, *13*, 114–134. [CrossRef]
38. Passos, C.S.; Carvalho, L.N.; Pontes, R.B., Jr.; Campos, R.R.; Ikuta, O.; Boim, M.A. Blood pressure reducing effects of *Phalaris canariensis* in normotensive and spontaneously hypertensive rats. *Can. J. Physiol. Pharmacol.* **2012**, *90*, 201–208. [CrossRef] [PubMed]
39. Chanput, W.; Theerakulkait, C.; Nakai, S. Antioxidative properties of partially purified barley hordein, rice bran protein fractions and their hydrolysates. *J. Cereal Sci.* **2009**, *49*, 422–428. [CrossRef]
40. Malomo, S.A.; Aluko, R.E. In vitro acetylcholinesterase-inhibitory properties of enzymatic hemp seed protein hydrolysates. *J. Am. Oil Chem. Soc.* **2016**, *93*, 411–420. [CrossRef]
41. Kchaou, M.; Ben Jannet, H.; Ben Salah, H.; Walha, A.; Allouche, N.; Salah, B.; Abdennabi, R. Antioxidant, antibacterial and antiacetylcholinesterase activities of *Phalaris canariensis* from tunisia. *J. Pharmacogn. Phytochem.* **2015**, *4*, 242–249.
42. Cavazos, A.; Gonzalez de Mejia, E. Identification of bioactive peptides from cereal storage proteins and their potential role in prevention of chronic diseases. *Compr. Rev. Food Sci. Food Saf.* **2013**, *12*, 364–380. [CrossRef]
43. Sabbione, A.C.; Nardo, A.E.; Añón, M.C.; Scilingo, A. Amaranth peptides with antithrombotic activity released by simulated gastrointestinal digestion. *J. Funct. Foods* **2016**, *20*, 204–214. [CrossRef]
44. Yu, G.; Wang, F.; Zhang, B.; Fan, J. In vitro inhibition of platelet aggregation by peptides derived from oat (*avena sativa* L.), highland barley (*Hordeum vulgare* linn. Var. Nudum hook. F.), and buckwheat (*fagopyrum esculentum* moench) proteins. *Food Chem.* **2016**, *194*, 577–586. [CrossRef] [PubMed]
45. Dia, V.P.; Bringe, N.A.; de Mejia, E.G. Peptides in pepsin-pancreatin hydrolysates from commercially available soy products that inhibit lipopolysaccharide-induced inflammation in macrophages. *Food Chem.* **2014**, *152*, 423–431. [CrossRef] [PubMed]

46. Nakurte, I.; Kirhnere, I.; Namniece, J.; Saleniece, K.; Krigere, L.; Mekss, P.; Vicupe, Z.; Bleidere, M.; Legzdina, L.; Muceniece, R. Detection of the lunasin peptide in oats (*Avena sativa* L.). *J. Cereal Sci.* **2013**, *57*, 319–324. [CrossRef]
47. Jeong, H.J.; Jeong, J.B.; Hsieh, C.C.; Hernández-Ledesma, B.; de Lumen, B.O. Lunasin is prevalent in barley and is bioavailable and bioactive in in vivo and in vitro studies. *Nutr. Cancer* **2010**, *62*, 1113–1119. [CrossRef] [PubMed]
48. Maldonado-Cervantes, E.; Jeong, H.J.; León-Galván, F.; Barrera-Pacheco, A.; De León-Rodríguez, A.; González de Mejia, E.; de Lumen, B.O.; Barba de la Rosa, A.P. Amaranth lunasin-like peptide internalizes into the cell nucleus and inhibits chemical carcinogen-induced transformation of nih-3t3 cells. *Peptides* **2010**, *31*, 1635–1642. [CrossRef] [PubMed]
49. Jeong, H.J.; Jeong, J.B.; Kim, D.S.; Park, J.H.; Lee, J.B.; Kweon, D.-H.; Chung, G.Y.; Seo, E.W.; de Lumen, B.O. The cancer preventive peptide lunasin from wheat inhibits core histone acetylation. *Cancer Lett.* **2007**, *255*, 42–48. [CrossRef] [PubMed]
50. Jeong, H.J.; Lee, J.R.; Jeong, J.B.; Park, J.H.; Cheong, Y.-k.; de Lumen, B.O. The cancer preventive seed peptide lunasin from rye is bioavailable and bioactive. *Nutr. Cancer* **2009**, *61*, 680–686. [CrossRef] [PubMed]
51. Nakurte, I.; Klavins, K.; Kirhnere, I.; Namniece, J.; Adlere, L.; Matvejevs, J.; Kronberga, A.; Kokare, A.; Strazdina, V.; Legzdina, L.; et al. Discovery of lunasin peptide in triticale (x *triticosecale wittmack*). *J. Cereal Sci.* **2012**, *56*, 510–514. [CrossRef]
52. Tapal, A.; Vegarud, G.E.; Sreedhara, A.; Hegde, P.; Inamdar, S.; Tiku, P.K. In vitro human gastro-intestinal enzyme digestibility of globulin isolate from oil palm (*Elaeis guineensis* var. *Tenera*) kernel meal and the bioactivity of the digest. *RSC Adv.* **2016**, *6*, 20219–20229. [CrossRef]
53. Sarwar Gilani, G.; Wu Xiao, C.; Cockell, K.A. Impact of antinutritional factors in food proteins on the digestibility of protein and the bioavailability of amino acids and on protein quality. *Br. J. Nutr.* **2012**, *108*, S315–S332. [CrossRef] [PubMed]
54. Newkirk, R.W.; Ram, J.I.; Hucl, P.; Patterson, C.A.; Classen, H.L. A study of nutrient digestibility and growth performance of broiler chicks fed hairy and hairless canary seed (*Phalaris canariensis* L.) products. *Poult. Sci.* **2011**, *90*, 2782–2789. [CrossRef] [PubMed]
55. Classen, H.; Cho, M.; Hucl, P.; Gomis, S.; Patterson, C.A. Performance, health and tissue weights of broiler chickens fed graded levels of hairless hulled yellow and brown canary seed (*Phalaris canariensis* L.). *Can. J. Anim. Sci.* **2014**, *94*, 669–678. [CrossRef]
56. Magnuson, B.A.; Patterson, C.A.; Hucl, P.; Newkirk, R.W.; Ram, J.I.; Classen, H.L. Safety assessment of consumption of glabrous canary seed (*Phalaris canariensis* L.) in rats. *Food Chem. Toxicol.* **2014**, *63*, 91–103. [CrossRef] [PubMed]
57. Thacker, P.A. Performance and carcass characteristics of growing-finishing pigs fed diets containing graded levels of canaryseed. *Can. J. Anim. Sci.* **2003**, *83*, 89–93. [CrossRef]
58. Rajamohamed, S.H.; Aryee, A.N.; Hucl, P.; Patterson, C.A.; Boye, J.I. In vitro gastrointestinal digestion of glabrous canaryseed proteins as affected by variety and thermal treatment. *Plant Foods Hum. Nutr.* **2013**, *68*, 306–312. [CrossRef] [PubMed]
59. Luallen, T. Utilizing starches in product development. In *Starch in Food*; Woodhead Publishing: Cambridge, UK, 2004; pp. 393–424.
60. Goering, K.J.; Schuh, M. New starches. Iii. The properties of the starch from *Phalaris canariensis*. *Cereal Chem.* **1967**, *44*, 532–538.
61. Irani, M.; Abdel-Aal, E.-S.M.; Razavi, S.M.A.; Hucl, P.; Patterson, C.A. Thermal and functional properties of hairless canary seed (*Phalaris canariensis* L.) starch in comparison with wheat starch. *Cereal Chem.* **2017**, *94*, 341–348. [CrossRef]
62. Abdel-Aal, E.-S.M.; Hucl, P.; Sosulski, F.W. Characteristics of canaryseed (*Phalaris canariensis* L.) starch. *Starch/Stärke* **1997**, *49*, 475–480. [CrossRef]
63. Lovegrove, A.; Edwards, C.H.; De Noni, I.; Patel, H.; El, S.N.; Grassby, T.; Zielke, C.; Ulmius, M.; Nilsson, L.; Butterworth, P.J.; et al. Role of polysaccharides in food, digestion, and health. *Crit. Rev. Food Sci. Nutr.* **2017**, *57*, 237–253. [CrossRef] [PubMed]

64. Lehmann, U.; Robin, F. Slowly digestible starch—Its structure and health implications: A review. *Trends Food Sci. Technol.* **2007**, *18*, 346–355. [CrossRef]
65. Irani, M.; Razavi, S.M.; Abdel-Aal el, S.M.; Hucl, P.; Patterson, C.A. Dilute solution properties of canary seed (*Phalaris canariensis*) starch in comparison to wheat starch. *Int. J. Biol. Macromol.* **2016**, *87*, 123–129. [CrossRef] [PubMed]
66. Irani, M.; Razavi, S.M.A.; Abdel-Aal, E.-S.M.; Taghizadeh, M. Influence of variety, concentration, and temperature on the steady shear flow behavior and thixotropy of canary seed (*Phalaris canariensis*) starch gels. *Starch/Stärke* **2016**, *68*, 1203–1214. [CrossRef]
67. Wang, S.; Li, C.; Copeland, L.; Niu, Q.; Wang, S. Starch retrogradation: A comprehensive review. *Compr. Rev. Food Sci. Food Saf.* **2015**, *14*, 568–585. [CrossRef]
68. Masatcioglu, T.M.; Sumer, Z.; Koksel, H. An innovative approach for significantly increasing enzyme resistant starch type 3 content in high amylose starches by using extrusion cooking. *J. Cereal Sci.* **2017**, *74*, 95–102. [CrossRef]
69. Raigond, P.; Ezekiel, R.; Raigond, B. Resistant starch in food: A review. *J. Sci. Food Agric.* **2015**, *95*, 1968–1978. [CrossRef] [PubMed]
70. Robinson, R.G. Chemical composition and potential uses of annual canarygrass. *Agron J.* **1978**, *70*, 797–800. [CrossRef]
71. American Dietetic Association and Dietitians of Canada. Position of the american dietetic association and dietitians of canada: Dietary fatty acids. *J. Am. Diet. Assoc.* **2007**, *107*, 1599–1611. [CrossRef]
72. Takagi, T.; Iida, T. Antioxidant for fats and oils from canary seed: Sterol and triterpene alcohol esters of caffeic acid. *J. Am. Oil. Chem. Soc.* **1980**, *57*, 326–330. [CrossRef]
73. Ben Salah, H.; Kchaou, M.; Ben Abdallah Kolsi, R.; Abdennabi, R.; Ayedi, M.; Gharsallah, N.; Allouche, N. Chemical composition, characteristics profiles and bioactivities of tunisian *Phalaris canariensis* seeds: A potential source of omega-6 and omega-9 fatty acids. *J. Oleo Sci.* **2018**, *67*, 801–812. [CrossRef] [PubMed]
74. Haard, N.F. *Fermented Cereals: A Global Perspective*; Food and Agriculture Organization of the United Nations: Rome, Italy, 1999; Available online: http://www.fao.org/docrep/x2184e/x2184e00.htm#con (accessed on 15 March 2017).
75. Welch, R.W. Fatty acid composition of grain from winter and spring sown oats, barley and wheat. *J. Sci. Food Agric.* **1975**, *26*, 429–435. [CrossRef] [PubMed]
76. Zhang, A.; Liu, X.; Wang, G.; Wang, H.; Liu, J.; Zhao, W.; Zhang, Y. Crude fat content and fatty acid profile and their correlations in foxtail millet. *Cereal Chem.* **2015**, *92*, 455–459. [CrossRef]
77. Frølich, W.; Nyman, M. Minerals, phytate and dietary fibre in different fractions of oat-grain. *J. Cereal Sci.* **1988**, *7*, 73–82. [CrossRef]
78. Ragaee, S.; Abdel-Aal, E.-S.M.; Noaman, M. Antioxidant activity and nutrient composition of selected cereals for food use. *Food Chem.* **2006**, *98*, 32–38. [CrossRef]
79. Abdel-Aal, E.-S.M.; Hucl, P.; Patterson, C.A.; Gray, D. Phytochemicals and heavy metals content of hairless canary seed: A variety developed for food use. *J. Food Sci. Technol.* **2011**, *44*, 904–910. [CrossRef]
80. Chen, Z.; Yu, L.; Wang, X.; Gu, Z.; Beta, T. Changes of phenolic profiles and antioxidant activity in canaryseed (*Phalaris canariensis* L.) during germination. *Food Chem.* **2016**, *194*, 608–618. [CrossRef] [PubMed]
81. Li, W.; Qiu, Y.; Patterson, C.A.; Beta, T. The analysis of phenolic constituents in glabrous canaryseed groats. *Food Chem.* **2011**, *127*, 10–20. [CrossRef]
82. Srinivasan, M.; Sudheer, A.R.; Menon, V.P. Ferulic acid: Therapeutic potential through its antioxidant property. *J. Clin. Biochem. Nutr.* **2007**, *40*, 92–100. [CrossRef] [PubMed]
83. Mellado-Ortega, E.; Hornero-MÈndez, D.M. Carotenoids in cereals: An ancient resource with present and future applications. *Phytochem. Rev.* **2015**, *14*, 873–890. [CrossRef]
84. Li, W.; Beta, T. An evaluation of carotenoid levels and composition of glabrous canaryseed. *Food Chem.* **2012**, *133*, 782–786. [CrossRef]
85. Thompson, L.U. Potential health benefits and problems associated with antinutrients in foods. *Food Res. Int.* **1993**, *26*, 131–149. [CrossRef]
86. Siró, I.; Kápolna, E.; Kápolna, B.; Lugasi, A. Functional food. Product development, marketing and consumer acceptance—A review. *Appetite* **2008**, *51*, 456–467. [CrossRef] [PubMed]

87. Umme Salma, V. Hemp seed and hemp milk: The new super foods? *Infant Child Adolesc. Nutr.* **2009**, *1*, 232–234. [CrossRef]
88. Šamec, D.; Urlić, B.; Salopek-Sondi, B. Kale (*Brassica oleracea* var. *acephala*) as a superfood: Review of the scientific evidence behind the statement. *Crit. Rev. Food Sci. Nutr.* **2018**, 1–37. [CrossRef]
89. van den Driessche, J.J.; Plat, J.; Mensink, R.P. Effects of superfoods on risk factors of metabolic syndrome: A systematic review of human intervention trials. *Food Funct.* **2018**. [CrossRef] [PubMed]
90. Jing, P.; Hu, X. Nutraceutical properties and health benefits of oats. In *Cereals and Pulses*; Wiley-Blackwell: Oxford, UK, 2012; pp. 21–36.

nutrients

MDPI

Article

A Pilot Study for the Detection of Cyclic Prolyl-Hydroxyproline (Pro-Hyp) in Human Blood after Ingestion of Collagen Hydrolysate

Yasutaka Shigemura [1,*], Yu Iwasaki [1], Mana Tateno [1], Asahi Suzuki [2], Mihoko Kurokawa [2], Yoshio Sato [1] and Kenji Sato [3]

1 Department of Nutrition, Faculty of Domestic Science, Tokyo Kasei University, 1-18-1 Kaga, Itabashi-ku, Tokyo 173-8602, Japan; k151907@tokyo-kasei.ac.jp (Y.I.); tateno-m@tokyo-kasei.ac.jp (M.T.); satouy@tokyo-kasei.ac.jp (Y.S.)

2 Q'sai Co., Ltd., 1-7-16 Kusagae, Chuo-ku, Fukuoka City 810-8606, Japan; a_suzuki@kyusai.co.jp (A.S.); kurokawa@kyusai.co.jp (M.K.)

3 Division of Applied Biosciences, Graduate School of Agriculture, Kyoto University, Kitashirakawa Oiwake-Cho, Kyoto 606-8502, Japan; kensato@kais.kyoto-u.ac.jp

* Correspondence: shigemura@tokyo-kasei.ac.jp; Tel.: +81-3-3961-5629

Received: 1 September 2018; Accepted: 20 September 2018; Published: 22 September 2018

Abstract: Levels of short linear hydroxyproline (Hyp)-containing peptides, such as prolyl-hydroxyproline (Pro-Hyp), increase in human blood after the ingestion of collagen hydrolysate, which has been associated with beneficial effects for human skin and joints. The present study demonstrates the presence of a novel food-derived collagen peptide, cyclic Pro-Hyp, in human blood after the ingestion of collagen hydrolysate. The cyclic Pro-Hyp levels in plasma samples were estimated by liquid chromatography mass spectrometry (LC-MS). Cyclic Pro-Hyp levels significantly increased in the plasma after ingestion of collagen hydrolysate, reaching a maximum level after 2 h and then decreasing. The maximum level of cyclic Pro-Hyp in plasma ranged from 0.1413 to 0.3443 nmol/mL, representing approximately 5% of linear Pro-Hyp in plasma after ingestion of collagen hydrolysate. Addition of cyclic Pro-Hyp in medium at 7 nmol/mL significantly enhanced the growth rate of mouse skin fibroblasts on collagen gel more extensively compared to linear Pro-Hyp.

Keywords: cyclic Pro-Hy; Pro-Hyp; collagen hydrolysate; collagen peptides; fibroblasts; mouse skin

---

1. Introduction

Collagen is the most abundant protein in the animal body and accounts for approximately 30% of all human proteins. This protein is present as a major extracellular matrix component in the skin, muscle, cartilage, bone, and tendons. The collagen molecule forms a triple helical structure and contains a unique amino acid, hydroxyproline (Hyp), which specifically exists in collagen [1]. The heat-denatured form of collagen is called gelatin. Gelatin has a collapsed triple helical structure and has been used in foods, pharmaceuticals, cosmetics, and photographic film at the industrial scale. It has been suggested that ingestion of gelatin improves conditions of joints, skin, nails, and hair [2–4]. The enzymatically degraded product of gelatin, referred to as "collagen hydrolysate" or "collagen peptide", has been developed in order to enhance the absorption and solubility of the molecule. Many recent studies have demonstrated that collagen hydrolysate ingestion also has beneficial effects on human joints and skin conditions [2,5–9]. Daily ingestion of collagen hydrolysate alleviates joint pain in athletes and patients with knee osteoarthritis [8,10]. Moreover, daily ingestion of collagen hydrolysate has also been shown to increase the moisture content of the epidermis in women during winter and to promote skin elasticity in women over the age of 50 [6,11]. A combination of daily ingestion of collagen hydrolysate and resistance training for 12 weeks increases muscle strength in sarcopenic patients [12]. These studies demonstrated that the ingestion of collagen hydrolysate can improve skin and joint condition as well as muscle condition, whereas no negative effects of collagen hydrolysate ingestion at 5–10 g/day for 12 weeks have been reported in human studies [13,14].

In 2005, Iwai et al. reported the discovery of Hyp-containing peptides, such as alanyl-hydroxyprolyl-glycine (Ala-Hyp-Gly), prolyl-hydroxyprolyl-glycine (Pro-Hyp-Gly), prolyl-hydroxyproline (Pro-Hyp), isoleucyl-hydroxyproline (Ile-Hyp), leucyl-hydroxyproline (Leu-Hyp), and phenilalanyl-hydroxyproline (Phe-Hyp) in human plasma after ingestion of collagen hydrolysate. They also found that Pro-Hyp was a major component among these food-derived Hyp-containing peptides [15]. Previous cell culture studies have reported on the bioactivities of Pro-Hyp. For example, Nakatani et al. reported that Pro-Hyp inhibited the mineralization of chondrocytes and modulates the expression of Runt-related transcription factor 1 (Runx1) and osteocalcin genes in a murine chondrocytic cell line [16]. Taga et al. reported that the Hyp-containing tripeptides Ala-Hyp-Gly and leucyl-hydroxyprolyl-glycine (Leu-Hyp-Gly) promoted the differentiation of MC3T3-E1 cells [17], and Ohara et al. reported that Pro-Hyp stimulated hyaluronic acid production in cultured synovium cells [13]. In addition, we have demonstrated that Pro-Hyp and hydroxyprolyl-glycine (Hyp-Gly) stimulated the growth of mouse skin fibroblasts on collagen gels [18,19]. These results partially support a mechanism whereby food-derived Hyp-containing peptides are bioactive in the human body and consequently have beneficial effects on human skin and joints after the ingestion of collagen hydrolysate.

Pro-containing dipeptides, such as prolyl-proline (Pro-Pro), prolyl-leucine (Pro-Leu), prolyl-isoleucine (Pro-Ile), prolyl-valine (Pro-Val), and prolyl-phenylalanine (Pro-Phe), have been demonstrated to form a cyclic structure by peptide bond, which is referred to as diketopiperazine [20]. Cyclic Pro-containing dipeptides exist in foods such as bread, beer, coffee, cacao, beer, and beer-brewing byproducts [21–24]. Taga et al. detected some of Hyp-containing cyclic dipeptides in ginger protease-degraded collagen hydrolysate under heating conditions [25]. Additionally, cyclic hydroxyprolyl-serine (Hyp-Ser) has been shown to alleviate hepatitis, and the cyclic forms of isoleucyl-proline (Ile-Pro), phenilalanyl-proline (Phe-Pro), Pro-Val, and leucyl-proline (Leu-Pro) have been found to exert antioxidant effects [26,27]. An in vitro study has reported the conversion of linear Pro-Hyp to cyclic Pro-Hyp, which has a blocked N-terminal region, by heating in alkaline conditions [28]. Cyclic Pro-Hyp might be generated in vivo during the digestion and absorption process of collagen hydrolysate, and may exert additional beneficial effects. However, to our best knowledge, there is no data on the presence of food-derived cyclic Pro-Hyp.

The objectives of the present study were to confirm the presence of cyclic Pro-Hyp in blood after ingestion of collagen hydrolysate in a pilot human study and to elucidate its biological activity.

2. Materials and Methods

2.1. Collagen Hydrolysate

Collagen hydrolysate that was prepared from porcine (*Sus scrofa domesticus*) skin gelatin by enzymatic hydrolysis was a kind gift from Qsai (Fukuoka, Japan); this product can be obtained commercially. The preparation mainly consisted of peptides with a molecular weight of 3000 Da.

2.2. Chemicals

A standard mixture of amino acids (Type H), Hyp, acetonitrile (high-performance liquid chromatography (HPLC)-grade), trifluoroacetic acid (TFA), and phenyl isothiocyanate (PITC) were purchased from Wako Chemicals (Osaka, Japan). All other reagents were of analytical grade or better. Pro-Hyp and Hyp-Gly were purchased from Bachem (Bubendort, Switzerland). An AG 50W-×8, ion exchanger resin was purchased from Bio-Rad Laboratories (Hercules, CA,

USA). The AccQ Tag was purchased from Waters (Milford, MA, USA), and consisted of the 6-aminoquinolyl-N-hydroxysuccinimidyl carbamate reagent (AccQ), acetonitrile, and 0.2 mM sodium borate buffer (pH 8.8). Dulbecco's modified Eagle's medium (DMEM) and Dulbecco's phosphate-buffered saline were purchased from Sigma Chemicals (St. Louis, MO, USA). Gentamicin was obtained from Invitrogen (Carlsbad, CA, USA), and a BWT S-1820, fetal bovine serum (FBS) was obtained from Biowest (Nuaillé, France). Calf acid-soluble type I collagen solution (0.3%) was purchased from Nippi (Tokyo, Japan), and the Cell Counting Kit-8 was purchased from Dojin Glocal (Kumamoto, Japan).

2.3. *Preparation of Cyclic Pro-Hyp*

Cyclic Pro-Hyp was prepared according to the method of Kibrick et al. Linear Pro-Hyp was heated in 0.02 M ammonia solution at 50 °C overnight [28]. Cyclic Pro-Hyp in heated samples was isolated using an LC-20 series HPLC system (Shimadzu, Kyoto, Japan). Cyclic Pro-Hyp was resolved on an Inertsil ODS-3 250 × 4.6 mm column (GL Science, Tokyo, Japan). Binary gradient elution was performed with 0.01% TFA (solvent A) and 60% acetonitrile (solvent B) at a flow rate of 1 mL/min. The column was equilibrated with 15% B. The gradient profile was as follows: 0–30 min, 15–75% B; 30–35 min, 75–100% B; 35–40 min, 100% B; 40–40.1 min, 100–15% B; and 40.1–50 min, 15% B. The column was maintained at 45 °C, and the absorbance at 214 nm was monitored. As shown in Figure 1, Pro-Hyp, peak 1 with $[M+H]^+$ ions of m/z 211.13, disappeared with the ammonia treatment and peak 2 with m/z corresponding to cyclic Pro-Hyp was generated. Cyclic peptide formation was calculated using the following equation. Cyclic formation (%) = 100 − (linear peptide peak area before heat treatment − linear peptide peak area after heat treatment)/linear peptide peak area before heat treatment × 100.

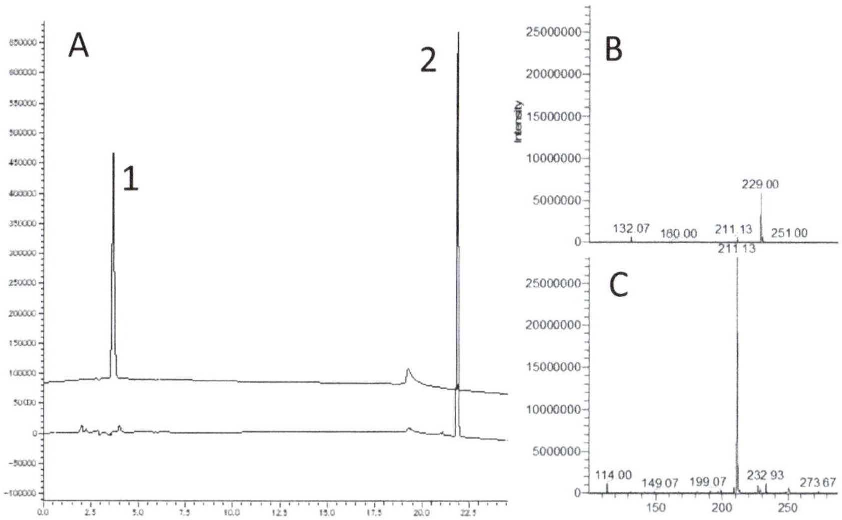

Figure 1. High-performance liquid chromatography (HPLC) and electrospray ionization mass spectrometry (ESI-MS) of linear and cyclic prolyl-hydroxyproline (Pro-Hyp). (**A**) The HPLC chromatogram peaks of (1) the linear Pro-Hyp and (2) after heating at 50 °C in 0.02 M ammonia solution. (**B**) Electrospray ionization mass spectra of peaks 1 and (**C**) 2 recovered from HPLC.

2.4. *Human Study*

The human studies were carried out according to a protocol described previously [15,29,30]. These studies were performed according to the Helsinki Declaration under the supervision of medical doctors and were approved by the experimental ethical committees of the Qsai Corporation (Fukuoka,

Japan). No negative effects were reported by collagen hydrolysate ingestion at 5–10 g/day for 12 weeks in human studies [13,14] and the safety of high-dose collagen hydrolysate ingestion (1.66 g/kg body weight) was also confirmed by animal experiments [31]. The volunteers were informed of the objectives of the present study and the potential risks of ingestion of collagen hydrolysate, such as diarrhea and abdominal pain. Before the experiment, five healthy female volunteers (age 40.8 ± 9.31 years, average body weight 63.6 ± 7.33 g) fasted for 12 h and then ingested the 5 g collagen hydrolysate dissolved in 200 mL water (Figure 2). Approximately 10 mL of venous blood were collected from the cubital vein before and 30, 60, 120, 240, 360, and 480 min after the ingestion. Plasma prepared from venous blood samples was then deproteinized by adding three volumes of ethanol [13,15], and the ethanol-soluble fraction was stored at −80 °C until analysis.

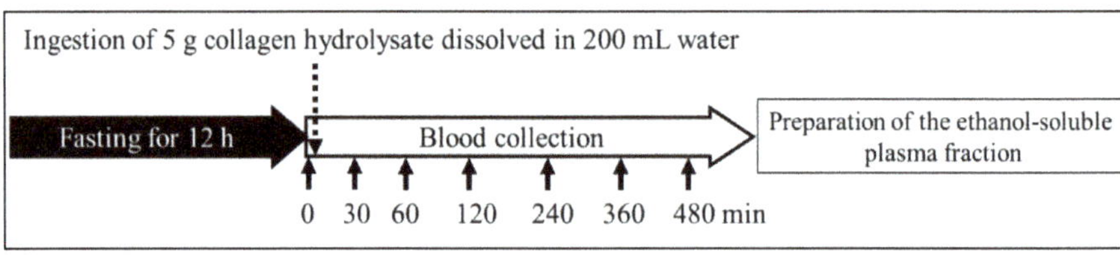

Figure 2. Design of the human study. Blood samples were collected before and after the ingestion of collagen hydrolysate.

2.5. Separation of Linear and Cyclic Pro-Hyp from Human Plasma by Strong-Cation Exchange Resin

Ethanol-soluble plasma fractions were treated with strong cation exchanger (AG50), (Figure 3). The N-terminus of the free peptides adsorbed to AG50 under acidic conditions, but those with a blocked N-terminal region did not. AG50 non-adsorbed and adsorbed plasma fractions were recovered as cyclic and linear peptide fractions, respectively.

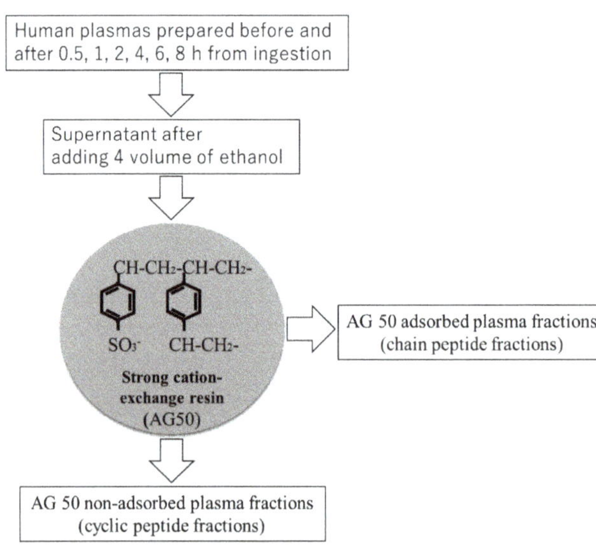

Figure 3. Diagram of the separation procedure for cyclic and linear peptide fractions from human plasma before and after ingestion of collagen hydrolysate.

2.6. Estimation of Hyp-Containing Peptide Concentration

Amino acid analysis was performed according to the method of Bidlingmeyer et al. with slight modifications [32,33]. Amino acids in the cyclic peptide fractions of plasma were derivatized with PITC, and the resulting phenyl thiocarbamoyl amino acids were resolved on a LiChro CART 250 × 4.0 mm column (Kanto Kagaku, Tokyo, Japan) using an LC-20 series HPLC system (Shimadzu). Binary gradient elution was performed with 150 mM ammonium acetate containing 5% acetonitrile (pH 6.0; solvent A) and 60% acetonitrile (solvent B) as the mobile phases at a flow rate of 0.5 mL/min. The column was equilibrated with 100% solvent A prior to the analysis. The gradient profile was as follows: 0–0.1 min, 0% B; 0.1–1.01 min, 0–10% B; 1.01–20 min, 10–47.5% B; 20–25 min, 47.5–100% B; 25–37 min, 100% B; 37–37.1 min, 100–0% B; and 37.1–50 min, 0% B. The column was maintained at 45 °C, and the absorbance of the eluate was monitored at 254 nm. The levels of Hyp-containing peptides in the ethanol-soluble fraction were estimated by subtracting the concentration of free Hyp from that of total Hyp in the HCl hydrolysate, as described previously [13,15,19,30].

2.7. Liquid Chromatograph–Mass Spectrometer (LC-MS) Analysis

LC-MS was carried out using an LC-MS-2020 equipped with a Prominence HPLC system (Shimadzu) in ESI-positive ion mode. An Inertsil ODS-3 column (150 × 2.1 mm; GL Science, Tokyo, Japan) was eluted with a binary gradient of 0.01% TFA (solvent A) and 100% acetonitrile (solvent B) at a flow rate of 0.2 mL/min. The column was equilibrated with 100% A. The gradient profile was as follows: 0–2.5 min, 0% B; 2.0–15.0 min, 0–28% B; 15.0–15.1 min, 28–60% B; 15.1–20.0 min, 60%; and 20.0–30.0 min, 0% B. The column was maintained at 45 °C, and the absorbance at 214 nm was monitored. The MS was operated with nebulizer gas flow of 1.5 L/min, drying gas flow of 15 L/min, ESI voltage of 1.8 kV, temperature of 250 °C. For detection of linear and cyclic Pro-Hyp in human plasma, linear and cyclic peptide fractions were derivatized with AccQ and analyzed under the same conditions.

2.8. Cell Culture

BALB/c mice were purchased from SLC Japan (Shizuoka, Japan). Fibroblasts were obtained from the skin of mice as described by Rittié et al., with slight modifications [18,34]. The abdominal skin was cut into square pieces (approximately 6–7 mm in width), and eight pieces were placed at the bottom of a culture dish (75 mm in diameter) such that they were not in contact with each other. Cultivation was carried out in 8 mL DMEM containing 584 mg/L L-glutamine, 0.01 mg/mL gentamicin, and 10% FBS in a humidified incubator at 37 °C under 5% CO_2. During cultivation, the medium was changed every 2 days. After cultivation for 2 weeks, the skin discs were removed, and fibroblasts were recovered using a 0.25% trypsin-ethylenediaminetetraacetic acid solution. The primary cultured fibroblasts were suspended to give a concentration of 5×10^4 cells/mL in DMEM containing 584 mg/L L-glutamine, 0.01 mg/mL gentamicin, 10% FBS, and the test component. The fibroblasts were then incubated on a collagen gel-coated plate as described previously with 7 nmol/mL linear or cyclic Pro-Hyp. The collagen solution (0.5%) was mixed with the same volume of the double-concentrated DMEM medium containing L-glutamine, gentamicin, and the test component in the absence of FBS. The mixture (100 µL) was then poured into the wells of 96-well plastic plates, and the plates were incubated in a humidified incubator for 24 h at 37 °C under 5% CO_2 to allow gelation. Growth of the cells on the gel after suitable intervals was estimated using Cell Counting Kit-8.

2.9. Statistical Analysis

The differences between the means were evaluated by analysis of variance, followed by Fisher's protected least significant difference method ($p < 0.05$) using Excel-Toukei 2010 (Social Survey Research Information Co., Ltd. Tokyo, Japan).

3. Results

3.1. Preparation of Cyclic Pro-Hyp

We prepared cyclic Pro-Hyp according to the method of Kibrick et al. by heating linear Pro-Hyp under alkaline conditions. As shown in Figure 1A, peaks 1 and 2 appeared in the HPLC chromatogram before and after heating of the Pro-Hyp sample, respectively. The $[M+H]^+$ ions were detected at m/z 229.00 and 211.13, respectively, corresponding to the molecular weight plus H+ of linear and cyclic Pro-Hyp, respectively (Figure 1B,C). The percentage of cyclic Pro-Hyp formation compared with total Pro-Hyp before heat treatment was 97.72% ± 0.79%, and the prepared cyclic Pro-Hyp was used as a standard cyclic peptide. Additionally, we examined the percentage of cyclic Hyp-Gly formation using the same technique as for preparation of cyclic Pro-Hyp; the results showed that the rate of Hyp-Gly formation was approximately half that of Pro-Hyp (43.01% ± 1.12%).

3.2. Hyp Concentration in Plasma Cyclic Peptide Fractions

To examine the presence of cyclic Hyp-containing peptides in human plasma, Hyp-containing peptide concentrations in plasma cyclic peptide fractions of five volunteers were estimated by HPLC. As shown in the chromatogram in Figure 4, Hyp peaks in hydrolyzed cyclic peptide fractions prepared from mixed plasma of five volunteers increased at 1, 2, and 4 h after ingestion; the concentrations of cyclic Hyp peptides in these samples were 2.62, 2.27, and 1.00 nmol/mL, respectively. This result was indicative of the presence of an increase in cyclic Hyp-containing peptides in human plasma after ingestion of collagen hydrolysate.

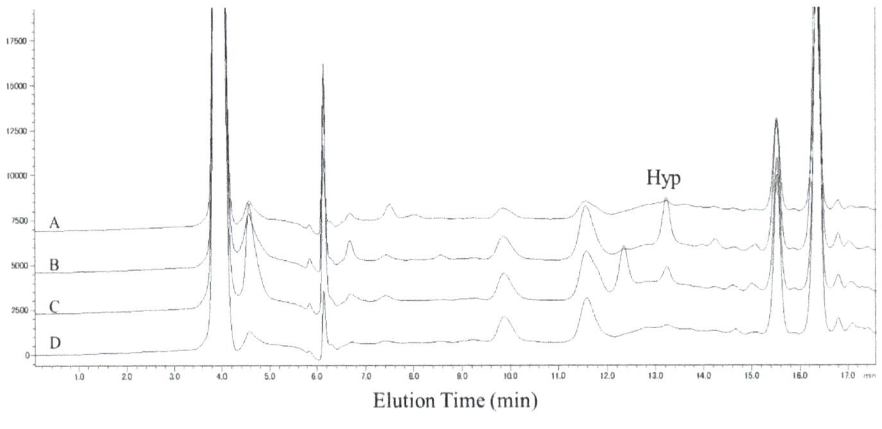

Figure 4. Amino acid analysis of the cyclic peptide fraction of mixed plasma samples from five volunteers. Cyclic peptide fractions prepared before (A) and at 1 (B), 2 (C), and 4 h (D) after ingestion of collagen hydrolysate were resolved by HPLC. Hydroxyproline peaks (Hyp) were observed in chromatograms of samples.

3.3. Changes in the Concentration of Cyclic Pro-Hyp in Human Plasma

Cyclic Pro-Hyp concentrations in the plasma of the volunteers began to increase after ingestion of collagen hydrolysate (Figure 5). The concentrations of cyclic Pro-Hyp reached a maximum after 2 h and then decreased after 4 h from ingestion of collagen hydrolysate. Differences in the maximum level of cyclic Pro-Hyp in the plasma among volunteers (0.1413–0.3443 nmol/mL) were observed, and the highest level was twice that of the lowest level, although the changes in concentrations within volunteers showed similar profiles. As shown in Figure 6, we estimated the average concentrations of linear and cyclic Pro-Hyp in human plasma after ingestion of collagen hydrolysate. The maximum levels of linear and cyclic Pro-Hyp were 3.867 and 0.2086 nmol/mL, respectively. The maximum concentration of cyclic Pro-Hyp was approximately 5% that of linear Pro-Hyp in human plasma. Changes in the concentrations of both peptides showed similar profiles, as significant increases were observed at 1 and 2 h after ingestion of collagen hydrolysate compared with that before ingestion.

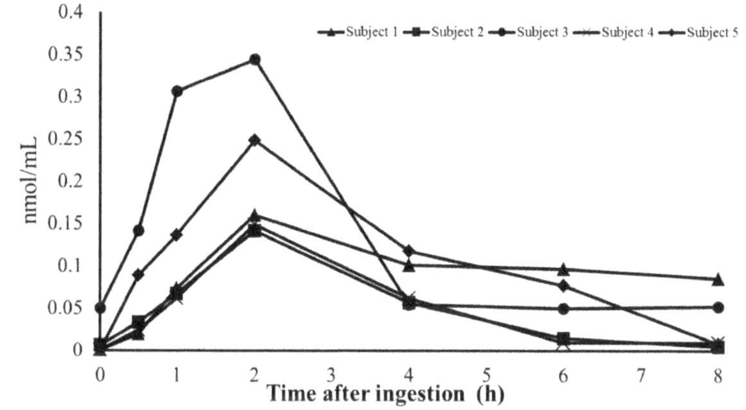

Figure 5. Changes in the concentration of cyclic Pro-Hyp in human plasma of five volunteers.

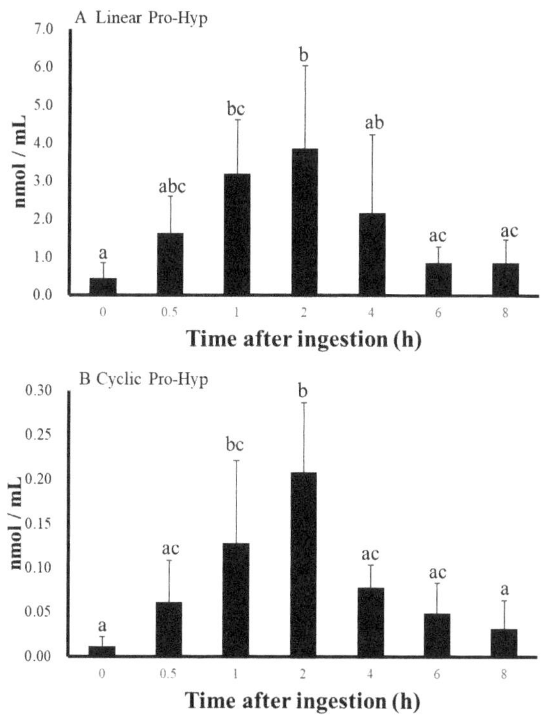

Figure 6. Changes in the average concentrations of linear (**A**) and cyclic (**B**) Pro-Hyp in human plasma of five volunteers. Data are shown as means ± SDs (n = 5). Different letters adjacent to data points indicate significant differences ($P < 0.05$).

3.4. Cell Culture

To examine the bio-activities of cyclic Pro-Hyp, we examined its effect on the growth of mouse skin fibroblasts on collagen gel (Figure 7). The growth rate of skin fibroblasts on the collagen gel after incubation for 1, 2, and 4 days was significantly enhanced in the presence of cyclic Pro-Hyp compared with that observed in control cells or in fibroblasts in the presence of Pro-Hyp.

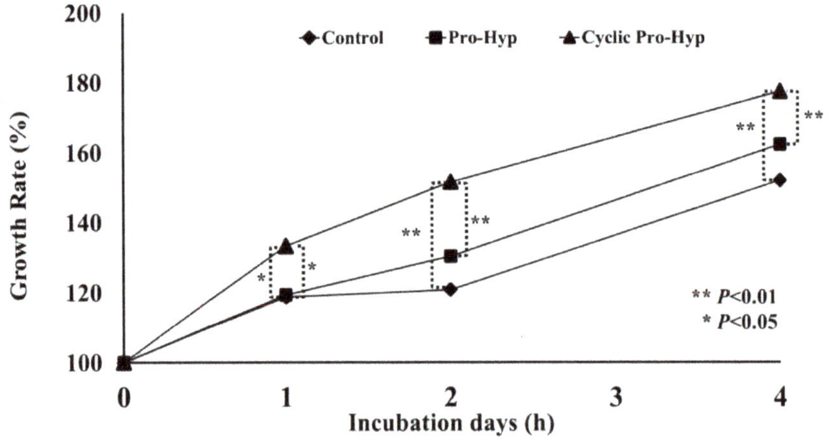

Figure 7. Growth rates of mouse skin fibroblasts on collagen gel. Growth rates were estimated after 0, 1, 2, and 4 days of incubation in the presence of linear (■) and cyclic (▲) Pro-Hyp or in the absence (●) of both peptides. ** and * indicate significant differences ($P < 0.01$ and $P < 0.05$, respectively).

4. Discussion

The present study is the first report describing the detection of cyclic Pro-Hyp from human plasma after ingestion of collagen hydrolysate. Taga et al. reported the presence of cyclic Ala-Hyp and cyclic Leu-Hyp in collagen hydrolysate prepared by enzymatic digestion of ginger protease and found that ingestion of collagen hydrolysate increased the levels of cyclic Hyp-containing peptides in mouse blood [25]. In contrast, the collagen hydrolysates used in the present study contained only 0.0104% cyclic Hyp-containing peptides. This result suggested that cyclic Pro-Hyp formation may occur after digestion of collagen hydrolysate or absorption in human blood. If cyclic Pro-Hyp formation occurs in human blood, the time at which the maximum level of cyclic Pro-Hyp was reached could be delayed compared with that of linear Pro-Hyp. Thus, changes in the concentrations of both types of Pro-Hyp peptides showed similar profiles, and cyclic Pro-Hyp formation may have occurred before absorption in human blood. However, it is also possible that cyclic Pro-Hyp formation could have occurred artificially during the experimental procedures, e.g., through heat drying in ethanol. Accordingly, we estimated the concentrations of cyclic Pro-Hyp before and after heating of linear Pro-Hyp in ethanol. The contents of cyclic Pro-Hyp in total Pro-Hyp before and after heating in ethanol were approximately 0.5582% and 0.6083%, respectively.

Because enhancement of cyclic Pro-Hyp formation during the experimental procedure was very low, cyclic Pro-Hyp, which was found in human blood in the present study, may not be an artificial cyclic peptide. Kwak et al. reported that lactic acid bacteria in foods can produce cyclic dipeptides [35,36]. Additionally, Liu et al. reported that cyclic Hyp-Ser JBP485 was absorbed by the intestine after oral administration by the intestinal peptide transporter 1 (PEPT1) [26,37]. In addition to these reports, the present results indicated that the digestion of collagen hydrolysate in digestive organs could produce cyclic Hyp-peptides and that the peptide could be absorbed via peptide transporter through the small intestine. In contrast, Taga et al. reported that cyclic Hyp-containing dipeptides could be produced by heating of linear Hyp-containing tripeptides [25]. This report also suggested the possibility for production of cyclic Hyp-containing dipeptides from the Hyp-containing tripeptides derived from digested collagen hydrolysate.

Notably, the concentration of cyclic Hyp-containing peptides in human plasma was higher than that of cyclic Pro-Hyp, and this result indicated that other cyclic Hyp-containing peptides may exist in the human blood after ingestion of collagen hydrolysate. Over 15 Hyp-containing linear peptides have been identified in human blood after ingestion of collagen hydrolysate [38]. Thus, the cyclic forms of these Hyp-containing peptides could be increased in human blood after ingestion of collagen hydrolysate. The present results showed that cyclic Hyp-Gly formation was significantly lower than total Pro-Hyp. Different rates of cyclic peptide formation between Pro-Hyp and Hyp-Gly may cause increases in the levels of cyclic Hyp peptides in human blood after ingestion of collagen hydrolysate. Although the detailed mechanisms mediating the formation of cyclic peptides after ingestion of collagen hydrolysate have not been clarified, previous studies have reported the occurrence of cyclic dipeptides in fermented food or/and enzyme-treated products; thus, enzymatic activities may be related to cyclic dipeptide formation [35,36,39]. Therefore, differences in the maximum levels of cyclic Pro-Hyp in the blood of individual volunteers could have occurred via different efficacies of digestive enzymes for the formation of cyclic Hyp-containing peptides or via absorption of these peptides by a peptide transporter.

Our previous study demonstrated that addition of 200 nmol/mL linear Pro-Hyp in cell culture medium significantly enhanced mouse skin fibroblasts on collagen gel compared with that in the absence of Pro-Hyp [18]. The present study revealed that 7 nmol/mL cyclic Pro-Hyp caused a significant increase in the growth rates of skin fibroblasts on collagen gel compared with the same concentration of linear Pro-Hyp. This result suggested that the increase in cyclic Pro-Hyp in human blood after ingestion of collagen hydrolysate could effectively enhance wound healing process in damaged skin tissues. Differences in both types of Pro-Hyp were observed with regard to its hydrophobicity, as shown by the different elution times for HPLC separation and in the different molecular structures of the molecules. Similarly, previous reports have shown that short peptides with high hydrophobicity exhibit high uptake by cells [40], and cyclic peptide formation could enhance cell incorporation of Pro-Hyp. Although the mechanisms mediating the enhancement of fibroblast growth have not been fully clarified, differences in hydrophobicity and incorporation of both types of Pro-Hyp could be related to growth enhancement of skin fibroblasts on collagen gel. However, the concentration of cyclic Pro-Hyp detected in human blood was significantly lower than that of linear Pro-Hyp after ingestion of collagen hydrolysate. Thus, in order to enhance the efficacy of collagen hydrolysate, it is necessary to promote the absorption of cyclic Pro-Hyp in human blood. Fermentation or treatment of food-derived enzymes could enhance the occurrence and absorption of cyclic Hyp-containing peptides in human blood. Additional studies on the formation of cyclic dipeptides using food-derived enzymes and the examination of its absorption in human blood are now in progress.

5. Conclusions

In summary, cyclic Pro-Hyp was detected in human plasma from five volunteers after ingestion of collagen hydrolysate. The maximum level was reached 2 h after ingestion of collagen hydrolysate, and the average concentration was 0.2086 nmol/mL. Cyclic Pro-Hyp enhanced the growth rate of mouse skin fibroblasts on collagen gel. These results suggested that the increase in cyclic Pro-Hyp in human blood after ingestion of collagen hydrolysate could effectively enhance the wound healing process in damaged skin tissues.

Author Contributions: data curation, Y.S., Y.I., M.T., and A.S.; formal analysis, Y.S. and Y.I.; investigation, Y.S. and A.S.; project administration, A.S., M.K., and Y.S.; resources, A.S. and M.K.; supervision, Y.S. and K.S.; writing—original draft, Y.S.; writing—review and editing, Y.S. and K.S.

Funding: This work was supported by a Grant-in-Aid for Scientific Research (C) (No. 17K00906) of The Ministry of Education, Culture, Sports, Science, and Technology, Japan.

Acknowledgments: The authors wish to acknowledge Dr. Tomoaki Kawaguchi of Fukuoka Industrial Technology Center, for his technical advice on preparing cyclic Pro-Hyp. Finally, we are grateful to the referees for useful comments.

Conflicts of Interest: The authors declare no conflict of interest.

References

1. Prockop, D.J. Collagens: Molecular Biology, Diseases, and Potentials for Therapy. *Annu. Rev. Biochem.* **1995**, *64*, 403–434. [CrossRef] [PubMed]
2. Moskowitz, R.W. Role of collagen hydrolysate in bone and joint disease. *Semin. Arthritis Rheum.* **2000**, *30*, 87–99. [CrossRef] [PubMed]
3. Tyson, T.L. The effect of gelatin on finger nails. *J. Investig. Dermatol.* **1950**, *14*, 323–325. [CrossRef] [PubMed]
4. Scala, J.; Hollies, N.R.S.; Sucher, K.P. Effect of daily gelatin ingestion on human scalp hair. *Nutr. Rep. Int.* **1976**, *13*, 579–592.
5. Kuwaba, K.; Koyama, Y.I.; Koikeda, T.; Tsukada, Y. Effects of collagen peptide ingestion on skin properties-placebo-controlled double-blind trial. *Jpn. Pharmacol. Ther.* **2014**, *42*, 995–1004.
6. Proksch, E.; Schunck, M.; Zague, V.; Segger, D.; Degwert, J.; Oesser, S. Oral intake of specific bioactive collagen peptides reduces skin wrinkles and increases dermal matrix synthesis. *Skin Pharmacol. Physiol.* **2014**, *27*, 113–119. [CrossRef] [PubMed]
7. Proksch, E.; Segger, D.; Degwert, J.; Schunck, M.; Zague, V.; Oesser, S. Oral supplementation of specific collagen peptides has beneficial effects on human skin physiology: A double-blind, placebo-controlled study. *Skin Pharmacol. Physiol.* **2013**, *27*, 47–55. [CrossRef] [PubMed]
8. Clark, K.L.; Sebastianelli, W.; Flechsenhar, K.R.; Aukermann, D.F.; Meza, F.; Millard, R.L.; Deitch, J.R.; Sherbondy, P.S.; Albert, A. 24-Week study on the use of collagen hydrolysate as a dietary supplement in athletes with activity-related joint pain. *Curr. Med. Res. Opin.* **2008**, *24*, 1485–1496. [CrossRef] [PubMed]
9. Kumar, S.; Sugihara, F.; Suzuki, K.; Inoue, N.; Venkateswarathirukumara, S. A double-blind, placebo-controlled, randomised, clinical study on the effectiveness of collagen peptide on osteoarthritis. *J. Sci. Food Agric.* **2014**, *95*, 702–707. [CrossRef] [PubMed]
10. Deal, C.L.; Moskowitz, R.W. Nutraceuticals as therapeutic agents in osteoarthritis. The role of glucosamine, chondroitin sulfate, and collagen hydrolysate. *Rheum. Dis. Clin. N. Am.* **1999**, *25*, 379–395. [CrossRef]
11. Matsumoto, H.; Ohara, H.; Itoh, K.; Nakamura, Y.; Takahashi, S. Clinical effect of fish type I collagen hydrolysate on skin properties. *ITE Lett.* **2006**, *7*, 386–390.
12. Zdzieblik, D.; Oesser, S.; Baumstark, M.W.; Gollhofer, A.; König, D. Collagen peptide supplementation in combination with resistance training improves body composition and increases muscle strength in elderly sarcopenic men: A randomised controlled trial. *Br. J. Nutr.* **2015**, *114*, 1237–1245. [CrossRef]
13. Ohara, H.; Iida, H.; Ito, K.; Takeuchi, Y.; Nomura, Y. Effects of Pro-Hyp, a collagen hydrolysate-derived peptide, on hyaluronic acid synthesis using in vitro cultured synovium cells and oral ingestion of collagen hydrolysates in a guinea pig model of osteoarthritis. *Biosci. Biotechnol. Biochem.* **2010**, *74*, 2096–2099. [CrossRef] [PubMed]
14. Trč, T.; Bohmová, J. Efficacy and tolerance of enzymatic hydrolysed collagen (EHC) vs. glucosamine sulphate (GS) in the treatment of knee osteoarthritis (KOA). *Int. Orthop.* **2011**, *35*, 341–348. [CrossRef] [PubMed]
15. Iwai, K.; Hasegawa, T.; Taguchi, Y.; Morimatsu, F.; Sato, K.; Nakamura, Y.; Higashi, A.; Kido, Y.; Nakabo, Y.; Ohtsuki, K. Identification of food-derived collagen peptides in human blood after oral ingestion of gelatin hydrolysates. *J. Agric. Food Chem.* **2005**, *53*, 6531–6536. [CrossRef] [PubMed]
16. Nakatani, S.; Mano, H.; Sampei, C.; Shimizu, J.; Wada, M. Chondroprotective effect of the bioactive peptide prolyl-hydroxyproline in mouse articular cartilage in vitro and in vivo. *Osteoarthr. Cartil.* **2009**, *17*, 1620–1627. [CrossRef] [PubMed]
17. Taga, Y.; Kusubata, M.; Ogawa-Goto, K.; Hattori, S.; Funato, N. Collagen-derived X-Hyp-Gly-type tripeptides promote differentiation of MC3T3-E1 pre-osteoblasts. *J. Funct. Foods* **2018**, *46*, 456–462. [CrossRef]
18. Shigemura, Y.; Iwai, K.; Morimatsu, F.; Iwamoto, T.; Mori, T.; Oda, C.; Taira, T.; Park, E.Y.; Nakamura, Y.; Sato, K. Effect of prolyl-hydroxyproline (Pro-Hyp), a food-derived collagen peptide in human blood, on growth of fibroblasts from mouse skin. *J. Agric. Food Chem.* **2009**, *57*, 444–479. [CrossRef] [PubMed]

19. Shigemura, Y.; Akaba, S.; Kawashima, E.; Park, E.Y.; Nakamura, Y.; Sato, K. Identification of a novel food-derived collagen peptide, hydroxyprolyl-glycine, in human peripheral blood by pre-column derivatisation with phenyl isothiocyanate. *Food Chem.* **2011**, *129*, 1019–1024. [CrossRef] [PubMed]
20. Deppermann, N.; Prenzel, A.H.G.P.; Beitat, A.; Maison, W. Synthesis of proline-based diketopiperazine scaffolds. *J. Org. Chem.* **2009**, *74*, 4267–4271. [CrossRef] [PubMed]
21. Ginz, M.; Engelhardt, U.H. Identification of proline-based diketopiperazines in roasted coffee. *J. Agric. Food Chem.* **2000**, *48*, 3528–3532. [CrossRef] [PubMed]
22. Ryan, L.A.M.; Fabio, D.B.; Arendt, E.K.; Koehler, P. Detection and quantitation of 2,5-diketopiperazines in wheat sourdough and bread. *J. Agric. Food Chem.* **2009**, *48*, 3528–3532. [CrossRef] [PubMed]
23. Poerschmann, J.; Koehler, R.; Weiner, B. Identification and quantification of 2,5-diketopiperazine platform biochemicals along with pyrazines and pyridinols in the dissolved organic matter phase after hydrothermal carbonization of brewer's spent grain. *Environ. Technol. Innov.* **2016**, *5*, 95–105. [CrossRef]
24. Gautschi, M.; Schmid, J.P.; Peppard, T.L.; Ryan, T.P.; Tuorto, R.M.; Yang, X. Chemical Characterization of Diketopiperazines in Beer. *J. Agric. Food Chem.* **1997**, *45*, 3183–3189. [CrossRef]
25. Taga, Y.; Kusubata, M.; Ogawa-Goto, K.; Hattori, S. Identification of Collagen-Derived Hydroxyproline (Hyp)-Containing Cyclic Dipeptides with High Oral Bioavailability: Efficient Formation of Cyclo(X-Hyp) from X-Hyp-Gly-Type Tripeptides by Heating. *J. Agric. Food Chem.* **2017**, *65*, 9514–9521. [CrossRef] [PubMed]
26. Liu, K.X.; Kato, Y.; Kaku, T.I.; Santa, T.; Imai, K.; Yagi, A.; Ishizu, T.; Sugiyama, Y. Hydroxyprolylserine derivatives JBP923 and JBP485 exhibit the antihepatitis activities after gastrointestinal absorption in rats. *J. Pharmacol. Exp. Ther.* **2000**, *294*, 510–515. [PubMed]
27. Takaya, Y.; Furukawa, T.; Miura, S.; Akutagawa, T.; Hotta, Y.; Ishikawa, N.; Niwa, M. Antioxidant constituents in distillation residue of Awamori spirits. *J. Agric. Food Chem.* **2007**, *55*, 75–79. [CrossRef] [PubMed]
28. Kibrick, A.C.; Hashiro, C.Q.; Schutz, R.S.; Walters, M.I.; Milhorat, A.T. Prolylhydroxyproline in urine: Its determination and observations in muscular dystrophy. *Clin. Chim. Acta* **1964**, *10*, 344–351. [CrossRef]
29. Shigemura, Y.; Kubomura, D.; Sato, Y.; Sato, K. Dose-dependent changes in the levels of free and peptide forms of hydroxyproline in human plasma after collagen hydrolysate ingestion. *Food Chem.* **2014**, *159*, 328–332. [CrossRef] [PubMed]
30. Shigemura, Y.; Suzuki, A.; Kurokawa, M.; Sato, Y.; Sato, K. Changes in composition and content of food-derived peptide in human blood after daily ingestion of collagen hydrolysate for 4 weeks. *J. Sci. Food Agric.* **2017**, *98*, 1944–1950. [CrossRef] [PubMed]
31. Wu, J.; Fujioka, M.; Sugimoto, K.; Mu, G.; Ishimi, Y. Assessment of effectiveness of oral administration of collagen peptide on bone metabolism in growing and mature rats. *J. Bone Miner. Metab.* **2004**, *22*, 547–553. [CrossRef] [PubMed]
32. Bidlingmeyer, B.A.; Cohen, S.A.; Tarvin, T.L. Rapid analysis of amino acids using pre-column derivatization. *J. Chromatogr.* **1984**, *336*, 93–104. [CrossRef]
33. Sato, K.; Tsukamasa, Y.; Imai, C.; Ohtsuki, K.; Shimizu, Y.; Kawabata, M. Improved method for identification and determination of epsilon.-(.gamma.-glutamyl)lysine cross-link in protein using proteolytic digestion and derivatization with phenyl isothiocyanate followed by high-performance liquid chromatography separation. *J. Agric. Food Chem.* **1992**, *40*, 806–810. [CrossRef]
34. Rittié, L.; Fisher, G.J. Isolation and culture of skin fibroblasts. *Methods Mol. Med.* **2005**, *117*, 83–98. [PubMed]
35. Kwak, M.K.; Liu, R.; Kwon, J.O.; Kim, M.K.; Kim, A.H.J.; Kang, S.O. Cyclic dipeptides from lactic acid bacteria inhibit proliferation of the influenza a virus. *J. Microbiol.* **2013**, *51*, 836–843. [CrossRef] [PubMed]
36. Kwak, M.K.; Liu, R.; Kim, M.K.; Moon, D.; Kim, A.H.J.; Song, S.H.; Kang, S.O. Cyclic dipeptides from lactic acid bacteria inhibit the proliferation of pathogenic fungi. *J. Microbiol.* **2014**, *52*, 64–70. [CrossRef] [PubMed]
37. Liu, Z.; Wang, C.; Liu, Q.; Meng, Q.; Cang, J.; Mei, L.; Kaku, T.; Liu, K. Uptake, transport and regulation of JBP485 by PEPT1 in vitro and in vivo. *Peptides* **2011**, *32*, 747–754. [CrossRef] [PubMed]
38. Taga, Y.; Kusubata, M.; Ogawa-Goto, K.; Hattori, S. Efficient Absorption of X-Hydroxyproline (Hyp)-Gly after Oral Administration of a Novel Gelatin Hydrolysate Prepared Using Ginger Protease. *J. Agric. Food Chem.* **2016**, *64*, 2962–2970. [CrossRef] [PubMed]

39. Bar-Or, D.; Slone, D.S.; Mains, C.W.; Rael, L.T. Dipeptidyl peptidase IV activity in commercial solutions of human serum albumin. *Anal. Biochem.* **2013**, *441*, 13–17. [CrossRef] [PubMed]
40. Matsumoto, R.; Okochi, M.; Shimizu, K.; Kanie, K.; Kato, R.; Honda, H. Effects of the properties of short peptides conjugated with cell-penetrating peptides on their internalization into cells. *Sci. Rep.* **2015**. [CrossRef] [PubMed]

nutrients

MDPI

Article

Purification and Identification of Angiotensin I-Converting Enzyme Inhibitory Peptides and the Antihypertensive Effect of *Chlorella sorokiniana* Protein Hydrolysates

Yu-Hsin Lin [1], Guan-Wen Chen [2,*], Chin Hsi Yeh [3], Helena Song [3] and Jenn-Shou Tsai [2]

1 Department of Food Technology and Marketing, Taipei University of Marine Technology, No. 212, Section 9, Yan Ping North Road, Taipei 111, Taiwan; yhlin@mail.tcmt.edu.tw
2 Department of Food Science, National Taiwan Ocean University, No. 2 Pei-Ning Road, Keelung 202, Taiwan; tsaijs@mail.ntou.edu.tw
3 Taiwan Chlorella Manufacturing Co., Ltd., 5 F, No. 71, Section 2, Nan-King East Road, Taipei 104, Taiwan; webmaster@taiwanchlorella.com.tw (C.H.Y.); helena@taiwanchlorella.com.tw (H.S.)
* Correspondence: chengw@mail.ntou.edu.tw; Tel.: +886-2-2462-2192 (ext. 5135)

Received: 26 August 2018; Accepted: 28 September 2018; Published: 1 October 2018

Abstract: Hot water was used to obtain *Chlorella sorokiniana* hot water extract (HWE). Subsequently, this byproduct was freeze-dried, hydrolysed at 50 °C using Protease N to obtain *C. sorokiniana* protein hydrolysates (PN-1), and then digested with a gastrointestinal enzyme (PN-1G). The inhibitory effects of the HWE and hydrolysates against angiotensin I-converting enzyme (ACE) were investigated. The soluble protein and peptide contents were 379.9 and 179.7 mg/g, respectively, for HWE and 574.8 and 332.8 mg/g, respectively, for PN-1. The IC_{50} values of the HWE, PN-1, and PN-1G on ACE were 1.070, 0.035, and 0.044 mg/mL, respectively. PN-1G was separated into seven fractions through size exclusion chromatography. The sixth fraction of the hydrolysate had a molecular weight between 270 and 340 Da, and the lowest IC_{50} value on ACE was 0.015 mg/mL. The amino acid sequences of the ACE-inhibitory peptides were Trp-Val, Val-Trp, Ile-Trp, and Leu-Trp, of which the IC_{50} values were 307.61, 0.58, 0.50, and 1.11 μM, respectively. Systolic blood pressure and diastolic blood pressure were reduced 20 and 21 mm Hg, respectively, in spontaneously hypertensive rats after 6 h of oral administration with a dose of 171.4 mg PN-1 powder/kg body weight.

Keywords: chlorella protein hydrolysate; angiotensin I-converting enzyme; spontaneously hypertensive rat; antihypertensive effect

1. Introduction

Hypertension has been identified as a cardiovascular risk factor and is often called a "silent killer" because people with hypertension can remain asymptomatic for years [1]. The prevalence of hypertension has reached epidemic levels, affecting 15 to 20% of adults worldwide [2]. One therapeutic approach to treating hypertension is inhibition of angiotensin I-converting enzyme (ACE) using synthetic drugs. ACE plays a key physiological role in blood pressure regulation of the renin–angiotensin system. ACE inhibitors such as captopril and enalapril [3,4] have been used as antihypertensive drugs [5,6]. However, such therapy can produce adverse effects, including coughing, loss of taste, angioedema, and skin rashes [7]. Hence, a trend has formed towards the development of natural ACE inhibitors.

Peptides are the most commonly studied natural compounds that inhibit ACE activity [8–11]. Therefore, to obtain ACE-inhibitory peptides, numerous studies have focused on the hydrolysis of food protein-based matrices such as fermented milk [12–14], shellfish [15,16], chicken [17], mushrooms [18], fish [19,20], and the following types of algae *Undaria pinnatifida*, *Chlorella vulgaris*, and *Spirulina platensis* [1,16,21–23]. Among these protein sources, protein from algae has received particular attention because of its potentially beneficial effects related to hypertension [24–26]. In addition, reports have noted that algae protein hydrolysate decreases blood pressure in spontaneously hypertensive rats (SHRs), which suggests that certain peptides possess potent antihypertensive effects comparable with those of pharmaceutical drugs [27–30]. After performing hydrolysis on *Porphyra yezoensis* by using pepsin, one study separated the primary ACE-inhibitory peptides Ile-Tyr, Ala-Lys-Tyr-Ser-Tyr, Leu-Arg-Tyr, and Met-Lys-Tyr [27]. The IC_{50} values of these peptides were 2.69, 1.52, 5.06, and 7.26 μM, respectively. After 1 h following oral administration of this hydrolysate to SHRs at a dose of 200 mg/kg body weight (BW), the SHRs' systolic blood pressure (SBP) was reduced by 53.0 mm Hg. Through the hydrolysis of *C. vulgaris* using Alcalase, an ACE-inhibitory peptide with an amino acid sequence of Ile-Gln-Pro and IC_{50} value of 5.77 μM was separated [30]. This tripeptide was then administered to SHRs via tube feeding. After 2 to 4 h, this tripeptide achieved the same blood pressure-lowering effect as captopril at the same dose [30]. In the *C. vulgaris* hydrolysate obtained through hydrolysis using pepsin, the sequence of the primary ACE-inhibitory peptide was Phe–Ala–Leu, and its IC_{50} value was 26.3 μM. This peptide fraction was administered to SHRs at a dose of 200 mg/kg BW. After 1 h following oral administration, the SBP of the SHRs was reduced by 49.9 mm Hg [21]. However, few studies have examined ACE-inhibitory peptides derived from protein hydrolysate of green algae. A review identified three studies [1,21,23] on ACE-inhibitory peptides from *Chlorella* sp; however, information regarding the ACE-inhibitory activity and antihypertensive effect of protein hydrolysate from *C. sorokiniana* is limited. ACE-inhibitory peptides prepared from *C. sorokiniana* are of great interest because of the abundance of proteins in this alga.

C. sorokiniana is a microalga within the green alga grouping and an edible single-cell microalga that does not cause side effects when consumed [1]. Green algae are composed of approximately 60% protein and have carbohydrate and lipid contents of 12 to 17% and 14 to 22%, respectively [31]. Hot water extracts (HWEs) of green algae are often used in dietary supplements and are commercially available. After hot water extraction, a substantial amount of green algae residue containing approximately 50% protein remains. This byproduct is a comparatively cheap protein source compared with most bioactive peptides deriving from expensive animal and plant proteins [1]. Algae protein waste is often used only as a protein source in animal feed. To better utilise *C. sorokiniana* protein waste, after hot water extraction, such waste should be initially freeze-dried and subsequently hydrolysed by using commercial enzymes, to produce some bioactive peptide substances. In this study, the inhibitory effects of *C. sorokiniana* protein waste on ACE were measured to compare the efficacy of the extracts and hydrolysates. The stability of the hydrolysates' ACE-inhibitory activity was examined by simulating gastrointestinal digestion. Furthermore, the ACE-inhibitory peptides of the hydrolysates following digestion by gastrointestinal protease were fractionated using gel filtration to determine their molecular weights (MWs), purified by reverse-phase high-performance liquid chromatography (RP-HPLC), and subjected to amino acid sequence analysis. The antihypertensive effect of the hydrolysates on SHRs was investigated through short-term oral administration.

2. Materials and Methods

2.1. Materials

C. sorokiniana was supplied by an aquaculture farm (Taiwan Chlorella Manufacturing Co., Taipei, Taiwan). Protamex with a nominal activity level of 1.5 AU/g was supplied by Novozymes (Novo Nordisk A/S Co., Bagsværd, Denmark). Protease N with a nominal activity level of 150,000 U/g was supplied by Amano Pharmaceutical Co. (Yokohama, Kanagawa, Japan). Pepsin, pancreatin, hippuryl-L-histidyl-L-leucine (HHL), ACE of rabbit lung, and other chemicals of analytical grade were obtained from Sigma Chemical Co. (St. Louis, MO, USA).

2.2. Preparation of Hot Water Extract and Hydrolysate of C. sorokiniana

Whole *C. sorokiniana* was mixed with tap water at a 1:10 (*w*/*w*) ratio and incubated at 90 °C for 30 min to simulate the commercial procedure. The resulting liquid was filtered through No. 2 filter paper (Toyo Roshi Kaisha, Tokyo, Japan), and lyophilised to become the HWE of *C. sorokiniana*. The residues were then collected and further lyophilised to a powder. Next, this powder was homogenised with deionised water at a ratio of 1:10 for 2 min and boiled for 10 min to produce *C. sorokiniana* homogenate. After this mixture had cooled to ambient temperature, the enzyme (Protamex or Protease N) was added to the substrate at ratios of 1:100 (*w*/*w*) and 2:100 (*w*/*w*). This reaction mixture was incubated at 50 °C for 5 h, and the protease was subsequently inactivated by incubation at 98 °C for 10 min. Centrifugation at 12,000× *g* (SCR 20BA, Hitachi Co. Ltd., Tokyo, Japan) for 20 min then produced a supernatant that was filtered through No. 2 filter paper; finally, the filtrate was collected and lyophilised to powder form in preparation for analysis or orally administered to SHRs via gastric intubation.

2.3. Chemical Analyses

The soluble protein contents of the HWE and hydrolysate were measured using the Folin–Lowry method [32,33] with bovine serum albumin as the standard. A total of 1 mL of an alkaline copper reagent was added to each sample, followed by 3 mL of Folin–Ciocalteu reagent (diluted 10-fold with deionised water) (Merck, KGaA, Darmstadt, Germany). Subsequently, the mixture was incubated at ambient temperature for 30 min and determined for the absorbance of the reaction mixture at 540 nm by using a spectrophotometer (Model UV-160A, Shimadzu, Kyoto, Japan).

2.4. Measurement of Peptide Content

The peptide content of the samples was measured by an ortho-phthaldialdehyde reagent with dipeptide (Leu-Gly) (Sigma, St. Louis, MO, USA) as a standard according to a modification of the method of Church et al. [34]. Prior to the measurement, the sample solution (30 mg/mL) was filtered through a 0.22-μm membrane, and the filtrate was passed through an ultrafiltration membrane (Millipore, Bedford, MA, USA) with an MW cut-off (MWCO) of 5000 Da. Then, 50 μL of the resulting permeate was mixed with 2 mL of the ortho-phthaldialdehyde reagent and incubated at ambient temperature for 2 min. The absorbance of the reaction mixture was subsequently determined using a spectrophotometer (UV-160A, Shimadzu, Taipei, Taiwan), which measured it as 340 nm.

2.5. In Vitro Assay for ACE-Inhibitory Activity

ACE-inhibitory activity was evaluated through RP-HPLC and assayed using the modified spectrophotometric method described by Cushman and Cheung [35] and Wu and Ding [36]. In brief, 15 mM HHL was dissolved in 100 mM Na-borate buffer (pH 8.3) supplemented with 300 mM NaCl. Rabbit lung ACE was dissolved in the same buffer at a concentration of 53.2 mU/mL. A mixture containing 75 μL of ACE solution and 75 μL of the sample with a 5000-Da MWCO membrane (Millipore, Burlington, MA, USA) was incubated at 37 °C for 10 min, to which was added 75 μL of HHL solution, and the mixture was incubated for a further 30 min. The reaction was halted by addition of 250 μL of 1 N hydrochloric acid, and 10 μL of this solution was injected directly into a Luna C_{18} analytical column (4.6 × 250 mm^2, particle size: 5 μm; Phenomenex, Torrance, CA, USA) to separate the substrate HHL and product hippuric acid (HA) liberated through hydrolysis of HHL. The column was eluted with a mobile phase of 0.1% trifluoroacetic acid in methanol and water (50/50, *v*/*v*) at a constant flow rate of 0.8 mL/min using a pump (model L-7100, Hitachi, Tokyo, Japan) and monitored at 228 nm using an ultraviolet (UV) spectrophotometer (UV-VIS detector 118, Gilson Medical Electronics, Villiers-le-Bel, France). Finally, inhibition activity was calculated using the following formula.

$$\text{Inhibition activity (\%)} = [(\text{Ec} - \text{Es})/(\text{Ec} - \text{Eb})] \times 100$$

where Ec is the absorbance with addition of the buffer instead of the test sample (control), Es is the absorbance when the sample was added to the reaction mixture (sample), and Eb is the absorbance when the stop solution was added before the reaction occurred (blank). The IC_{50} value was defined as the concentration of peptide in milligrams per millilitre required to reduce 50% of the absorbance peak height of the HA (50% inhibition of ACE), which was determined through regression analysis of ACE inhibition (%) versus the log 10 (peptide concentration, mg/mL) curve and constructed using at least six separate analyses to calculate the concentration. Captopril (positive control) exhibited the highest significant ACE-inhibitory activity (IC_{50} value = 0.0069 μM). All data presented in this paper are the average of three repeats or mean ± standard deviation (SD).

2.6. In Vitro Gastrointestinal Digestion

Digestion was simulated in vitro with slight modifications to previously published methods [36]. A 3.5% PN-1 (*w*/*v*) (control group) was redissolved in 0.1 M KCl-HCl (pH 2.0) buffer with pepsin at an enzyme-to-protein ratio of 1:25 (*w*/*w*) for 4 h at 37 °C, after which the reaction was halted through heating in a boiling water bath for 10 min. Subsequently, the reaction mixture was neutralised to pH 7.0 with 2M NaOH solution. The neutralised suspension (50 mL) was centrifuged (10,000× *g*, 30 min) to produce a supernatant that was subsequently used to determine ACE-inhibitory activity. The remaining neutralised suspension was then digested with pancreatin (E:S = 1:25 (*w*/*w*)) at 37 °C for 4 h. The enzyme was inactivated by boiling water for 10 min and then centrifuged at 10,000× *g* for 30 min. The resulting supernatant was used to determine ACE-inhibitory activity. In addition, this supernatant was collected and lyophilised to powder form in preparation for analyses.

2.7. Size Exclusion Chromatography

The lyophilised hydrolysate that exhibited the highest ACE-inhibitory activity was fractionated through gel filtration chromatography on a Sephadex G-15 column (1.6 × 90 cm^2; Amersham Pharmacia Biotech AB, Uppsala, Sweden) and then equilibrated with deionised water. The hydrolysate powder (200 mg) was then dissolved in 10 mL of deionised water; the resulting solution was passed through the 5000-Da MWCO membrane, and the filtrate of 2 mL was directly injected into the column and eluted with deionised water at a constant flow rate of 0.5 mL/min. Resultant fractions of 5 mL each were collected, and the absorbance of each fraction at 280 nm was determined. Notably, the MW standards for calibration of gel filtration were bacitracin (MW 1422 Da), penta-L-phenylalanine (MW 753.9 Da), and tryptophan (MW 204.2 Da).

2.8. Purification of ACE-Inhibitory Peptide

Purification of ACE-inhibitory peptide from protein hydrolysate was performed by following the method described by Chen et al. with minor modifications [12]. The aforementioned fraction from gel filtration with the highest inhibition of ACE was collected, lyophilised, and further purified through RP-HPLC (L-7100, Hitachi) using an analytical C_{18} column (Synergi 4 μ Hydro-RP 80A, 10 × 250 mm^2; particle size: 4 μm; Phenomenex, Torrance, CA, USA). Solution A was deionised water containing 0.1% trifluoroacetic acid, and solvent B was acetonitrile solution. Elution was performed at ambient temperature with a linear gradient from 0% to 40% of solvent B within 120 min. The flow rate was set at 1.5 mL/min, and the sample load volume was 500 μL. The absorbance of the resultant eluate was monitored at 220 nm by using a UV spectrophotometer (UV-VIS detector 118, Gilson Medical Electronics, Middleton, WI, USA) connected to a data station (715 system controller, Gilson Medical Electronics). The peaks were collected via repeated chromatography, and then each peak purity was confirmed as a single component by using a reversed-phase C_{12} column (Joupiter 4 μm Proteo 90 A, 250 × 4.6 mm^2, Phenomenex) with linear gradients from 0 to 40% acetonitrile solution within 120 min at a flow rate of 1.5 mL at ambient temperature. The absorbance of elution was monitored at 220 nm. Finally, the peaks exhibiting the highest ACE-inhibitory activity were collected and lyophilised, and their amino acid sequences were identified.

2.9. Sequence Analysis

The sequence of the peptide was identified by following the method described by Lin et al. with slight modifications [20]. Samples were first prepared prior to sequencing analysis. The PN-1G concentration was increased from 20 to 100 mg/mL and separated by gel filtration chromatography. The fraction F was collected through triplicate chromatography. Three combined collections were lyophilised and then dissolved in 0.5 mL of deionised water. The resulting solution was further purified on an RP-HPLC column (ODS C_{18}) using the aforementioned method. Each peak was collected five times through repeated chromatography and then confirmed as a single component with an RP-HPLC C_{12} column using the aforementioned method. The five collected mixtures were then lyophilised, and their ACE-inhibitory activities and amino acid sequences were analysed. Next, the sequences of ACE-inhibitory peptides were identified through automated Edman degradation using a Procise 492 protein sequencer (Perkin-Elmer Co. Ltd., Applied Biosystem Inc., Foster City, CA, USA) [20]. Finally, the amino acid sequences of identified peptides were synthesised through solid-phase peptide synthesis. Synthetic peptides were used as the standard for qualitative analysis of these peptides in algae protein hydrolysates, followed by use of an RP-HPLC C_{12} column through the aforementioned method. The amino acid sequence alignment of *C. sorokiniana* proteins (e.g., succinate dehydrogenase (ubiquinone) iron-sulphur subunit, mitochondrial [accession number: A0A2P6TTG2]; photosystem II protein D [accession number: W8SIR2]; and ribokinase [accession number: A0A2P6TU56]) was performed using the UniProt database [37]. To confirm identical sequences, the pairwise sequence alignment tools available [38].

2.10. Animals and In Vivo Measurement of Blood Pressure

All animal experiments were executed in accord with the guidelines for the Care and Use of Laboratory Animals under a protocol approved by the Institutional Animal Care and Use Committee of National Taiwan Ocean University, Keelung, Taiwan. The approval number for the ethical clearance was 96,023. Eighteen male SHRs aged 7 weeks were purchased from the National Laboratory Animal Center, Taipei, Taiwan. The SHRs were housed in cages with a maintained light–dark cycle of 12 h. The constant temperature and humidity in the animal room were controlled at 23 ± 1 °C and 55% ± 5%, respectively. The SHRs were fed a standard laboratory diet (Rodent Laboratory Chow Diet 5001, PMI Nutrition International, Brentwood, MO, USA). Tap water was freely available to the rats for eight weeks before the beginning of the experimental period. At the age of 15 weeks, the SHRs (body weight = 350 ± 5 g, SBP = 173.0 ± 4.2 mm Hg, diastolic blood pressure (DBP) = 150.0 ± 3.7 mm Hg) were divided into two experimental groups (both $n = 6$) that were respectively administered PN-1 dissolved in 2 mL of saline by gastric intubation at doses of 30 and 60 mg of powder/rat BW (350 g, equivalent to 85.7 and 171.4 mg of powder/kg BW or 10 and 20 mg peptide/rat BW). Equal volumes of saline were given to the control group ($n = 6$) during the trial. The SBP and DBP of each SHR were measured at 2, 4, 6, 8, and 24 h after oral administration. Each rat was placed in a thermostatic box at 45 °C for 5 min to determine the SBP, DBP, and heart rate by using the tail-cuff method (BP-98, Softron, Tokyo, Japan). The results are shown as means and SDs.

2.11. Statistical Analysis

Changes in blood pressures are expressed as the difference in SBP and DBP before and after oral administration of PN-1 containing 30 and 60 mg of peptide/rat BW. Data are given as mean ± SD except for the yield of *C. sorokiniana* protein hydrolysates, size exclusion chromatography, and RP-HPLC chromatography, which are reported as the averages of three samples. An analysis of variance for the results of the aforementioned experiments was conducted using the SAS [39] general linear model procedure. Multiple mean comparisons were performed using Duncan's multiple range test.

3. Results and Discussion

3.1. Soluble Protein Content, Peptide Content, Yield, and IC_{50}

The residue of the HWE of *C. sorokiniana* underwent hydrolysis using Protamex and Protease N. Table 1 presents the effects of the hydrolysis on soluble protein, peptide content, yield, and ACE-inhibitory activity. The results revealed that compared with HWE, hydrolysates subjected to protease hydrolysis had higher yields and higher soluble protein and peptide content. Moreover, as the amount of protease added increased, so did the protein and peptide compositions. Specifically, the hydrolysates of Protease N (PN-1 and PN-2) had higher yields and higher soluble protein and peptide contents than did those of Protamex hydrolysates (PX-1 and PX-2). PN-1 had yields and soluble protein and peptide contents that were 1.5, 1.4, and 1.3 times that of PX-1, respectively, and those of PN-2 were 1.1, 1.2, and 1.1 times that of PX-2, respectively. The soluble protein contents of PN-1 and PN-2 were 1.5 and 1.6 times that of HWE, respectively; the peptide contents of PN-1 and PN-2 were 1.8 and 1.9 times that of HWE, respectively; and the yields of PN-1 and PN-2 were 7.0 and 7.8 times that of HWE, respectively (Table 1). The IC_{50} of HWE was 1.070 mg/mL. However, of all the hydrolysates derived from the *C. sorokiniana* residues, PN-1 had the most satisfactory ACE-inhibitory effect, and its IC_{50} value was 0.035 mg/mL (Table 1).

Table 1. Effect of treatment on soluble protein and peptide content, yield, and angiotensin I-converting enzyme (ACE) IC_{50} of *C. sorokiniana* protein hydrolysates.

Sample	Soluble Protein (mg/g)	Peptide Content (mg/g)	Yield [1]	IC_{50} [2] (mg/mL)
HWE [3]	379.9 ± 1.5	179.7 ± 2.1	4.0	1.070 ± 0.020
PX-1 [4]	482.0 ± 2.2	260.4 ± 2.0	19.1	0.043 ± 0.001
PX-2 [5]	566.6 ± 3.5	298.6 ± 2.0	22.7	0.043 ± 0.002
PN-1 [6]	574.8 ± 2.3	332.8 ± 3.0	28.1	0.035 ± 0.002
PN-2 [7]	610.6 ± 3.8	341.6 ± 3.1	31.2	0.042 ± 0.001

Each value represents the average of three samples. [1] Yield: (1-dry weight of sample after treatment/dry weight of sample) × 100%. [2] The concentration of an inhibitor required to inhibit 50% of ACE activity. [3] HWE: the hot water extract of *C. sorokiniana*. [4] PX-1: hydrolysate from Protamex hydrolysis at 1% (the enzyme-to-protein ratio was 1:100 *w/w*) for 5 h. [5] PX-2: hydrolysate from Protamex hydrolysis at 2% (the enzyme-to-protein ratio was 2:100 *w/w*) for 5 h. [6] PN-1: hydrolysate from protease N hydrolysis at 1% (the enzyme-to-protein ratio was 1:100 *w/w*) for 5 h. [7] PN-2: hydrolysate from protease N hydrolysis at 2% (the enzyme-to-protein ratio was 2:100 *w/w*) for 5 h.

These results show that use of PN-1 in the mass processing of plants can reduce the amount of enzymes used in this process, thereby lowering cost. Therefore, this study focused on PN-1.

3.2. In Vitro Stability of *C. sorokiniana*–Derived ACE-Inhibitory Peptides

In vitro gastric digestion provides a practical and easy process to imitate oral administration of bioactive peptides. The ACE-inhibitory activity of *C. sorokiniana*-derived peptides decreased markedly after increasing IC_{50} from 0.035 to 0.044 mg peptide/mL through hydrolysis with pepsin and pancreatin, which simulated stomach and small intestine digestion (Table 2). This may be because (1) after the rehydrolysis of pepsin and pancreatin the ACE-inhibitory peptides also underwent rehydrolysis or (2) the proportion of ACE-inhibitory peptides decreased, leading to an increase of IC_{50} and an inferior ACE-inhibitory effect. The main ACE-inhibitory peptide obtained from manchego cheese through purification was α_{S2}-CN f 205-208 (VRYL). Subsequently, this peptide underwent hydrolysis with digestive enzymes (i.e., pepsin, chymotrypsin, and trypsin), after which its IC_{50} value increased from 0.009 to 0.03 mg/mL. The inhibitory capacity of ACE decreased because the hydrophobic amino acid leucine at the carboxy terminal of VRYL underwent hydrolysis and produced VRY [40]. This outcome showed that ACE-inhibitory peptides are released through hydrolysis by proteolytic enzymes and can survive or maintain their active form even following gastrointestinal digestion.

Table 2. Effect of gastrointestinal protease hydrolysis on ACE-inhibitory activity of PN-1.

Protease	IC_{50} (mg Peptide/mL)
Control	0.035 ± 0.002
Pepsin [1]	0.044 ± 0.001
Pepsin + Pancreatin [2]	0.044 ± 0.001

Each value represents the average of three samples. [1] Hydrolysed for 4 h. [2] Pepsin hydrolysed for 4 h followed by pancreatin hydrolysed for 4 h.

3.3. Isolation and Purification of ACE-Inhibitory Peptide

In this study, the ACE inhibitory effect of PN-1 exhibited a decreasing trend (its IC_{50} value increased from 0.035 to 0.044 mg/mL) after it was enzymatically hydrolysed in the stomach and intestines. This result indicates that enzymes in the stomach and intestine can rehydrolyse ACE inhibitory active peptide sequences in PN-1 mixtures. To purify and identify possible active peptides generated by PN-1 in the stomach and intestines of SHRs, we selected PN-1G to perform purification and identification. The MW distribution of the ACE-inhibitory peptides in PN-1 after digestion by gastrointestinal proteases (PN-1G) was fractionated by size exclusion chromatography on a Sephadex G-15 column. Seven fractions were separated and designated as A–G (Figure 1), and their MWs ranged from 1400 to 200 Da. The peptide concentrations of fractions A–G were 0.210, 0.027, 0.025, 0.064, 0.057, 0.034, and 0.053 mg/mL, respectively (Table 3). Although fraction A had the highest ACE-inhibitory proportion and peptide content, the data for effective ACE inhibition (inhibitory efficiency ratio (IER) = inhibition (%)/peptide concentration (mg/mL)) indicated that fractions B, C, E, and F exhibited superior inhibition than did the other peaks, ranging between 1130% and 2230% per mg/mL. The IC_{50} value for ACE was further analysed; the results revealed that of all the fractions, fraction F was the most effective at inhibiting ACE activity, and its IC_{50} value was 0.0150 mg/mL (Table 3). Compared with PN-1 after digestion by gastrointestinal proteases, the ACE inhibition capacity of fraction F markedly improved, with its IC_{50} value being reduced to approximately one-third of that of PN-1G. The MW of fraction F was 270 to 340 Da, indicating that it was a di- or tripeptide. The highest ACE-inhibitory effect was similar to that of the potent inhibitory tripeptides found in *C. vulgaris*, *S. platensis*, and *U. pinnatifida* [21,30,41].

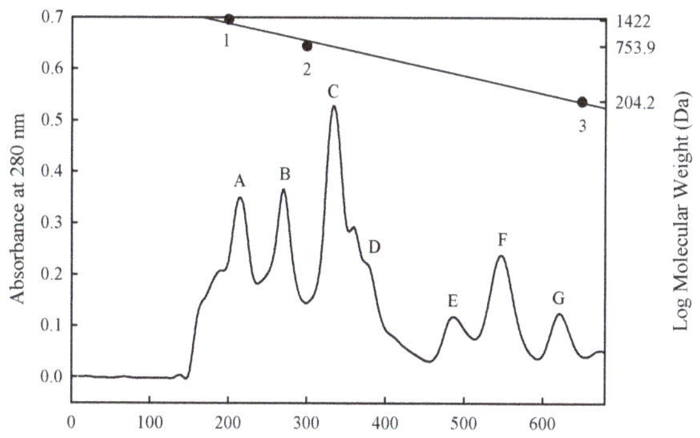

Figure 1. Sephadex G-15 column chromatography of peptides separated from PN-1 after digestion by gastrointestinal proteases. ● Standard materials: bacitracin (1422 Da); penta-L-phenylalanine (753.9 Da); and L-tryptophan (204.2 Da).

Table 3. ACE IC_{50} of the size exclusion chromatographic fractions obtained from PN-1 after digestion by gastrointestinal proteases.

Fraction	Molecular Weight (Da)	Inhibition (%)	Peptide Content (mg/mL)	IER [1] (%/mg/mL)	IC_{50} (mg/mL)
A	1400–1180	74.0	0.210	350	— [2]
B	1180–910	30.6	0.027	1130	0.0450
C	910–740	58.2	0.025	2230	0.0187
D	680–590	48.0	0.064	750	—
E	460–370	73.2	0.057	1280	0.0160
F	340–270	68.6	0.034	2020	0.0150
G	200–250	40.0	0.053	760	—

Each value represents the average of three samples. [1] IER: inhibitory efficiency ratio = % inhibition/peptide content. [2] Undetected.

The most active peptide of fraction F was further purified on an RP-HPLC column (ODS C_{18}). The elution profiles of the peptides are shown in Figure 2. Ten major peaks were observed and labelled according to the eluted order of 1 to 10. These 10 peaks were collected separately through repeated chromatography, and each peak was confirmed as a single component by an RP-HPLC C_{12} column with the same gradients comprising 0 to 40% acetonitrile solution. In addition, the IER values of the F_1–F_{10} peaks were measured. The results revealed that the F_7, F_8, F_9, and F_{10} peaks had relatively strong ACE-inhibitory effects, with IERs of 5425%, 8613%, 9510%, and 8770% per mg/mL, respectively (Table 4). Finally, peaks F_7, F_8, F_9, and F_{10} were collected separately, lyophilised, and further analysed to determine their amino acid sequences.

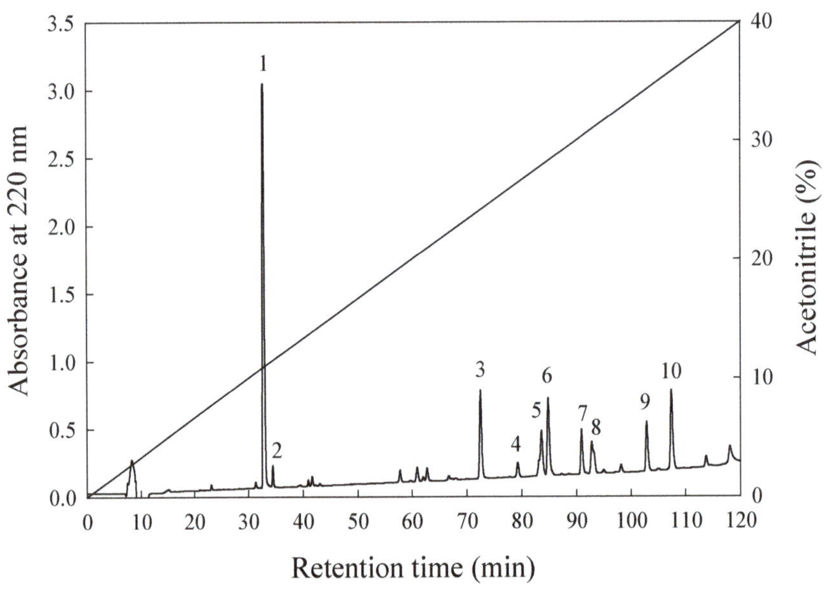

Figure 2. Elution profile of fraction F from Figure 1 by reversed phase-high performance liquid chromatography (RP-HPLC). Column: Synergi 4u Hydro-RP 80A (10 × 250 mm^2; particle size: 4 μm; Phenomenex); elution A (deionised water containing 0.1% trifluoroacetic acid) and B (100% acetonitrile containing 0.1% trifluoroacetic acid); mobile phase: a linear gradient from 0% to 40% of B within 120 min; flow rate of 1.5 mL/min at room temperature, and detection at 220 nm.

Table 4. ACE IER of peaks isolated from fraction F of PN-1G.

Peak	ACE Inhibitory (%)	Peptide Content (mg/mL)	IER (%/mg/mL)
F_1	14.3	0.01	1430
F_2	19.1	0.01	1910
F_3	41.2	0.02	2060
F_4	36.8	0.01	3680
F_5	72.4	0.02	3621
F_6	75.7	0.03	2523
F_7	54.3	0.01	5425
F_8	86.1	0.01	8613
F_9	95.1	0.01	9510
F_{10}	87.7	0.01	8770

Each value represents the average of three samples. IER: inhibitory efficiency ratio = % inhibition/peptide content.

3.4. Amino Acid Sequences and ACE-Inhibitory Activity

The amino acid sequences and IC_{50} values for the peptides from peaks F_7, F_8, F_9, and F_{10} are shown in Table 5. The peptide sequences of the F_7, F_8, F_9, and F_{10} peaks were Trp–Val, Val–Trp, Ile–Trp, and Leu–Trp, respectively, and the IC_{50} values of the F_7, F_8, F_9, and F_{10} peaks were 307.61, 0.58, 0.50, and 1.11 μM, respectively (equivalent to 0.0933, 0.00018, 0.00016, and 0.00035 mg/mL, respectively). These isolates were identified as a part of the amino acid sequence of succinate dehydrogenase (ubiquinone) iron-sulphur subunit, mitochondrial residues 2031–2032, 552–553, 2736–2737, and 3738–3739, respectively [37]. Sekiya et al. [42] reported that food-derived peptides with IC_{50} values between 100 and 500 μM have potential as antihypertensive agents. Compared with the *C. sorokiniana* protein hydrolysate (0.044 mg/mL), which did not undergo purification, the IC_{50} values of Val-Trp, Ile-Trp, and Leu-Trp were approximately 244, 275, and 126 times lower, respectively. In addition, research on ACE-inhibitory peptides has identified Val–Trp, Ile–Trp, and Leu–Trp in various protein hydrolysates such as the hydrolysates of wakame (*U. pinnatifida*), fish sauce, sake lees, dried bonito, ovalbumin, and salmon; the IC_{50} values ranged between 0.48 and 31.3 μM [43–46], 0.7 and 4.7 μM [44,47–49], and 6.76 and 50.12 μM [47,50,51], all of which were similar to the IC_{50} value of the purified peptide from PN-1G. The IC_{50} value for Trp-Val prepared in this study through purification was lower than the value obtained by Ono et al. (500.5 μM) [49]. However, similar to their results, when the IC_{50} values of Trp–Val and its reverse sequence were compared in the present study, the N-terminal Trp-containing dipeptides exhibited lower ACE-inhibitory activity than did the C-terminal-residue Trp-containing dipeptides, and the IC_{50} value increased from 0.58 to 307.61 μM. These results agree with the importance of amino acids at the C-terminal of dipeptides, as reported by Ono et al. [49]. Studies have reported that the ACE inhibition mode of peptides with Trp as the C-terminal residue—namely Val–Trp, Ile–Trp, and Leu–Trp—showed noncompetitive inhibition, whereas reversed sequence peptides with Trp at the N-terminal exhibited competitive inhibition [49,51]. In addition, Val–Trp, Ile–Trp, and Leu–Trp exhibited excellent ACE inhibition, which may have been because the carboxy terminals of these peptide sequences were all Trp-containing aromatic amino acids, whereas the nitrogen terminals were all branched-chain hydrophobic amino acids. This result is consistent with some previous studies [52]. Wu et al. [50] used *Z* descriptors to investigate the quantitative structure–activity relationship of 58 ACE dipeptides. They found that ACE inhibition was greatly affected by the three-dimensional chemical properties and hydrophobicity of C-terminal amino acids. Dipeptides with hydrophobic amino acids at the C-terminal, such as trypotophan, phenylalanine, and tyrosine, have stronger ACE-inhibitory activity. The identification results were consistent with the systematic induction results of Li et al. [53] and Cheung et al. [54] with respect to the properties of ACE-inhibitory peptides. In addition, Xiao et al. [55] further used flexible molecule docking technology to elucidate ACE active sites. The results demonstrated that hydrogen bonds; hydrophilic, hydrophobic, and electrostatic interactions; and coordinate bonds existed between the active pockets of the C-domain and Val–Trp and Ile–Trp. The interaction of the N-domain with the dipeptides was similar to that of the C-domain, which had fewer hydrogen bonds and no electrostatic interactions. However, further investigations regarding the relationship between the inhibitory mechanism and dipeptide structure are necessary.

Table 5. Peptide sequences and IC_{50} of various peaks (F_7 to F_{10}) from PN-1G.

Peak	Sequence	IC_{50} (μM)
F_7	Trp–Val	307.61 ± 0.01
F_8	Val–Trp	0.58 ± 0.02
F_9	Ile–Trp	0.50 ± 0.01
F_{10}	Leu–Trp	1.11 ± 0.02

Although these peptides have been reported in other foods, to date, no reports have revealed that these peptides arise from *C. sorokiniana* protein waste. Compared with salmon, Antarctic krill, and other foods that have been utilised to develop functional foods for the prevention of hypertension, *C. sorokiniana* protein waste is a cheap food source that can provide high additive value.

3.5. Antihypertensive Effect of *C. sorokiniana* Protein Hydrolysate

In short-term administration, *C. sorokiniana* protein hydrolysate (PN-1) containing 30 and 60 mg of peptide/rat BW (350 g; equivalent to 85.7 and 171.4 mg powder/kg BW) was administered to SHRs. Saline was used as a control that had negligible effects on SBP. SBP decreased significantly between 4 and 6 h after PN-1 administration and recovered to its initial level after 24 h. At 6 h after feeding, SBP reached its lowest point, namely 11.1 ± 2.8 mm Hg lower than that of the controls for the SHRs administered 30 mg/rat BW and 20.0 ± 3.2 mm Hg lower than that of the controls for the SHRs administered 60 mg/rat BW. A similar trend was observed for DBP, for which the values of the two experimental groups were 14.4 ± 5.3 and 21.0 ± 2.6 mm Hg lower than that of the controls, respectively (Figure 3). Other studies have examined the antihypertensive effects of ACE inhibitors on SHRs through short-term administration [56]. Upstream chum salmon (*Oncorhynchus keta*) muscle with thermolysin exhibited a potent antihypertensive effect in SHRs at 500 and 2000 mg of hydrolysate/kg BW at 4 h after oral administration, which resulted in decreases in SBP of 28 and 38 mm Hg, respectively. However, the main ACE-inhibitory peptides separated from the salmon hydrolysate were Val–Trp, Ile–Trp, and Leu–Trp. In addition, single oral administration of these three peptides (purified from brown seaweed—wakame) has been reported in detail by Sato et al. [41,51]. Results for Val–Trp, Ile–Trp, and Leu–Trp in SHRs revealed that a dose of 1 mg/kg BW exerted a blood pressure-lowering effect. Similar results revealed that a single dose of peptide fraction from *C. vulgaris* significantly reduced SBP to 49.9 mm Hg at 1 h, and the antihypertensive effect continued for 4 h after oral administration [21].

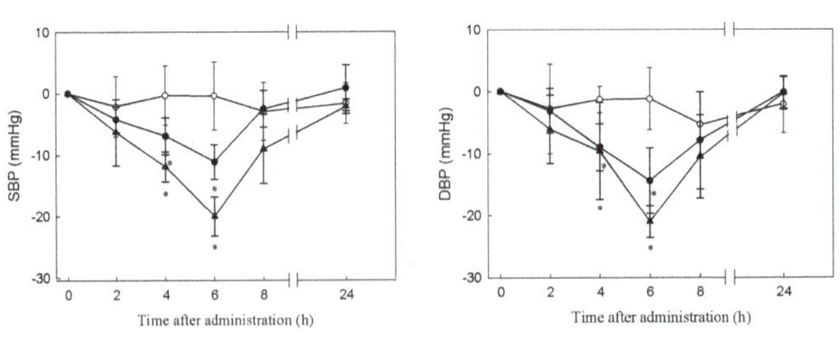

Figure 3. Changes in blood pressure of SHRs after oral administration of PN-1. (**a**) SBP; (**b**) DBP. —○—, 0.9% NaCl in water as control; —●—, 30 mg of *C. sorokiniana* protein hydrolysate powder with 0.9% NaCl; —▲—, 60 mg of *C. sorokiniana* protein hydrolysate powder with 0.9% NaCl. Each point represents a mean value (n = 6) and the vertical bars represent the standard errors. *: significant difference from the control, $p < 0.05$.

4. Conclusions

Residues of *C. sorokiniana* after hot water extraction were hydrolysed using Protease N 1% for 5 h. The IC_{50} of this hydrolysate (PN-1) to ACE was 0.035 mg/mL. PN-1 was administered to the SHRs through 30 and 60 mg of powder/350 g; after 6 h following oral administration, the SBPs of the two experimental groups were respectively 11.1 and 20.1 mm Hg lower than that of the control group, and the DBPs of the two experimental groups were 14.4 and 21.0 mmHg lower than that of the control group, respectively. Four inhibitory peptides were isolated from the hydrolysate that exhibited high ACE-inhibitory activity, and their amino acid sequences were Trp–Val, Val–Trp, Ile–Trp, and Leu–Trp, with IC_{50} values of 307.61, 0.58, 0.50, and 1.11 μM, respectively. These findings revealed ACE-inhibitory activity in vitro and antihypertensive activity in vivo. These findings suggest that an ACE inhibitor derived from *C. sorokiniana* protein hydrolysate could be utilised to develop functional foods for prevention of hypertension. In addition, this research provides evidence that small peptides from *C. sorokiniana* insoluble protein have potential for application because of their bioactivities.

Author Contributions: G.-W.C., J.-S.T., C.H.Y., and H.S. proposed and designed the experiment. G.-W.C. and Y.H.L. all participated in the experiment. Y.H.L., G.-W.C., and J.-S.T. analysed the data and composed the manuscript. G.-W.C. revised the manuscript and was responsible for supervising the research.

Funding: This research was funded by [the National Science Council, Taiwan, Republic of China] grant number [NSC98-2321-B-019-002].

Acknowledgments: This study was supported by Taiwan Chlorella Manufacturing Co., Ltd.

Conflicts of Interest: The authors declare no conflicts of interest.

References

1. Sheih, I.C.; Fang, T.J.; Wu, T.K. Isolation and characterisation of a novel angiotensin I-converting enzyme (ACE) inhibitory peptide from the algae protein waste. *Food Chem.* **2009**, *115*, 279–284. [CrossRef]
2. Wang, J.; Hu, J.; Cui, J.; Bai, X.; Du, A.Y.; Miyaguchi, Y.; Lin, B. Purification and identification of a ACE inhibitory peptide from oyster proteins hydrolysate and the antihypertensive effect of hydrolysate in spontaneously hypertensive rats. *Food Chem.* **2008**, *111*, 302–308. [CrossRef] [PubMed]
3. Ondetti, M.A. Design of specific inhibitors of angiotensin-converting enzyme: New class of orally active antihypertensive agents. *Science* **1977**, *196*, 441–444. [CrossRef] [PubMed]
4. Sawayama, T.; Itokawa, A.; Shimada, K.; Doi, Y.; Kimura, Y.; Nishimura, H. Synthesis of 1-[(S)-3-acetylthio-2-methylpropanoyl]-L-phenylalanine (Alacepril) and one of its active metabolites, the desacetyl derivative (DU-1227). *Chem. Pharm. Bull.* **1990**, *38*, 1767–1771. [CrossRef]
5. Julius, S.; Nesbitt, S.D.; Egan, B.M.; Weber, M.A.; Michelson, E.L.; Kaciroti, N.; Black, H.R.; Grimm, R.H.; Messerli, F.H.; Oparil, S.; et al. Feasibility of treating prehypertension with an angiotensin-receptor blocker. *N. Engl. J. Med.* **2006**, *354*, 1685–1697. [CrossRef] [PubMed]
6. Bhuyan, B.J.; Mugesh, G. Synthesis, characterization and antioxidant activity of angiotensin converting enzyme inhibitors. *Org. Biomol. Chem.* **2011**, *9*, 1356–1365. [CrossRef] [PubMed]
7. Al Shohaib, S.; Raweily, E. Acute tubular necrosis due to captopril. *Am. J. Nephrol.* **2000**, *20*, 149–152. [CrossRef] [PubMed]
8. Bhuyan, B.J.; Mugesh, G. Antioxidant activity of peptide-based angiotensin converting enzyme inhibitors. *Org. Biomol. Chem.* **2012**, *10*, 2237–2247. [CrossRef] [PubMed]
9. Samarakoon, K.W.; O-Nam, K.; Ko, J.Y.; Lee, J.H.; Kang, M.C.; Kim, D.; Lee, J.B.; Lee, J.S.; Jeon, Y.J. Purification and identification of novel angiotensin-I converting enzyme (ACE) inhibitory peptides from cultured marine microalgae (*Nannochloropsis oculata*) protein hydrolysate. *J. Appl. Phycol.* **2013**, *25*, 1595–1606. [CrossRef]
10. Yamada, A.; Sakurai, T.; Ochi, D.; Mitsuyama, E.; Yamauchi, K.; Abe, F. Novel angiotensin I-converting enzyme inhibitory peptide derived from bovine casein. *Food Chem.* **2013**, *141*, 3781–3789. [CrossRef] [PubMed]
11. Pan, S.; Wang, S.; Jing, L.; Yao, D. Purification and characterisation of a novel angiotensin-I converting enzyme (ACE)-inhibitory peptide derived from the enzymatic hydrolysate of Enteromorpha clathrata protein. *Food Chem.* **2016**, *211*, 423–430. [CrossRef] [PubMed]

12. Chen, G.W.; Tsai, J.S.; Sun, P.B. Purification of Angiotensin I-converting enzyme inhibitory peptides and antihypertensive effect of milk produced by protease-facilitated lactic fermentation. *Int. Dairy J.* **2007**, *17*, 641–647. [CrossRef]
13. Chen, G.W.; Tsa, J.S.; Sun, P.B. Cardiovascular effects of whey from prozyme 6-facilitated lactic acid bacteria fermentation of milk. *J. Food Biochem.* **2007**, *31*, 639–655. [CrossRef]
14. Tsai, J.S.; Chen, T.J.; Pan, B.S.; Gong, S.D.; Chung, M.Y. Antihypertensive effect of bioactive peptides produced by protease-facilitated lactic acid fermentation of milk. *Food Chem.* **2008**, *106*, 552–558. [CrossRef]
15. Tsai, J.S.; Lin, T.C.; Chen, J.L.; Pan, B.S. The inhibitory effect of freshwater clam (*Corbicula fluminea*, Muller) muscle protein hydrolysates on angiotensin I converting enzyme. *Process Biochem.* **2006**, *41*, 2276–2281. [CrossRef]
16. Tsai, J.S.; Chen, J.L.; Pan, B.S. ACE-inhibitory peptides identified from the muscle protein hydrolysate of hard clam (*Meretrix lusoria*). *Process Biochem.* **2008**, *43*, 743–747. [CrossRef]
17. Terashima, M.; Baba, T.; Ikenmoto, N.; Katayama, M.; Morimoto, T.; Matsumura, S. Novel angiotensin-concerting enzyme (ACE) inhibitory peptides derived from boneless chicken leg meat. *J. Agric. Food Chem.* **2010**, *58*, 7432–7436. [CrossRef] [PubMed]
18. Jang, J.H.; Jeong, S.C.; Kim, J.H.; Lee, Y.H.; Ju, Y.C.; Lee, J.S. Characterisation of a new antihypertensive angiotensin I-converting enzyme inhibitory peptide from *Pleurotus cornucopiae*. *Food Chem.* **2011**, *127*, 412–418. [CrossRef] [PubMed]
19. Wijesekara, I.; Qian, Z.J.; Ryu, B.; Ngo, D.H.; Kim, S.K. Purification and identification of antihypertensive peptides from seaweed pipefish (*Syngnathus schlegeli*) muscle protein hydrolysate. *Food Res Int.* **2011**, *44*, 703–707. [CrossRef]
20. Lin, H.C.; Alashi, A.M.; Aluko, R.E.; Sun, P.B.; Chang, Y.W. Antihypertensive properties of tilapia (Oreochromis spp.) frame and skin enzymatic protein hydrolysates. *Food Nutr. Res.* **2018**, *61*. Available online: https://www.tandfonline.com/doi/abs/10.1080/16546628.2017.1391666 (accessed on 20 August 2018). [CrossRef] [PubMed]
21. Suetsuna, K.; Chen, J.R. Identification of antihypertensive peptides from peptic digest of two microalgae, *Chlorella vulgaris* and *Spirulina platensis*. *Mar. Biotechnol.* **2001**, *3*, 305–309. [CrossRef] [PubMed]
22. Olivares-Molina, A.; Fernández, K. Comparison of different extraction techniques for obtaining extracts from brown seaweeds and their potential effects as angiotensin I-converting enzyme (ACE) inhibitors. *J. Appl. Phycol.* **2016**, *28*, 1295–1302. [CrossRef]
23. Xie, J.; Chen, X.; Wu, J.; Zhang, Y.; Zhou, Y.; Zhang, L.; Tang, Y.J.; Wei, D. Antihypertensive effects, molecular docking study, and isothermal titration calorimetry assay of angiotensin I-converting enzyme inhibitory peptides from *Chlorella vulgaris*. *J. Agric. Food Chem.* **2018**, *66*, 1359–1368. [CrossRef] [PubMed]
24. Okamoto, K.; Suzuki, T.; Ito, H.; Mitachi, Y.; Morita, N. *Spontaneous Hypertension: Its Pathogenesis and Complications*, 2nd ed.; DHEW Publication: Washington, WA, USA, 1976; pp. 1177–1179.
25. Murakami, T.; Okamoto, K.; Ogaki, M.; Iizuka, Y. Effect of *Chlorella* on blood pressure, cerebral stroke lesions, hypertensive vascular change and life-span in spontaneously hypertensive rats. *J. Jpn. Soc. Nutr. Food Sci.* **1987**, *40*, 351–359. [CrossRef]
26. Miyakoshi, M.; Tanaka, M.; Miyazawa, K.; Nara, H.; Takemoto, Y.; Maki, T.; Fukui, S.; Antoku, E.; Shinpo, K.; Shimizu, K. Study of *Chlorella* producted from the Chikugo area. *Clin. Rep.* **1980**, *14*, 3931–3941.
27. Suetsuna, K. Purification and identification of angiotensin I–converting enzyme inhibitors from the red alga *Porphyra yezoensis*. *J. Mar. Biotechnol.* **1998**, *6*, 163–167. [PubMed]
28. Suetsuna, K. Separation and identification of angiotensin I–converting enzyme inhibitory peptides from peptic digest of *Hizikia fusiformis* protein. *Nippon Suisan Gakk.* **1998**, *64*, 862–866. [CrossRef]
29. Suetsuna, K.; Nakano, T. Identification of an antihypertensive peptide from peptic digest of wakame (*Undaria pinnatifida*). *J. Nutr. Biochem.* **2000**, *11*, 450–454. [CrossRef]
30. Lu, J.; Ren, D.F.; Xue, U.L.; Sawano, Y.; Miyakawa, T.; Tanokura, M. Isolation of an antihypertensive peptide fome alcalase digest of Spirulina platensis. *J. Agric. Food Chem.* **2010**, *58*, 7166–7171. [CrossRef] [PubMed]
31. Spolaore, P.; Joannis-Cassan, C.; Duran, E.; Isambert, A. Commercial applications of microalgae. *J. Biosci. Bioeng.* **2006**, *101*, 87–96. [CrossRef] [PubMed]
32. Lowry, O.H.; Resebrough, N.J.; Farr, A.L.; Randall, R.J. Protein measurement with the folin phenol reagent. *J. Biol. Chem.* **1951**, *193*, 265–275. [PubMed]

33. Cooper, T.G. Spectrophotometry. In *The Tools of Biochemistry*, 1st ed.; Wiley-Interscience: Hoboken, NJ, USA, 1977; pp. 53–55. ISBN 0471171166.
34. Church, F.C.; Swaisgood, H.E.; Porter, H.D.; Catignani, G.L. Spectrophotometric assay using *o*-phthaldialdehyde for determination of proteolysis in milk and isolated milk proteins. *J. Dairy Sci.* **1983**, *66*, 1219–1227. [CrossRef]
35. Cushman, D.W.; Cheung, H.S. Spectrophotometric assay and properties of the angiotensin-converting enzyme of rabbit lung. *Biochem. Parmacol.* **1971**, *20*, 1637–1648. [CrossRef]
36. Wu, J.; Ding, X. Characterization of inhibition and stability of soy-protein-derived angiotensin I-converting enzyme inhibitory peptides. *Food Res. Int.* **2002**, *35*, 367–375. [CrossRef]
37. UniProt Database. Available online: http://www.uniprot.org (accessed on 15 May 2018).
38. Pairwise Sequence Alignment Software. Available online: https://www.ebi.ac.uk/Tools/psa/ (accessed on 15 May 2018).
39. SAS Institute Inc. *SAS/STAT User's Guide*; SAS Institute Press: Cary, NC, USA, 1988; p. 584.
40. Ruiz, J.Á.G.; Ramos, M.; Recio, J. Angiotensin converting enzyme inhibitory activity of peptides isolated from Manchego cheese. Stability under simulated gastrointestinal digestion. *Int. Dairy J.* **2004**, *14*, 1075–1080. [CrossRef]
41. Sato, M.; Oba, T.; Yamaguchi, T.; Nakano, T.; Kahara, T.; Funayama, K.; Kobayashi, A.; Nakano, T. Antihypertensive effects of hydrolysates of wakame (*Undar pinnatifida*) and their angiotensin-I-converting enzyme inhibitory activity. *Ann. Nutr. MeTab.* **2002**, *46*, 259–267. [CrossRef] [PubMed]
42. Sekiya, S.; Kobayashi, Y.; Kita, E.; Imamura, Y.; Toyama, S. Antihypertensive effects of tryptic hydrolysate of casein on normotensive and hypertensive volunteers. *J. Jpn. Soc. Nutr. Food Sci.* **1992**, *45*, 513–517. [CrossRef]
43. Ben, H.Y.; Labidi, A.; Arnaudin, I.; Bridiau, N.; Delatouche, R.; Maugard, T.; Piot, J.M.; Sannier, F.; Thiéry, V.; Bordenave-Juchereau, S. Measuring angiotensin-I converting enzyme inhibitory activity by micro plate assays: Comparison using marine cryptides and tentative threshold determinations with captopril and losartan. *J. Agric. Food Chem.* **2013**, *61*, 10685–10690.
44. Okamoto (Kainuma), A.; Matsumoto, E.; Iwashita, A.; Yasuhara, T.; Kawamura, Y.; Koizumi, Y.; Yanagida, F. Angiotensin I-converting enzyme inhibitory action of fish sauce. *Food Sci. Technol. Int.* **1995**, *1*, 101–106. [CrossRef]
45. Saito, S.; Wanezaki (Nakamura), K.; Kawato, A.; Imayasu, S. Structure and activity of angiotensin I converting enzyme inhibitory peptides from sake and sake lees. *Biosci. Biotechnol. Biochem.* **1994**, *58*, 1767–1771. [CrossRef] [PubMed]
46. Xu, Y.; Bao, T.; Han, W.; Zheng, X.; Wang, J. Purification and identification of an angiotensin I-converting enzyme inhibitory peptide from cauliflower byproducts protein hydrolysate. *Process Biochem.* **2016**, *51*, 1299–1305. [CrossRef]
47. Fujita, H.; Yokoyama, K.; Yoshikawa, M. Classification and antihypertensive activity of angiotensin I-converting enzyme inhibitory peptides derived from food proteins. *J. Food Sci.* **2000**, *65*, 564–569.
48. Martin, M.; Wellner, A.; Ossowski, I.; Henle, T. Identification and quantification of inhibitors for angiotensin-converting enzyme in hypoallergenic infant milk formulas. *J. Agric. Food Chem.* **2008**, *56*, 6333–6338. [CrossRef] [PubMed]
49. Ono, S.; Hosokawa, M.; Miyashita, K.; Takahashi, K. Inhibition properties of dipeptides from salmon muscle hydrolysate on angiotensin I-converting enzyme. *Int. J. Food Sci. Technol.* **2006**, *41*, 383–386. [CrossRef]
50. Wu, J.; Aluko, R.E.; Nakai, S. Structural requirements of angiotensin I-converting enzyme inhibitory peptides: Quantitative structure–activity relationship study of di- and tripeptides. *J. Agric. Food Chem.* **2006**, *54*, 732–738. [CrossRef] [PubMed]
51. Sato, M.; Hosokawa, T.; Yamaguchi, T.; Nakano, T.; Muramoto, K.; Kahara, T.; Funayama, K.; Kobayashi, A.; Nakano, T. Angiotensin I-converting enzyme inhibitory peptides derived from wakame (*Undaria pinnatifida*) and their antihypertensive effect in spontaneously hypertensive rats. *J. Agric. Food Chem.* **2002**, *50*, 6245–6252. [CrossRef] [PubMed]
52. He, R.; Ma, H.; Zhao, W.; Qu, W.; Zhao, J.; Luo, L.; Zhu, W. Modeling the QSAR of ACE-inhibitory peptides with ANN and its applied illustration. *Int. J. Pept.* **2012**. [CrossRef] [PubMed]
53. Li, G.H.; Le, G.W.; Shi, Y.H.; Shrestha, S. Angiotensin-I-converting enzyme inhibitory peptides derived from food proteins and their physiological and pharmacological effects. *Nutr. Res.* **2004**, *24*, 469–486. [CrossRef]

54. Cheung, H.S.; Wang, F.L.; Ondetti, M.A.; Sabo, E.F.; Cushman, D.W. Binding of peptide substrates and inhibitors of angiotensin-converting enzyme. *J. Biol. Chem.* **1980**, *255*, 401–407. [PubMed]
55. Xiao, G.; Yanhan, H.; Jing, L.; Jing, L.; Zhu, S.; Fei, H. Binding modes between C-domain selective angiotensin-converting enzyme (ACE) inhibitory dipeptides and ACE domains. *Food Sci.* **2017**, *38*, 160–166. [CrossRef]
56. Ono, S.; Hosokawa, M.; Miyashita, K.; Takahashi, K. Isolation of peptides with angiotensin I-converting enzyme inhibitory effect derived from hydrolysate of upstream chum salmon muscle. *J. Food Sci.* **2003**, *68*, 1611–1614. [CrossRef]

nutrients

MDPI

Article

Suppressive Effect of the α-Amylase Inhibitor Albumin from Buckwheat (*Fagopyrum esculentum* Moench) on Postprandial Hyperglycaemia

Kazumi Ninomiya [1], Shigenobu Ina [2], Aya Hamada [2], Yusuke Yamaguchi [2], Makoto Akao [2], Fumie Shinmachi [2], Hitoshi Kumagai [1] and Hitomi Kumagai [2,*]

[1] Department of Food Science and Nutrition, Kyoritsu Women's University, 2-2-1 Hitotsubashi, Chiyoda-ku, Tokyo 101-8347, Japan; kninomiya@kyoritsu-wu.ac.jp (K.N.); kumagai@kyoritsu-wu.ac.jp (H.K.)

[2] College of Bioresource Sciences, Nihon University, 1866 Kameino, Fujisawa-shi, Kanagawa 252-0880, Japan; carlosshige@yahoo.co.jp (S.I.); hama-aya527@snow.ocn.ne.jp (A.H.); yamaguchi.yusuke@nihon-u.ac.jp (Y.Y.); makao01@brs.nihon-u.ac.jp (M.A.); shinmachi.fumie@nihon-u.ac.jp (F.S.)

* Correspondence: kumagai@brs.nihon-u.ac.jp; Tel.: +81-466-84-3946

Received: 1 September 2018; Accepted: 12 October 2018; Published: 15 October 2018

Abstract: Inhibiting starch hydrolysis into sugar could reduce postprandial blood glucose elevation and contribute to diabetes prevention. Here, both buckwheat and wheat albumin that inhibited mammalian α-amylase in vitro suppressed blood glucose level elevation after starch loading in vivo, but it had no effect after glucose loading. In contrast to the non-competitive inhibition of wheat α-amylase inhibitor, buckwheat albumin acted in a competitive manner. Although buckwheat α-amylase inhibitor was readily hydrolysed by digestive enzymes, the hydrolysate retained inhibitory activity. Together with its thermal stability, this suggests its potential use in functional foods that prevent diabetes.

Keywords: buckwheat; albumin; α-amylase inhibitor; diabetes; hyperglycaemia

1. Introduction

Diabetes mellitus (DM) has a major impact on health worldwide, with the number of patients estimated to be 422 million in 2014 according to the latest survey that was conducted by World Health Organization (WHO) [1] (p. 25). DM is called a "silent killer" because patients often experience no obvious symptoms until they suddenly develop lesions, such as retinopathy, nephropathy, neuropathy, and angiopathy [1] (p. 13). These complications sometimes lead to blindness, renal failure, and food ulcer, which seriously affect health-related quality of life of patients. One factor contributing to prevention of DM and its complications is controlling the elevation in postprandial blood glucose levels by consuming an appropriate diet. Ingestion of a substance that inhibits polysaccharide hydrolysis is an effective means to suppress the elevation of blood glucose levels [2]. Therefore, α-amylase inhibitor (α-AI) has been attracting attention for its potential to prevent and treat DM.

Cereals often contain a high concentration of α-AI albumin proteins in seeds to resist against animals, like insects [3], including well-studied examples in cereals, such as wheat (*Triticum aestivum* L.), rice (*Oryza sativa* L.), barley (*Hordeum vulgare* L.), rye (*Secale cereal* L.), maize (*Zea mays* L.), and kidney beans (*Phaseolus vulgaris* L.) [4–12]. In particular, α-AIs from wheat and kidney beans strongly inhibit mammalian α-amylases and delay the hydrolysis of starch to reducing sugars [13–15]. Wheat α-AI inhibits α-amylase from both insects and mammals, suppressing blood glucose elevation in rats, dogs, and humans [16–18]. In addition, wheat α-AI shows considerable resistance to digestion by pepsin and trypsin, as well as thermal stability [19], and is therefore expected to maintain its inhibitory activity even after sterilization processes. Wheat α-AI has already been used as a functional component to suppress the elevation of blood glucose level in Food for Specified Health Uses (FoSHU) in Japan [20]. On the other hand, rice α-AI has strong resistance to hydrolysis by digestive enzymes and inhibits α-amylase from insects, but does not inhibit that from mammals [21]. However, we have shown that rice α-AI suppresses blood glucose elevation even after glucose loading, indicating a starch-independent mechanism, such as adsorbing glucose in the small intestine [21]. Both wheat and rice α-AIs are water-soluble albumin proteins that are tasteless and odourless and can therefore be included in almost any kind of food. Because rice α-AI suppresses postprandial hyperglycaemia through a different mechanism than that of wheat α-AI, simultaneous intake of these α-AIs may show a synergistic effect in suppressing blood glucose elevation. Furthermore, the different characteristics of rice α-AI as compared with wheat α-AI motivated us to discover other cereal α-AI proteins for anti-hyperglycaemic applications.

Buckwheat (*Fagopyrum esculentum* Moench) also contains a proteinaceous α-AI albumin fraction that is known to inhibit porcine pancreatic α-amylase [22,23]. Buckwheat flour has been used as an ingredient mainly for noodles and pancakes in Asian and European countries. Since many people in these countries have experience of eating buckwheat, buckwheat α-AI is considered to be acceptable as a food additive for anti-hyperglycaemia. However, the detailed characteristics of buckwheat α-AI and its effect in vivo have not yet been investigated. Therefore, in this study, we examined the suppressive effect of buckwheat α-AI on postprandial hyperglycaemia and characterised its enzyme-inhibition mechanism, digestibility, and thermal stability, the latter being an important property in food processing.

2. Materials and Methods

2.1. Materials

Buckwheat flour (Tomizawa Shoten Co., Ltd., Tokyo, Japan), wheat flour (Nisshin Flour Milling Inc., Tokyo, Japan), and mealworms were purchased from a local market. α-Amylases from the human pancreas and saliva and porcine pancreas were obtained from Sigma-Aldrich (St. Louis, MO, USA), and 2-chloro-4-nitrophenyl-α-D-maltotrioside (G3-CNP), the substrate for α-amylase, was from Oriental Yeast (Tokyo, Japan). α-Amylase from mealworms was prepared, as described by Buonocore and Poerio, with some modifications [24]. Pepsin from porcine stomach mucosa and trypsin from bovine pancreas were obtained from Wako Pure Chemical Industries (Osaka, Japan). All other chemicals used were of reagent grade.

2.2. Preparation of Buckwheat and Wheat α-AIs

Buckwheat and wheat α-AIs were prepared according to the method that was described by Feng et al., with some modifications [7]. Buckwheat flour or wheat flour was mixed with 5 times its weight of 25 mM 4-(2-hydroxyethyl)piperazine-1-ethanesulfonic acid (HEPES) buffer at pH 6.9 for 3 h at 4 °C and then centrifuged at 15,000× *g* for 15 min at 4 °C. The supernatant was heated at 80 °C for 20 min to denature non-heat-stable proteins and centrifuged at 15,000× *g* for 15 min at 4 °C. The clear supernatant was subjected to ammonium sulphate fractionation; the protein fraction precipitating at 40% $(NH_4)_2SO_4$ was collected by centrifugation at 15,000× *g* for 60 min at 4 °C. The precipitate was dialysed against distilled water to re-solubilise the protein and centrifuged at 15,000× *g* for 15 min at 4 °C. After lyophilisation of the supernatant, about 15 mg of protein dissolved in 20 mL of distilled water was applied to a Sephadex G-50 column (φ2.5 × 100 cm) (GE Healthcare UK Ltd., Buckinghamshire, UK) and equilibrated and eluted with distilled water at a flow rate of 0.2 mL/min, the absorbance of the eluate being measured continuously at 280 nm. Fractions (5 mL) were collected and the α-amylase inhibitory activity in each fraction was measured (see Section 2.3 below). The fractions showing more than 90% inhibitory activity against α-amylase from porcine pancreas were collected and lyophilised. α-AI powder was stored at −20 °C until use.

2.3. Measurement of α-Amylase Inhibitor Activity

The α-amylase inhibitory activity was measured, as described by Foo and Bais, with some modifications [25]. The inhibitory activity against α-amylase from mammals was determined by measuring the absorbance of 2-chloro-nitrophenol (CNP) at 405 nm produced from the cleavage of G3-CNP by α-amylase in the presence or absence of α-AI. The standard α-amylase inhibition assay was carried out by preincubating 25 μL of 1.6 U/μL α-amylase solution with 25 μL of 1 μg/μL cereal α-AI solution for 30 min at 37 °C in 20 mM HEPES buffer at pH 6.9 containing 50 mM NaCl and 3 mM $CaCl_2$. The reaction was initiated by the addition of 50 μL of G3-CNP and incubated for 10 min at 37 °C. The enzyme reaction was terminated by the addition of 100 μL of 10% (*v*/*v*) Tris solution, after which the absorbance at 405 nm of the 2-chloro-4-nitrophenol that was produced by the reaction was measured. The control mixture was prepared by replacing the α-AI solution with 20 mM HEPES buffer at pH 6.9 containing 50 mM NaCl and 3 mM $CaCl_2$. The inhibitory activity against α-amylase from mealworms was measured by the same procedure except that the buffer used was 20 mM acetate buffer at pH 5.4 containing 100 mM NaCl and the incubating temperature was 25 °C. The α-amylase inhibitory activity was expressed as percent inhibition relative to control using the following equation.

$$\text{Inhibition percent (\%)} = (\text{Ac} - \text{Ai})/\text{Ac} \times 100 \quad (1)$$

where Ai and Ac are enzyme activities with and without an inhibitor, respectively.

2.4. Animals

Male Wistar rats seven weeks of age were purchased from Japan SLC (Shizuoka, Japan). The rats were acclimatised for a period of 7 days. Throughout the acclimatisation and subsequent study periods, rats were maintained in controlled environment of 23 ± 1 °C and 55% humidity under a 12-h light/dark cycle with light from 8:00 to 20:00. All rat experiments were performed in accordance with the Guidelines for Animal Experiments of the College of Bioresource Science of Nihon University (Approval numbers: AP11B012 and AP12B059).

2.5. Oral Starch and Glucose Tolerance Tests

The oral starch tolerance test (OSTT) and oral glucose tolerance test (OGTT) were conducted according to the methods described by Ina et al. [21] with some modifications. The OSTT and OGTT were carried out under non-anaesthesia conditions. After seven rats in each group were fasted overnight for 14 h, 300 mg/kg of buckwheat α-AI or wheat α-AI was orally administered as a mixture with phosphate-buffered saline containing 1 g/kg body weight soluble starch or glucose. Then, blood was taken from the tail vein at 0, 15, 30, 45, and 90 min. Blood glucose levels were measured with the Dexter-ZII meter (Bayer, Osaka, Japan) and plasma insulin was measured by ELISA (Rat Insulin ELISA Kit (U-E type); Shibayagi, Gunma, Japan). The area under the curve (AUC) was calculated for blood glucose and plasma insulin according to the methods that were described by Wolever and Jenkins [26].

2.6. Analysis of In Vitro Digestibility by Digestive Enzymes

Hydrolysates were prepared in vitro by pepsin and trypsin, as described by Ma and Xiong and Iwami et al., with some modifications [27,28]. First, 10 mg of α-AI suspended in 1 mL of 0.1 mg/mL pepsin in HCl adjusted to pH 2.0 was incubated at 37 °C for 2 h. After the pepsin was inactivated by neutralisation with 1 mL of 4% (*w*/*v*) $NaHCO_3$, 1 mL of 1 mg/mL trypsin in 50 mM Tricine buffer at pH 8.0 was added and the mixture was incubated at 37 °C for 2, 4, or 6 h. The enzymatic hydrolysis was stopped by heating the sample solution at 100 °C for 5 min. The degree of hydrolysis was evaluated by the analysis of residual amylase inhibitory activity (see Section 2.3 above) and sodium dodecyl sulphate-polyacrylamide gel electrophoresis (SDS-PAGE). SDS-PAGE was carried out by the method of Laemmli [29]. After electrophoresis, the gels were stained for protein with 0.025% (*w*/*v*) Coomassie Brilliant Blue R-250 solution (Wako Pure Chemical Industries, Osaka, Japan).

2.7. Glycoprotein Staining

After SDS-PAGE, the fractionated protein was transferred electrophoretically to a polyvinylidene fluoride (PVDF) membrane (ProBlott, Applied Biosystem, Foster City, CA, USA). The membrane was washed three times with TPBS (phosphate-buffered saline containing 0.05% Tween 20) and immersed in a periodic-acid solution (TPBS containing 0.05% periodic acid). After washing three times with TPBS, the membrane was immersed in a biotin-hydrazide solution (25 μg/mL (+)-Biotin hydrazide (B7639, SIGMA-ALDRICH JAPAN, Tokyo, Japan)) dissolved in dimethyl sulfoxide. Then, the membrane was washed three times with TPBS and it was immersed in a horseradish peroxidase (HRP)-conjugated streptavidin solution (HRP-conjugated streptavidin (Funakoshi Co., Ltd., Tokyo, Japan) diluted with TPBS. The membrane was washed three times again with TPBS. To detect sugar chain bound to buckwheat α-AI, chemiluminescent reagent (Amersham™ ECL™ Western Blotting Analysis System, RPN2109, GE Healthcare UK Ltd., Buckinghamshire, UK) was used. The resulting light emission was detected using a gel imaging system (ChemiDoc MP, BioRad, Hercules, CA, USA).

2.8. Kinetic Analysis of α-Amylase Inhibition

The inhibitory activity of buckwheat α-AI against α-amylase from porcine pancreas was measured, as described by Seri et al. with some modifications [30] and compared with that of wheat α-AI. The α-amylase inhibitory activities of 0.05, 0.15, 0.25, and 0.35 mg/mL buckwheat and wheat α-AI were measured and the data were plotted according to the Lineweaver-Burk method [31].

2.9. Thermal Stability Analysis

The thermal stability of α-AI was evaluated by measuring the inhibitory activity against α-amylase from porcine pancreas after heating. α-AI was dissolved in 1 mL of distilled water to 0.1% (*w*/*w*) and boiled at 100 °C for 10, 30, 60, or 120 min. After cooling to room temperature, α-amylase inhibitory activity was measured as previously described in Section 2.3. The percent of unheated α-AI inhibitory activity remaining after heat treatment was defined as thermal stability, and was calculated as follows.

$$\text{Thermal stability (\%)} = \text{IAh}/\text{IAn} \times 100 \quad (2)$$

where IAh and IAn are α-amylase inhibitor activity of heated α-AI and that of non-heated α-AI, respectively.

2.10. Statistical Analysis

The data were represented as mean ± standard error (S.E.) The values were evaluated by one-way analysis of variance followed by the post-hoc Tukey-Kramer multiple range test.

3. Results

3.1. α-Amylase Inhibitory Activity

The inhibitory activity of buckwheat and wheat α-AI against α-amylase from several sources is shown in Figure 1. Wheat α-AI strongly inhibited α-amylase from human saliva (99.5%), human pancreas (99.3%), porcine pancreas (99.4%), and mealworm (97.6%). On the other hand, buckwheat α-AI also strongly inhibited α-amylase from porcine pancreas (97.9%) and mealworm (93.2%), but it showed somewhat decreased inhibition of α-amylase from human pancreas (68.7%) and only very weak inhibition of that from human saliva (10.2%).

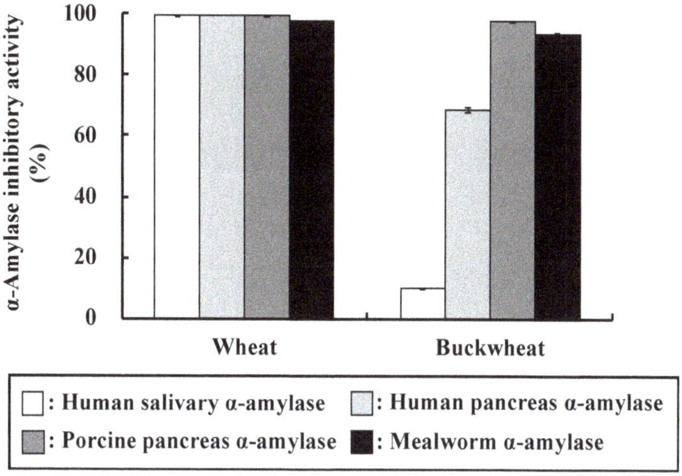

Figure 1. α-Amylase inhibitory activity of wheat and buckwheat α-AIs. Each value is the mean of three experiments with standard error (S.E.) shown as a vertical bar.

3.2. Oral Starch and Glucose Tolerance Test

The effect of buckwheat and wheat α-AIs on blood glucose and plasma insulin levels after starch loading was examined in normal rats. The postprandial blood glucose levels 15 min after starch loading of rats administered buckwheat and wheat α-AIs were 12% and 15% lower, respectively, than those of the rats used as a control group (Figure 2). At the same time point after starch loading, the postprandial plasma insulin levels of rats that were administered buckwheat and wheat α-AIs were 85% and 70% lower, respectively, than those of control rats (Figure 3). When the same experiment was conducted with glucose loading rather than starch loading, buckwheat, and wheat α-AIs did not suppress postprandial blood glucose elevation (Figure 4) or plasma insulin level (Figure 5).

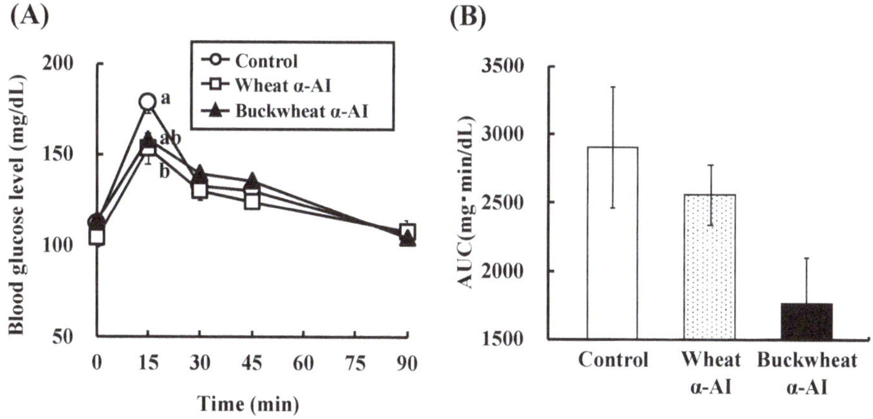

Figure 2. Effect of wheat and buckwheat α-amylase inhibitors (α-AIs) on (**A**) blood glucose level and (**B**) glucose area under the curve (AUC) after oral starch tolerance test using Wistar rats. Each value is the mean of 6–7 experiments with S.E. shown as a vertical bar. Values with different letters are significantly different at $p < 0.05$.

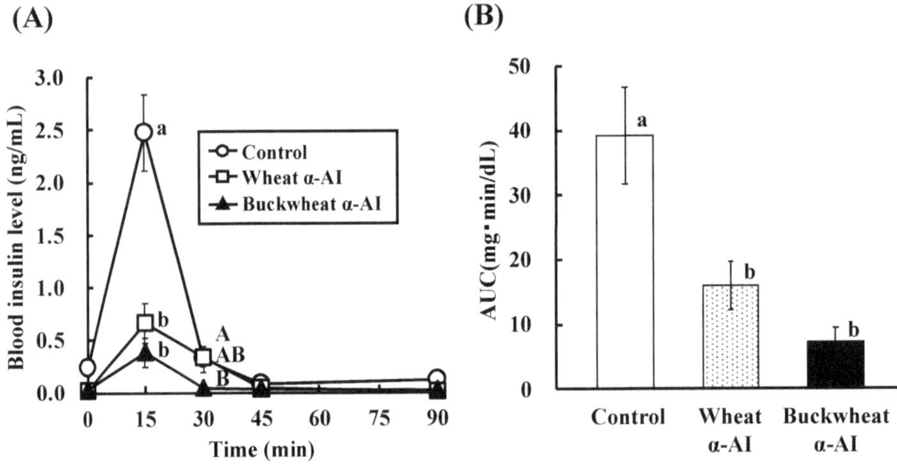

Figure 3. Effect of wheat and buckwheat α-AIs on (**A**) plasma insulin level and (**B**) insulin AUC after oral starch tolerance test using Wistar rats. Each value is the mean of seven experiments with S.E. shown as a vertical bar. Values with different letters are significantly different at $p < 0.05$.

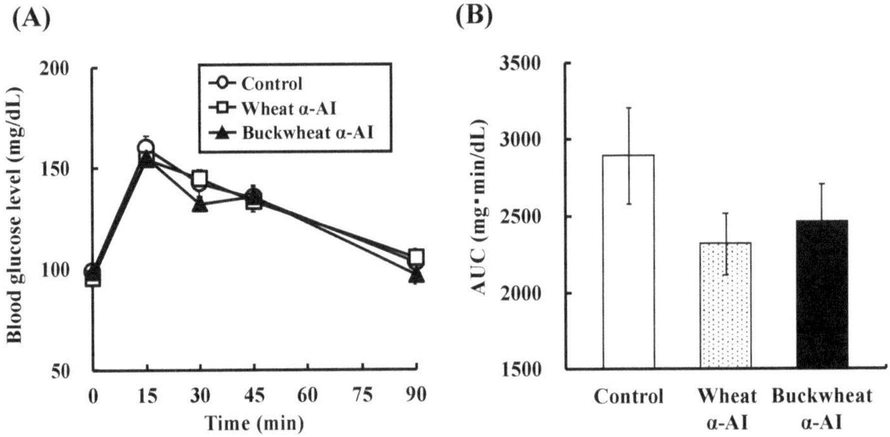

Figure 4. Effect of wheat and buckwheat α-AIs on (**A**) blood glucose level and (**B**) glucose AUC after oral glucose tolerance test using Wistar rats. Each value is the mean of seven experiments with S.E. shown as a vertical bar.

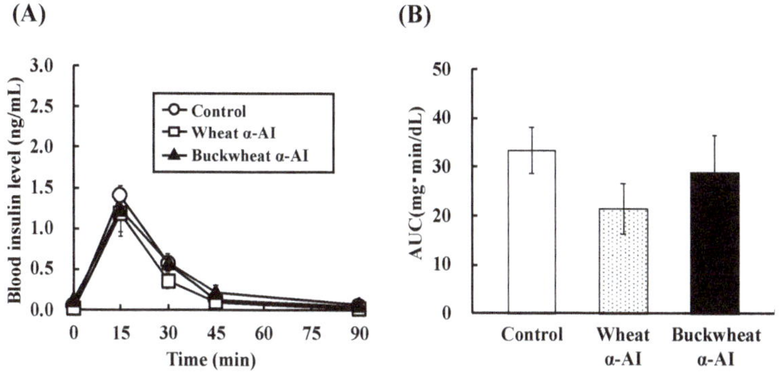

Figure 5. Effect of wheat and buckwheat α-AIs on (**A**) plasma insulin level and (**B**) insulin AUC after oral glucose tolerance test using Wistar rats. Each value is the mean of seven experiments with S.E. shown as a vertical bar.

3.3. *In Vitro Digestibility and Glycoprotein Staining*

The in vitro protein digestibility of α-AI was examined using sequential digestion by pepsin and trypsin. The 14-kDa wheat protein showed high resistance to digestion (Figure 6A), whereas the buckwheat protein was mostly hydrolysed to peptides that were smaller than 6.5 kDa, indicating that buckwheat α-AI is not resistant to digestive enzymes. The remaining α-amylase inhibitory activity of buckwheat and wheat α-AIs was examined after treatment by digestive enzymes (Figure 7). Although buckwheat α-AI was hydrolysed by digestive enzymes, it retained high inhibitory activity against α-amylase (91.4%). On the other hand, the α-amylase inhibitory activity of wheat α-AI decreased to 55.9% of its original level after treatment by pepsin and trypsin in spite of its resistance to digestion.

Buckwheat α-AI of higher molecular weight (> 29 kDa) was stained with glycoprotein-staining reagent. On the other hand, glycoprotein was hardly detected in bovine serum albumin, which was used as a negative control.

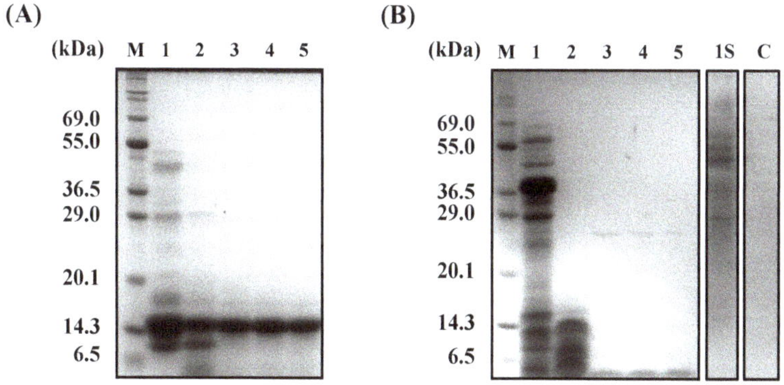

Figure 6. SDS-PAGE of wheat and buckwheat α-AIs before and after treatment with digestive enzymes and glycoprotein staining. (**A**) Wheat α-AI; (**B**) Buckwheat α-AI. (M) Marker; (1) Undigested; (2) Digested by pepsin for 2 h; (3) Digested by pepsin for 2 h followed by digestion with trypsin for 2 h; (4) Digested by pepsin for 2 h followed by digestion with trypsin for 4 h; and, (5) Digested by pepsin for 2 h followed by digestion with trypsin for 6 h; (1S) Undigested and stained with glycoprotein-staining reagent; (C) Bovine serum albumin stained with glycoprotein-staining reagent.

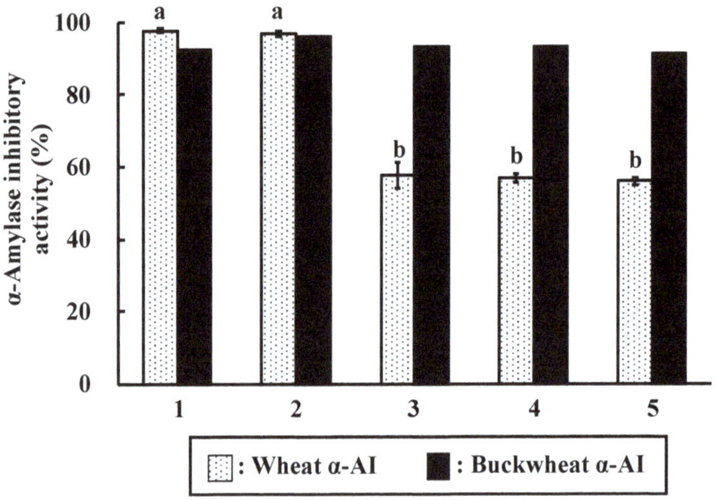

Figure 7. α-Amylase inhibitory activity of wheat and buckwheat α-AIs after digestion. (1) Undigested; (2) Digested by pepsin for 2 h; (3) Digested by pepsin for 2 h followed by digestion with trypsin for 2 h; (4) Digested by pepsin for 2 h followed by digestion with trypsin for 4 h; and, (5) Digested by pepsin for 2 h followed by digestion with trypsin for 6 h. Values with different letters are significantly different at $p < 0.05$.

3.4. Kinetic Analysis of α-Amylase Inhibition

Lineweaver-Burk plots were generated to assess the enzyme kinetics of wheat (Figure 8A) and buckwheat (Figure 8B) α-AIs. The plots of wheat α-AI intersected on the same abscissa section. On the other hand, the plots of buckwheat α-AI intersected on the same ordinate section.

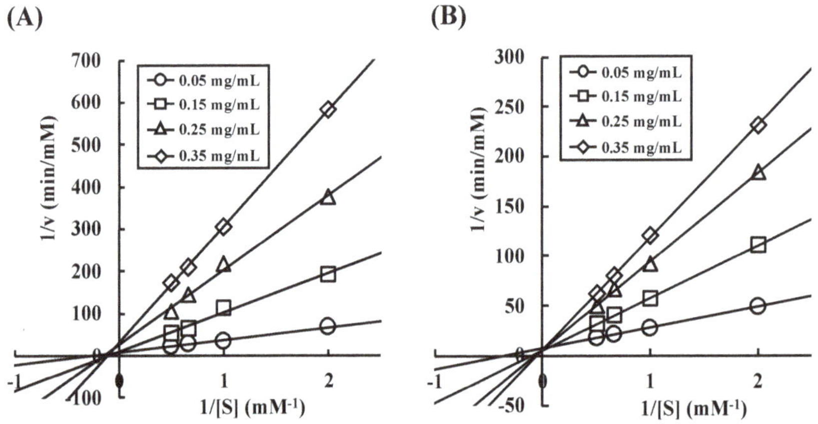

Figure 8. Kinetic analysis of the inhibitory activity against α-amylase from porcine pancreas. (**A**) Wheat α-AI; and, (**B**) Buckwheat α-AI.

3.5. Thermal Stability

To characterise the heat stability of buckwheat and wheat α-AIs, the inhibitory activity against porcine pancreatic α-amylase was measured after heating at 100 °C for 10–120 min (Figure 9). Both wheat and buckwheat α-AIs maintained high inhibitory activity even after heating at 100 °C for 120 min (98.2% and 75.4%, respectively).

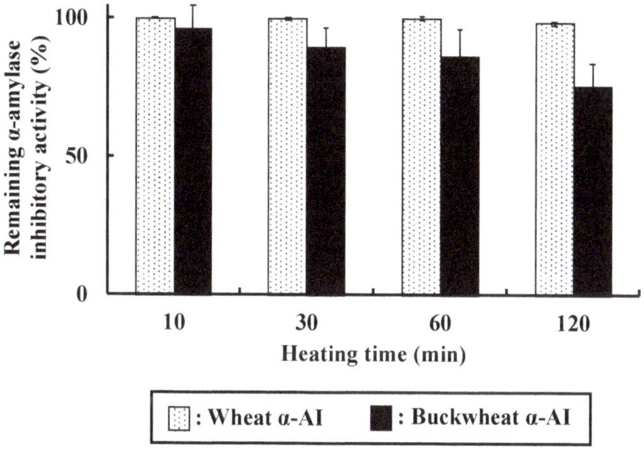

Figure 9. Thermal stability of wheat and buckwheat α-AIs. Each value is the mean of 2–3 experiments with S.E. shown as a vertical bar.

4. Discussion

This study demonstrated for the first time that buckwheat α-AI suppressed postprandial blood glucose elevation in rats. Wheat α-AI has already been reported to inhibit α-amylase from both insects and mammals [4–6,19], and it has a suppressive effect on blood glucose elevation [16–18]. As a result of its thermal stability [19], which allows it to retain activity even after sterilisation, wheat α-AI has already been used as a functional component in FoSHU in Japan [20]. In the present study, the α-amylase inhibitory activity and suppressive effect on postprandial hyperglycaemia of buckwheat α-AI were compared with those of wheat α-AI. In addition, the thermal stability of buckwheat α-AI was evaluated as a means to predict its stability during the sterilisation and cooking processes necessary to produce food products.

Various cereals contain α-AIs, some of which inhibit α-amylase from mammals and others that from insects only. As shown in Figure 1, wheat α-AI inhibited α-amylase from human saliva, human pancreas, porcine pancreas, and mealworms. We have reported that rice α-AI inhibits α-amylase from mealworms, but it does not inhibit α-amylase from human saliva, human pancreas, and porcine pancreas [21]. α-AI from barley, rye, maize, and kidney bean are also reported to inhibit α-amylase from mealworms [8–12]. On the other hand, buckwheat α-AI inhibited α-amylase from human pancreas, porcine pancreas, and mealworms, but did not inhibit that from human saliva (Figure 1), which is similar to the results of Feng et al., Ikeda et al., and Buonocore et al. [7,23,24]. These results imply that the mechanisms of substrate recognition of α-amylases from human saliva and pancreas are different and the structures of buckwheat and wheat α-AIs are not identical. Although the in vitro α-amylase inhibitory activity of buckwheat α-AI was about 30% less than that of wheat, these results encouraged us to investigate the suppressive effect of buckwheat α-AI on hyperglycaemia in vivo.

In OSTT, buckwheat α-AI suppressed the elevation in blood glucose and plasma insulin levels slightly more strongly than wheat α-AI (Figures 2 and 3), while neither α-AI suppressed the elevation upon OGTT (Figures 4 and 5). The results for wheat α-AI were similar to those of Puls and Keup [16].

We have reported that rice α-AI suppresses blood glucose elevation both on OSTT and OGTT. Because rice α-AI does not inhibit α-amylase from mammals but is not hydrolysed by digestive enzymes, its suppressive effect on blood glucose elevation after glucose loading is assumed to be due to the adsorption of glucose molecules onto its indigestible structure in the small intestine in a similar action as that of dietary fibre [21]. Because buckwheat α-AI inhibited α-amylase from mammals in vitro, as shown in Figure 1, its effect on postprandial hyperglycaemia after starch loading can likely be attributed to inhibiting the hydrolysis of starch to reducing sugars, similar to the mechanism of wheat α-AI.

Although the in vitro α-amylase inhibitory activity of buckwheat α-AI was less than that of wheat α-AI (Figure 1), the in vivo anti-hyperglycemic effect of buckwheat α-AI was higher than that of wheat α-AI (Figures 2 and 3). To explain these contradictory phenomena, we evaluated the α-amylase inhibitory activity after digestion in vitro. The α-amylase inhibitory activity of wheat α-AI decreased to 60% after treatment with pepsin followed by trypsin (Figure 7), though the protein showed resistance to digestion (Figure 6). On the other hand, although buckwheat α-AI was hydrolysed to low-molecular-weight peptides by digestive enzymes (Figure 6), it retained almost 100% α-amylase inhibitory activity even after digestion (Figure 7). These results suggest that the wheat α-AI was partially digested in vivo, reducing the suppressive effect on hyperglycaemia, while the hydrolysate of buckwheat α-AI possessed high α-amylase inhibitory activity. This may explain why buckwheat α-AI showed a more potent suppressive effect on hyperglycaemia in spite of its weaker α-amylase inhibitory activity in vitro when compared with wheat α-AI.

There are two hypotheses that explain the phenomenon of buckwheat α-AI hydrolysate having α-amylase inhibitory activity: (1) a certain peptide sequence shows α-amylase inhibitory activity, or (2) sugar chain covalently bound to some peptide shows α-amylase inhibitory activity. To explore these two possibilities, we investigated the enzyme-inhibition mechanism of wheat and buckwheat α-AIs. In Figure 8, the Lineweaver-Burk plots of wheat α-AI intersected at the same point on the abscissa, indicating that wheat α-AI inhibited the activity of α-amylase from porcine pancreas in a non-competitive manner, as previously reported [32]. On the other hand, the plots of buckwheat α-AI intersected at the same point on the ordinate, indicating that buckwheat α-AI inhibited α-amylase activity in a competitive manner. Because sugars commonly fit the active site of α-amylase and peptides are unlikely to be recognised as a substrate, glycopeptides produced from buckwheat α-AI would be the competitive inhibitors. Some researchers reported glycoproteins that were obtained from plants inhibit α-amylase in a competitive manner [33–35]. In addition, glycoproteins larger than 29 kDa were detected in undigested buckwheat α-AI (Figure 6B). Considering that free sugars should have been removed during the preparation of buckwheat α-AI and most buckwheat albumin was hydrolysed to be peptides smaller than 6.5 kDa, glycopeptides that were produced by digestive enzymes from glycoproteins present in buckwheat α-AI might have exhibited α-amylase inhibitory activity. Therefore, as the mechanisms of α-amylase inhibitory activity of buckwheat and wheat α-AIs differed with each other, these would be proteins of different structure and molecular weight.

Both wheat and buckwheat α-AIs maintained high α-amylase inhibitory activity after heating, as shown in Figure 9. Oneda et al. reported that wheat α-AI showed high thermal stability [19], consistent with our results showing that it retained more than 98% of α-amylase inhibitory activity even after heating at 100 °C for 120 min, probably due to intramolecular disulphide bonds. The α-amylase inhibitory activity of buckwheat α-AI gradually decreased but it was still 75% after heating at 100 °C for 120 min. This result is consistent with our assumption that sugar chain in buckwheat α-AI shows α-amylase inhibitory activity and thus retained the activity, even after denaturation by heating. The thermal stability of buckwheat α-AI is high enough to be used in food products that undergo sterilisation.

5. Conclusions

In conclusion, buckwheat α-AI suppressed postprandial hyperglycaemia after starch loading by inhibiting α-amylase activity in a competitive manner. Buckwheat α-AI retained its inhibitory activity against α-amylase, even after digestion and heating. Therefore, it is a good candidate for use as a functional component in FoSHU, such as foods to suppress the elevation of blood glucose levels and prevent diabetes.

Author Contributions: K.N., S.I. and H.K. (Hitomi Kumagai) designed the study. K.N. and A.H. conducted the research. K.N., S.I., Y.Y., H.K. (Hitoshi Kumagai) and H.K. (Hitomi Kumagai) analyzed the data. K.N., Y.Y., H.K. (Hitoshi Kumagai) and H.K. (Hitomi Kumagai) wrote the manuscript. M.A. and F.S. assisted with data preparation and analyses. H.K. (Hitoshi Kumagai) and H.K. (Hitomi Kumagai) had primary responsibility for final content. All authors read and approved the final manuscript.

Funding: This research received no external funding.

Conflicts of Interest: The authors declare no conflict of interest.

References

1. *Global Report on Diabetes*; World Health Organization: Geneva, Switzerland, 2016; pp. 13, 25.
2. Van de Laar, F.A.; Lucassen, P.L.; Akkermans, R.P.; van de Lisdonk, E.H.; Rutten, G.E.; van Weel, C. α-Glucosidase inhibitors for patients with type 2 diabetes. *Diabetes Care* **2004**, *28*, 154–163. [CrossRef]
3. Svensson, B.; Fukuda, K.; Nielsen, P.K.; Bønsager, B.C. Proteinaceous α-amylase inhibitors. *Biochim. Biophys. Acta* **2004**, *1696*, 145–156. [CrossRef] [PubMed]
4. Silano, V.; Pocchiari, F.; Kasarda, D.D. Physical characterization of α-amylase inhibitors from wheat. *Biochim. Biophys. Acta* **1973**, *317*, 139–148. [CrossRef]
5. O'Donnell, M.D.; McGeeney, K.F. Purification and properties of an α-amylase inhibitor from wheat. *Biochim. Biophys. Acta* **1976**, *422*, 159–169. [CrossRef]
6. Petrucci, T.; Rab, A.; Tomasi, M.; Silano, V. Further characterization studies of the α-amylase protein inhibitor of gel electrophoretic mobility 0.19 from the wheat kernel. *Biochim. Biophys. Acta* **1976**, *420*, 288–297. [CrossRef]
7. Feng, G.H.; Chen, M.; Kreamer, K.J.; Reeck, G.R. Alpha-amylase inhibitors from rice: Fractionation and selectivity toward insect, mammalian, and bacterial alpha-amylases. *Cereal Chem.* **1991**, *68*, 516–526.
8. Weselake, R.J.; MacGregor, A.W.; Hill, R.D. An endogenous α-amylase inhibitor in barley kernels. *Plant Physiol.* **1983**, *72*, 809–812. [CrossRef] [PubMed]
9. Granum, P.E. Purification and characterization of an α-amylase inhibitor from rye (secale cereal) flour. *J. Food Biochem.* **1978**, *2*, 103–120. [CrossRef]
10. Iulek, J.; Franco, O.L.; Silva, M.; Slivinski, C.T.; Bloch, C., Jr.; Rigden, D.J.; Grossi de Sá, M.F. Purification, biochemical characterization and partial primary structure of a new α-amylase inhibitor from *Secale cereale* (rye). *Int. J. Biochem. Cell Biol.* **2000**, *32*, 1195–1204. [CrossRef]
11. Blanco-labra, A.; Iturbe-chiñas, F.A. Purification and characterization of an α-amylase inhibitor from maise (zea maize). *J. Food Biochem.* **1981**, *5*, 1–17. [CrossRef]
12. Marshall, J.J.; Lauda, C.M. Purification and properties of phaseolamin, an inhibitor of α-amylase, from the kidney bean, phaseolus vulgaris. *J. Biol. Chem.* **1975**, *250*, 8030–8037. [PubMed]
13. Kodama, T.; Miyazaki, T.; Kitamura, I.; Suzuki, Y.; Namba, Y.; Sakurai, J.; Torikai, Y.; Inoue, S. Effects of single and long-term administration of wheat albumin on blood glucose control: Randomized controlled clinical trials. *Eur. J. Clin. Nutr.* **2005**, *59*, 384–392. [CrossRef] [PubMed]
14. Tormo, M.A.; Gil-Exojo, I.; Romero de Tejada, A.; Campillo, E. Hypoglycaemic and anorexigenic activities of an α-amylase inhibitor from white kidney beans (*Phaseolus vulgaris*) in Wistar rats. *Br. J. Nutr.* **2004**, *92*, 785–790. [CrossRef] [PubMed]
15. Tormo, M.A.; Gil-Exojo, I.; Romero de Tejada, A.; Campillo, E. White bean amylase inhibitor administered orally reduces glycaemia in type 2 diabetic rats. *Br. J. Nutr.* **2006**, *96*, 539–544. [CrossRef] [PubMed]
16. Puls, W.; Keup, U. Influence of an α-amylase inhibitor (BAY d 7791) on blood glucose, serum insulin and NEFA in starch loading test in rats, dogs and man. *Diabetologia* **1973**, *9*, 97–101. [CrossRef] [PubMed]

17. Koike, D.; Yamadera, K.; Dimagno, E.P. Effect of a wheat amylase inhibitor on canine carbohydrate digestion, gastrointestinal function, and pancreatic growth. *Gastroenterology* **1995**, *108*, 1221–1229. [CrossRef]
18. Lankisch, M.; Layer, P.; Rizza, R.A.; DiMagno, E.P. Acute postprandial gastrointestinal and metabolic effects of wheat amylase inhibitor (WAI) in normal, obese, and diabetic humans. *Pancreas* **1998**, *17*, 176–181. [CrossRef] [PubMed]
19. Oneda, H.; Lee, S.; Inouye, K. Inhibitory effect of 0.19 α-amylase inhibitor from wheat kernel on the activity of porcine pancreas α-amylase and its thermal stability. *J. Biochem.* **2004**, *135*, 421–427. [CrossRef] [PubMed]
20. Arai, S.; Yasuoka, A.; Abe, K. Functional food science and food for specified health use policy in Japan: State of the art. *J. Lipid Res.* **2008**, *19*, 69–73. [CrossRef] [PubMed]
21. Ina, S.; Ninomiya, K.; Mogi, T.; Hase, A.; Ando, T.; Matsukaze, N.; Ogihara, J.; Akao, M.; Kumagai, H.; Kumagai, H. Rice (*Oryza sativa japonica*) Albumin Suppresses the elevation of blood glucose and plasma insulin levels after oral glucose loading. *J. Agric. Food Chem.* **2016**, *64*, 4882–4890. [CrossRef] [PubMed]
22. Ikeda, K.; Shida, K.; Kishida, M. α-Amylase inhibitor in buckwheat seed. *Fagopyrum* **1994**, *14*, 3–6.
23. Ikeda, K.; Kishida, M. Digestibility of proteins in buckwheat seed. *Fagopyrum* **1993**, *13*, 21–24.
24. Buonocore, V.; Poerio, R. Affinity column purification of amylases on protein inhibitors from wheat kernel. *J. Chromatogr.* **1975**, *114*, 109–114. [CrossRef]
25. Foo, A.Y.; Bais, R. Amylase measurement with 2-chloro-4-nitrophenyl maltotrioside as substrate. *Clin. Chim. Acta* **1998**, *272*, 137–147. [CrossRef]
26. Wolever, T.M.; Jenkins, D.J. The use of the glycemic index in predicting the blood glucose response to mixed meals. *Am. J. Clin. Nutr.* **1986**, *43*, 167–172. [CrossRef] [PubMed]
27. Ma, Y.; Xiong, Y.L. Antioxidant and bile acid binding activity of buckwheat protein in vitro digests. *J. Agric. Food Chem.* **2009**, *57*, 4372–4380. [CrossRef] [PubMed]
28. Iwami, K.; Sakakibara, K.; Ibuki, F. Involvement of post-digestion 'hydrophobia' peptides in plasma cholesterol-lowering effect of dietary plant proteins. *Agric. Biol. Chem.* **1986**, *50*, 1217–1222. [CrossRef]
29. Laemmli, U.K. Cleavage of structural proteins during the assembly of the head of bacteriophage T4. *Nature* **1970**, *227*, 680–685. [CrossRef] [PubMed]
30. Seri, K.; Sanai, K.; Matsuo, N.; Kawakubo, K.; Xue, C.; Inoue, S. L-Arabinose selectively inhibits intestinal sucrose in anuncompetitive manner and suppresses glycemic response after sucrose ingestion in animals. *Metabolism* **1996**, *45*, 1368–1374. [CrossRef]
31. Lineweaver, H.; Burk, D. The determination of enzyme dissociation constants. *J. Am. Chem. Soc.* **1934**, *56*, 658–666. [CrossRef]
32. O'Connor, C.M.; McGeeney, K.F. Interaction of human α-amylases with inhibitors from wheat flower. *Biochim. Biophys. Acta* **1981**, *658*, 397–405. [CrossRef]
33. Gadge, P.P.; Wagh, S.K.; Shaikh, F.K.; Tak, R.D.; Padul, M.V.; Kachole, M.S. A bifunctional α-amylase/trypsin inhibitor from pigeonpea seeds: Purification, biochemical characterization and its bio-efficacy against *Helicoverpa armigera*. *Pest Biochem. Physiol.* **2015**, *125*, 17–25. [CrossRef] [PubMed]
34. Gibbs, B.F.; Alli, I. Characterization of a purified α-amylase inhibitor from white kidney beans (*Phaseolus vulgaris*). *Food Res. Int.* **1998**, *31*, 217–225. [CrossRef]
35. Maskos, K.; Huber-Wunderlich, M.; Glockshuber, R. RBI, a one-domain α-amylase/trypsin inhibitor with completely independent binding sites. *FEBS Lett.* **1996**, *397*, 11–16. [CrossRef]

nutrients

MDPI

Review

Food-Derived Bioactive Peptides in Human Health: Challenges and Opportunities

Subhadeep Chakrabarti [1,†], Snigdha Guha [2,†] and Kaustav Majumder [2,*]

[1] Bureau of Nutritional Sciences, Food Directorate, Health Products and Food Branch, Health Canada, Ottawa, ON K1A 0K9, Canada; subhadee@ualberta.ca

[2] Department of Food Science and Technology, University of Nebraska-Lincoln, Lincoln, NE 68588-6205, USA; sguha3@unl.edu

[*] Correspondence: kaustav.majumder@unl.edu; Tel.: +1-(402)-472-3510; Fax: +1-(402)-472-4474

[†] These authors contributed equally.

Received: 16 October 2018; Accepted: 9 November 2018; Published: 12 November 2018

Abstract: Recent scientific evidence suggests that food proteins not only serve as nutrients, but can also modulate the body's physiological functions. These physiological functions are primarily regulated by some peptides that are encrypted in the native protein sequences. These bioactive peptides can exert health beneficial properties and thus are considered as a lead compound for the development of nutraceuticals or functional foods. In the past few decades, a wide range of food-derived bioactive peptide sequences have been identified, with multiple health beneficial activities. However, the commercial application of these bioactive peptides has been delayed because of the absence of appropriate and scalable production methods, proper exploration of the mechanisms of action, high gastro-intestinal digestibility, variable absorption rate, and the lack of well-designed clinical trials to provide the substantial evidence for potential health claims. This review article discusses the current techniques, challenges of the current bioactive peptide production techniques, the oral use and gastrointestinal bioavailability of these food-derived bioactive peptides, and the overall regulatory environment.

Keywords: bioactive peptides; enzymatic hydrolysis; fermentation; peptide absorption; oral bioavailability; functional foods

1. Introduction

The physicochemical roles of proteins in foods, apart from serving as dietary nutrients, are being increasingly acknowledged. Many of these physicochemical roles of naturally occurring dietary proteins are carried out by peptide sequences encrypted inside the parent protein, which exert their actions when released, either enzymatically, during food processing, or by microbial fermentation [1,2]. Bioactive peptides are defined as peptide sequences within a protein that exert a beneficial effect on body functions and/or positively impact human health, beyond its known nutritional value [3]. These peptides can regulate important bodily functions through their myriad activities, including antihypertensive, antimicrobial, antithrombotic, immunomodulatory, opioid, antioxidant, and mineral binding functions [4–7].

Different activities of the bioactive peptides are governed by the sequence of the amino acids, as they would interact with other proteins in the body and modulate natural processes [8]. Although the structure and functional relationship of bioactive peptides are not well established, most of them share some common properties. For instance, most of these peptides contain 2 to 20 amino acids and are generally rich in hydrophobic amino acids [3,9]. Thus, over the last few years, there has been an increased scientific interest in finding distinct bioactive peptide sequences that can reduce or prevent the risk of chronic diseases and provide immune protection [2]. Thus, the use of bioactive peptides has gained much interest as nutraceuticals [10] and functional foods [11]. As a result, much research has been dedicated recently to the processing and generation of bioactive peptides from food products, and the previously under-utilized protein-rich by-products of the food industries [12,13]. The bioactivity of these peptides could be tested through in vitro bio-chemical assays, cell culture, in vivo studies via animal models, and human clinical trials. While the research related to the development of food-derived bioactive peptide-based nutraceuticals is gaining momentum, the ability to translate these new findings into practical or commercial use remains delayed. The major reasons behind this delay are (1) lack of scalable and consistent methods of producing bioactive peptides from different food or non-food sources; (2) general lack of understanding of gastrointestinal stability or absorption of these peptides; (3) lack of knowledge of their mechanisms of actions, and (4) lack of proper clinical trials to provide substantial evidence for potential health claims. Thus, the scope of this review includes the challenges pertaining to manufacturing/processing, oral use and/or bioavailability, and the regulatory environment governing use of bioactive peptides.

2. Production of Bioactive Peptides

A diverse array of plant and animal food proteins has been used for extracting bioactive peptides [7]. The most widely used animal proteins are from eggs, milk (casein and whey), and meat proteins. Bioactive peptides from plant sources are typically from soy, oat, pulses (chickpea, beans, peas, and lentils), canola, wheat, flaxseed, and hemp seed. Furthermore, proteins from marine sources have also been used, for instance, fish, squid, salmon, sea urchin, oyster, seahorse, and snow crab [3,9]. In the manufacturing process, food proteins from various sources are first digested with an enzyme, and then the biological activity of the whole hydrolysate is evaluated, followed by a series of activity-guided purification and identification, so as to find the most potent sequence. However, the activity-guided identification and purification of bioactive peptides is time-consuming, and often studies do not provide enough rational behind the selection of enzymes. To overcome these issues, a quantitative structure–activity relationship (QSAR) and bioinformatics based in-silico method is often used to predict the yield of bioactive peptides from food protein sources [14]. However, this method works best only when we have the complete sequence of a food protein and the structure and functional properties of the peptides are known. Unfortunately, there is lack of understanding of such structure–functional properties and hence, researchers are still using the traditional activity-guided methods to search for bioactive peptides from food proteins. The following section highlights the basic bioactive production techniques.

2.1. *Production Methods*

Bioactive peptides from food proteins can be produced either by enzymatic hydrolysis (using proteolytic enzymes from either plants or microbes), hydrolysis with digestive enzymes (simulated gastrointestinal digestion), or by fermentation using starter cultures. Some studies also used a combination of these methods to produce peptides with a biological activity [2]. Furthermore, bioactive peptides can also be synthesized chemically, as the amount of these peptides found in the nature is very low, and there is a constant increasing commercial interest of producing synthetic bioactive peptide [15]. However, it is doubtful if purely synthetic peptides would be considered as food or nutrients, and fit within the scope of this review. Therefore, in this review, we primarily discuss the enzymatic hydrolysis and fermentation, and briefly introduce the chemical synthesis process for producing bioactive peptides.

2.1.1. Enzyme Hydrolysis

In the enzymatic hydrolysis method, the protein of interest is subjected to enzymatic treatment at a specific pH and temperature. The advantages of this method are that it is easy to scale up and generally has a shorter reaction time than microbial fermentation [1]. For instance, in a study by Gobbetti et al., angiotensin converting enzyme (ACE)-inhibitory peptides were generated from the fermentation of milk, using the strains *Lactobacillus lactis* ssp. *cremoris* and *Lactobacillus delbrueckii* ssp. *bulgaricus*, each for 72 h separately [16]. This was in contrast to the study by El-Fattah et al., where bioactive peptides with ACE-inhibitory activities were produced from the hydrolysis of milk using protease (*Aspergillus oryzae*) for only 1 h [17]. More than one protease can also be used one after the other to generate shorter peptides, however, the temperature and pH would need to be optimized for each of the proteases [1]. Furthermore, the choice of protease used and the time of enzymatic hydrolysis could be important in deciding the type of peptides generated. For example, rice proteins hydrolyzed with bacillolysin showed a stronger anti-inflammatory and anti-tyrosinase activities compared with those hydrolyzed by subtilisin [18]. On the other hand, samples hydrolyzed with leucyl and papain aminopeptidase and cysteine endopeptidase showed the least activity [18]. Similarly, different enzymes generated bioactive peptide-rich hydrolysates from bovine muscle and porcine plasma with divergent taste profiles, as observed in a recent study [19]. Several studies have also used in-vitro simulated gastrointestinal digestion technique to produce bioactive peptides from food proteins [20–23]. In such methods, the researchers have tried to identify the activity of the peptides that may be produced in our body after consuming a particular food or food-protein.

2.1.2. Fermentation

Fermentation involves the culturing of microorganisms, such as yeasts, fungi, or bacteria, on the protein of interest in order to hydrolyze the protein into shorter peptides with their own enzymes. The bacteria usually needs to be in the exponential growth phase before they are harvested, washed, and added to glucose containing sterile distilled water, which ultimately serves as the starting inoculum for the protein substrate [24,25]. The degree of hydrolysis depends on the fermentation time, microbial strain, and the protein source. For instance, Ahn et al. showed that the ACE-inhibitory activity of whey protein derived peptides fermented with *Lactobacillus brevis* was stronger than those fermented with *L. casei*, *L. lactis*, *L. plantarum*, and *L. acidophilus* [26]. Similarly, Sanjukta et al. demonstrated that soybean proteins fermented by *Bacillus subtilis* MTCC5480 produced a higher degree of hydrolysis compared with *B. subtilis* MTCC1747 [27]. Co-cultures using different combinations of bacteria, yeasts, and fungi can also be used to modulate the hydrolysis processes [28].

2.2. Production Issues

The classical approach of producing bioactive peptides is to find a suitable protein source, followed by its hydrolysis, using either enzymes or by microbial fermentation, so as to generate peptides with a potential bioactivity. This would be followed by the identification of the peptide sequences and confirmation of the bioactivity. However, much of the published literature on bioactive peptides have not taken a systematic approach to optimize the multiple parameters affecting the production and purification of these peptides [29]. Hanke and Ottens suggested that "one factor at a time" and "trial and error" methods are obsolete and are being taken over by systemic design of experiments (DOE) approaches. DOE methods require the knowledge of the critical process parameters (CPP) that would affect the critical quality attributes (CQA) [30]. Certain CPPs, with respect to the production of bioactive peptides, requires knowledge of the starting material (protein content of a food and seasonal variabilities), the enzyme (optimal temperature and pH, purity, specific activity, and substrate specificity), and finally the process conditions (time, temperature, and enzyme to substrate ratio). On the other hand, certain CQAs may be recognized for the peptide fractions or the protein hydrolysates [29]. For example, Cheung and Li-Chan applied a Taguchi's L_{16} (4^5) fractional factorial design to study the effect four CPPs on three CQAs (degree of hydrolysis, ACE-inhibitory effect, and bitterness) of the protein hydrolysate obtained from the by-products of shrimp processing. The use of this DOE approach enabled the assessment of the protein hydrolysates using only 16 unique experiments, which were generated under conditions linked with the combination of the four CPPs. This was in contrast to the use of either a full factorial design with 256 unique experiments, or a one-factor-at a time experiment, where one factor is changed, keeping the other three constant. However, the use of Taguchi's methods and other DOE approaches are more beneficial in other disciplinary sectors, while its recognition in the field of food-derived bioactive peptides has been limited [31].

Furthermore, Kopf-Bolanz et al. suggested that processing can affect the peptide profiles and cause protein degradation when present in food matrices such as dairy products [32]. During thermal processing, besides Maillard reactions, oxygen- and carbon-based radicals can be generated, which could lead to the oxidation of proteins, peptides, and carbohydrates [33]. A number of studies have been reported for food-derived bioactive peptides from the hydrolysis of protein isolates or protein concentrates in isolation, rather than a direct hydrolysis of the whole food [34,35]. However, it is critical to consider the food matrix, which may also influence the hydrolysis reaction. Foods contain many naturally occurring compounds, such as lipids, carbohydrates, and secondary metabolites (like quinones), which interacts with the proteins in the matrix, and thus can affect the type of peptides generated upon hydrolysis. Schiff base reactions between reducing sugars and peptides are well established. Peptides undergo reactions with reactive oxygen species, oxidized lipids, and aldehydes, as well as decarboxylation, deamination, and nitration reactions. All of these could potentially affect the availability of the peptides within the food matrix [33]. For instance, in a study by Lacroix and Li-Chan, the whey protein constituents were hydrolyzed individually by pepsin. Among them, α-lactalbumin hydrolysate showed the highest dipeptidyl peptidase IV (DPP-IV) inhibitory activity, although the specific peptides responsible for the inhibition were not identified. However, in a subsequent study, in order to identify the peptides responsible for the DPP-IV inhibition, it was found that the most potent anti-DPP-IV peptides were from β-lactoglobulin rather than α-lactalbumin. This suggests that co-existence of different proteins in a particular food matrix might induce conformational changes during commercial production, which might in turn affect the susceptibility and accessibility of the peptide bonds during digestion [29].

In-silico prediction methods, such as QSAR, use knowledge of the activity and structure of peptides present in the databases and literature. It can be used to predict the sequences of the peptides likely to have any bioactivities, their structural–functional relationships, specific location of the peptides within the parent protein, and the possible mechanism of action [36]. However, even though there is much data on food peptides and the enzymes required to release them from the source proteins, the majority describe the endogenous bioactive peptides, which are of physiological relevance, instead of those that are obtained from food [37]. Furthermore, the information that is available in the databases often involves well-characterized and purified proteolytic enzymes, in comparison with the commercially used enzymes for food processes, which are less substrate specific and of variable purity [38].

2.3. Commercialization Challenges and Quality Assurance

Once the peptides are produced, either through classical ways or by in-silico methods, the next step is to confirm the bioactivity of the peptides. However, unlike synthetic drug molecules, which are single entities, the target bioactive peptides isolated from foods are usually a mixture of peptides. The purification of these peptides to 99% purity would not only increase the cost to unacceptable levels and reduce the yields, but would also eliminate any beneficial additive or synergistic effects with other peptides present in the whole hydrolysate. Furthermore, bioactive peptides are generally hydrophobic, and thus they are less soluble at higher concentrations. Indeed, Li-Chan suggested preparing formulations of several different bioactive peptides, each having a low concentration, but conferring similar bioactivity levels, to address this problem [29].

Food proteins are often hydrolyzed using enzymes such as trypsin, pepsin, chymotrypsin, bromelain, ficain, or papain. Although there are several advantages to using enzymatic hydrolysis, such as the absence of residual toxic chemicals and organic solvents in the final product, the use of the enzymes on an industrial scale highly increases the cost of the production. One solution to that is to use cheaper enzyme sources such as by-products of the meat industry (i.e., pancreases of animal origin) [39]. Secondly, a mixture of peptides is generated during in vitro enzymatic hydrolysis, depending on the complexity of the starting material. This in turn makes the process of purification time-consuming and challenging; in some cases, each of the peptide may require a complex purification protocol [40].

On the other hand, naturally occurring peptides have many advantages compared with the peptides produced by enzymatic hydrolysis, as these peptides are perceived to be safe [40,41]. However, the lack of technology at a larger scale and very expensive purification techniques are some of the limitations for the commercialization of extracting naturally occurring bioactive peptides from food sources [40]. Thus, research should focus on addressing the above-mentioned challenges associated with production methods for commercial applications of these food-derived bioactive peptides.

3. Oral Use of Bioactive Peptides: Challenges and Considerations

As these peptides are derived from food, they are generally considered more "natural"; hence, perceptions of acceptance are likely to be higher. Yet, their use as orally ingested products also presents special challenges and consequences.

3.1. *Taste*

The oral intake of food and medicinal products is fundamentally dependent on taste. Taste is often the body's first response to an orally ingested substance. We eat things that taste good and reject those with bitter or other unpleasant tastes. It is believed to be an evolutionary response, developed over millennia to avoid toxic or rancid substances [42]. As such, it is vital for orally taken products to have a favorable taste profile. Protein hydrolysates and individual peptides often fail on these grounds, as a significant number of these products are bitter, which may limit their acceptability [43,44]. A number of studies have identified factors such as increasing molecular weight, presence of hydrophobic amino acids at the C-terminal, presence of certain amino acid sequences, and degree of electrical charge with a propensity towards bitterness (reviewed in [45]). However, the molecular mechanisms of bitterness and its regulation are not completely understood; hence, the modification rather than prevention of the bitter taste may be a more feasible option in many instances.

Traditionally, bitterness modification (also called "debittering") has been approached through methods to reduce levels of these bitter-tasting peptides. One of the procedures involves the further hydrolysis of the product (bioactive peptide or protein hydrolysate, generated by initial enzymatic hydrolysis) by enzymes, to reduce the content of any bitter-tasting peptides [46–48]. While reasonably effective, this process can be expensive because of the costs of additional enzymes, and it also risks inadvertently destroying the very bioactive properties that made the preparation valuable in the first place. The alternative option has been to "screen out" bitter peptides from a complex mixture involving one or more techniques, such as gel separation, alcohol extraction, chromatography on silica gel, and isoelectric precipitation (reviewed in [49]). While each of these methods has its benefits, the time and expense added to a commercial production scheme are often considerable. Besides, the lack of a comprehensive structure–activity relationship between taste and molecular structure further impedes on the successful application of such a method to a growing array of bioactive peptides derived from a range of food proteins.

An alternative approach is to modify, modulate, or mask the offending taste, instead of trying to screen it out using the addition of taste-modifying agents, such as various sugars, salts, and nucleotides, as suggested by Leksrisompong et al. [50]. Starter cultures of *Lactobacillus* added to the proteins during hydrolysis have been touted as another taste modifying agent that could be acceptable because of their widespread use in fermented food products since ancient times [11,49]. Deamidation, the removal of amino groups by specific enzymes, is another option that has been shown to increase umami-tasting peptides, which also contributes to the masking of an existing bitter taste [51]. Interestingly, a recent study demonstrated that specific peptides from beef protein hydrolysates could block the bitter taste receptor T2R4 and directly inhibit bitter taste perception instead of simply masking it [52]. This is an exciting discovery of bioactive peptide/s blocking bitter taste sensation (which could be derived from other bioactive peptides), and further exemplifies the versatility of these peptides in offering novel solutions to persistent problems.

3.2. Digestion

Orally ingested substances are metabolized by various digestive enzymes, starting in the oral cavity, continuing in the stomach, and finally in the small and large intestines. A number of proteolytic enzymes are present in the human body, and their actions can irreversibly alter the peptide profile of such products. Indeed, many bioactive peptide preparations were initially produced by mimicking the digestive environment in the gastrointestinal (GI) tract, with protease treatment yielding the "active" peptides out of the native protein structure (reviewed in [3,7,53]). Being generated through simulated digestion, some bioactive peptides, such as the egg protein derived tripeptide IRW, are naturally resistant to digestive enzymes [54]. This is a huge advantage in delivering bioactives through the oral route, as a lack of digestion in the GI tract ensures increased bioavailability and a better chance of exerting a significant effect on the body's physiology. On the other hand, some peptides such as LKPNM, derived from enzymatic digestion of bonito fish protein, are further metabolized into their active components in the GI tract (LKP, an anti-hypertensive tripeptide is released from LKPNM), which then exert the intended biological action upon absorption into the systemic circulation. This could be considered analogous to a pro-drug, which undergoes metabolism to yield the active ingredient [55].

The skeptic may now question the need to generate peptides (or hydrolysates) through in vitro enzymatic procedure, as all orally ingested proteins are digested anyway in the GI tract. While a definitive yes/no answer is unlikely, it is plausible response is that an industrial scale digestive method may generate a different profile of bioactive peptides, which could then be characterized through chemical and biological assays to define their physiologic effects. The use of different enzymes can yield bioactive peptides from the same source protein with diverse biological functions, which could be tailored to different physiological (and potentially pathological) needs. This could be due to the different enzymes cleaving the same source protein at different sites, as well as the subsequent digestion of initially generated peptides, both of which contribute towards the generation of distinct peptide repertoires. Indeed, a study by Offengenden et al. used a range of commercially available enzymes, used singly or in combination, to generate a number of chicken collagen hydrolysates with different actions on proliferation, extracellular matrix deposition, and resistance to inflammation in osteoblastic cells [56]. Similar studies have been done on hydrolyzed proteins sourced from egg and milk proteins [57,58]. Another potential benefit is the unmasking of specific bioactive sequences, which may not be accessed/generated/released under normal digestive processes. For example, a study by Jahandideh et al. showed that enzymatically pre-digested fried egg preparations significantly reduced blood pressure in spontaneously hypertensive rats, while the lack of such pre-digestion completely abolished this antihypertensive effect [59].

Finally, protein hydrolysates containing an array of peptides may undergo GI tract digestion to yield a different set of peptides, the biological effects of which are still incompletely understood. Surprisingly, a study of casein (a milk protein) hydrolysates in infant formula has shown a reduced variety of casein peptides compared to formula with intact casein. However, the functional significance of these differences remain unclear [60]. Indeed, comparison studies of infant formula with intact and (extensively) hydrolyzed protein have shown similar effects on growth and tolerance, suggesting the possibility of a functional overlap and/or redundancy among different casein peptides [61].

3.3. Absorption

Absorption from the GI tract is essential for a bioactive peptide to exert any systemic biological actions downstream. Traditionally, it was believed that all peptides and proteins were digested down to their constituent amino acids, and only these amino acids were capable of absorption across the intestinal epithelial barrier. Indeed, the absorption of larger entities such as peptides and proteins were only considered as pathological phenomena, and a key culprit in food allergies! However, it is apparent now that many peptides do cross the intestinal epithelium under normal conditions, enter into the circulation, and exert systemic effects (reviewed in [61,62]).

Several mechanisms have been postulated to explain the intestinal uptake of peptides from the GI lumen, as detailed in the review by Lundquist et al. [63]. Briefly, the key mechanisms are as follows: paracellular transport through intercellular tight junctions; direct penetration of the epithelial cell membranes; endocytosis/phagocytosis by cells; and last, but not least, active transport by specific carrier proteins. Each of these mechanisms may occur alone or in association with others, while the same peptide may utilize one or more different approaches, adding to the complexity. A number of approaches have been tried in order to estimate and enhance the intestinal absorption of proteins and peptides, a brief overview of such potential solutions will be given here.

Paracellular transport is mediated through one or more tight junction proteins [64]. Two different approaches have been tested to increase peptide absorption by modulating the permeability of these junctions. The use of absorption enhancers, either covalently bound to the bioactive peptide or just used in conjunction, can enhance the uptake of the bioactive molecules [65,66]. However, this increased permeability is hard to modulate, and uncontrolled permeability changes could lead to localized inflammation and long-term damage to the intestinal epithelium [67]. An alternative method is targeting the myosin light chain phosphorylation process, which regulates cellular shape changes and intercellular junction integrity. Under physiological conditions, the myosin light chains are held in a state of equilibrium between its phosphorylated and dephosphorylated forms. The myosin light chain kinase phosphorylates its target, while the myosin light chain phosphatase exerts an opposite effect by dephosphorylating it. A higher level of phosphorylation would "open up" the intracellular tight junctions, allowing for greater access to peptides [68,69]. Thus, the transient inhibition of myosin light chain phosphatase, which shifts the balance towards increased phosphorylation, has been touted as an alternative approach to enhance peptide transport through tight junctions, but its clinical efficacy is yet to be verified [63].

The direct penetration of the cell membrane is a property of many peptides, and some bioactive peptides may utilize this mechanism to cross the intestinal epithelium on their own [70]. In addition, highly cell-permeable peptides, such as HIV-Tat and Penetratin, could be covalently conjugated to various bioactive peptides for a more efficient delivery [71,72]. However, further research may be needed to determine the nature of the membrane crossing abilities and the factors (peptide composition as well as external issues like pH and presence of minerals) that modulate such actions [73].

Endocytosis and/or transcytosis by epithelial cells could be enhanced if bioactive peptides are encapsulated within the carrier molecules known to be targets of such processes [74]. A number of approaches such as the use of liposomes or nanomaterials have been investigated for this purpose. Typically, such microencapsulation helps to protect the bioactive peptide inside, while addition of other molecules on the outer surface of the particles helps with its adhesion, localization, and eventual uptake by the intended target cells [75]. A number of different approaches have been utilized to enhance the intestinal uptake, including use of bacterial toxins, antibody fragments, and polysaccharides [76–78].

Finally, many peptides are selectively transported by specific transporters such as Pept1, an active transporter of oligopeptides. Studies undertaken by several research groups have demonstrated the key regulatory roles played by these transporter proteins on the transport of exogenous bioactive peptides [79–81]. Hence, the pharmacological modulation of these molecules may offer one of the more plausible avenues for regulating peptide absorption in the GI tract (reviewed in [82,83]). Future therapeutic approaches could involve modulation at the level of these transporters, allowing for further fine tuning of the intestinal uptake of the beneficial peptides [84].

In summary, the absorption of intact peptides, either alone or as part of a protein hydrolysate, is an exciting area of research that is critical for the successful oral use of these compounds. As an examination of the specific mechanisms and therapeutic approaches in greater detail is beyond the scope of this article, the interested reader is referred to two excellent reviews by Muheem et al. and Lundquist et al. [62,63].

3.4. Local Effects

Peptides do not necessarily need to be absorbed from the GI tract in order to exert biological effects. The GI tract is a large organ by itself, and local actions of bioactive peptides is an area of growing interest. Chronic diseases of the GI tract, especially inflammatory bowel diseases (IBD) in all their various manifestations, are a major cause of morbidity in the developed world. Current pharmacological treatments offer limited benefits at best, and require a lifelong adherence to therapeutic regimens, with their attendant cost and side-effects. As such, alternative therapies are an attractive idea to manage these diseases, and there exists the potential for locally-acting peptides (and protein hydrolysate preparations), given orally, to step into the void. A large number of food peptides have already been validated for their anti-inflammatory and anti-oxidant properties [5], which make them, either alone or in combination, theoretically well-suited for management of IBD cases [85,86]. While clinical data in humans is still lacking, a study in cats demonstrated the efficacy of commercially available hydrolyzed protein preparation in resolving pre-existing IBD [87]. Similarly, a recent study showed the beneficial effects of an egg shell membrane hydrolysate to attenuate the experimental GI tract inflammation in mice, further supporting the therapeutic potential of orally taken peptides acting in situ [88].

In conclusion, the oral use of bioactive peptides and protein hydrolysates offer a number of unique advantages and challenges that require further efforts in research and development targeted towards different aspects such as palatability, digestion, and sites of action. The development of these peptides for health promoting and therapeutic purposes would have to take into account these factors when devising strategies for oral usage.

4. Regulatory Environment for Bioactive Peptides

The regulatory environment includes the laws, regulations, and licensing systems that govern the manufacture, import, export, and sale of regulated products. In the context of biomedical and food industries, it involves various aspects of foods, drugs, and other products with effects on health and nutrition. Most advanced economies have robust regulatory regimens that ensure the safety and (where applicable) efficacy of such products, in order to protect the well-being of their citizens [89]. Given the novelty and potential health and nutritional roles of food derived bioactive peptides and protein hydrolysates, it is critical to understand and engage with the regulatory system/s in place in order to successfully translate the discoveries from the laboratory to the real world. While regulatory regimens do vary across different national and regional jurisdictions [90–93], certain common themes observed are discussed here.

4.1. Food or Drug?

The first issue is whether a product is a food or a drug. As bioactive peptides are obtained from food proteins and are purported to have health benefits, this could be more complicated than it seems at first glance. For example, if a peptide is derived from milk and reduces high blood pressure, is it a food, drug, or both? However, national regulatory systems are quire decisive about the food versus drug classification, and a product could be placed as either a food or a drug with little overlap between them.

The general principle is to focus on their intended use. If a product is taken as a food (i.e., the primary use is to gain sustenance and/or nutrition), it should be considered a food. On the other hand, if the primary use is to mitigate a disease or improve a bodily function, it is a drug. The latter category includes both natural health products and pharmaceuticals, as mentioned later. Indeed, the Canadian Food and Drugs Act (F&D Act) clearly defines "food" and "drug" based on their intended usage profile [94].

However, it can be argued that in some instances, the food/drug dichotomy is less clear cut and there are a number of product categories that straddle the divide, despite being legally defined as either "food" or "drug". As a growing number and variety of natural products become available for general use, it may be reasonable to consider such products as part of a food-to-drug continuum, with traditional foods at one end and dietary supplements (or, natural health products) and/or pharmaceuticals on the other.

4.2. Traditional Foods

While the concept of bioactive peptides is relatively new; many such products have been in widespread use since time immemorial. Across different cultures and continents, people have used foodstuff like yoghurt/cheese/kefir (milk protein derived peptides), pickles (peptides from fermented fruit or vegetable proteins), and fermented soybean products (tempeh, tofu, and natto), which are rich sources of food peptides, many with well-known bioactive properties [95,96]. Being widely known for their culinary use and regarded as safe to eat, these products have the least regulatory requirements. As long as these are prepared in a sanitary environment and use food grade chemicals (e.g., enzymes and processing aids), no special action is needed.

4.3. Novel Foods

This category includes foods that lack a history of safe use or those that have undergone novel processing methods that significantly change their nutritional or safety aspects. The Canadian Food and Drug Regulations (FDR) describing novel foods also include genetically modified organisms under its aegis [97]. For bioactive peptides and hydrolysates, the first sub-category may involve an unusual (or less widely known/used) protein source, while the second sub-category may involve the use of "new" enzymes, bacteria (for fermentation), and any number of chemical/physical methods used to generate, protect, or preserve an array of peptides. One or more applications may be needed to seek approval for usage and the consequent marketing of foods containing such ingredients. In Canada, novel food applications may involve the final food product, or it may pertain to a processing aid or a bacterial strain. In the United States, both foods and food-making processes can be covered under "generally recognized as safe" (GRAS), a process used to allow for both novel products and procedures [98,99].

4.4. Functional Foods

While traditional and novel foods are widely sold, there are restrictions on health-related claims pertaining to these products. There is a growing tendency within both the scientific and industry communities to promote the concept of a "functional food", that is, a food endowed with specific health/medical functions over and above its nutritional role [95,100,101]. Indeed, a recent search on PubMed for "functional food" merited over 4000 hits, compared to ~2500 for "bioactive peptides" and ~1100 for "protein hydrolysates" (personal observation, May 2018). Despite the wide usage of this term, its legal validity remains unclear. Countries like Canada and the United States do not provide any legal status for "functional food", although Health Canada had defined such a product [102]. In contrast, Japan has long maintained a regulated category of "food for specific health uses" (FOSHU), which may be the closest approximation to functional foods as a legal concept [102–104]. Outside Japan, such usage has remained uncommon, and so this may not be a viable regulatory option for bioactive peptide-based products in most markets in the near future.

4.5. Food for Special Uses

There are a number of special regulatory requirements for foods for special uses, which may involve those for medical conditions (e.g., low-energy, high-energy, and low in particular amino acids) or those intended for vulnerable populations. The commonest example is infant formula (for those aged 0–12 months). Most jurisdictions use stringent regulatory standards to protect infants' nutritional needs; as such, it is one of the common regulated foods sold all over the world. Globally, infant formula is regulated by Codex Alimentarius standards (e.g., Codex STAN72-1981), under the auspices of the World Health Organization (WHO) and the Food and Agriculture Organization (FAO) [105]. Nationally, many countries follow these international standards, while others, such as Canada and the United States, use their own standards for infant formula [97,106]. Given the putative role of hydrolysis in reducing the allergenicity of milk proteins, milk protein derived bioactive peptides are already a key component of many infant formulae sold across the world [107,108]. Indeed, this may well be one of the major instances of enzymatically pre-digested food proteins being used in a mass-marketed product. With the rising interest in both hypoallergenic and vegan diets, it is likely that peptide-rich plant protein hydrolysates (e.g., those from soy or rice proteins) would become an alternative source for bioactive peptides in these products [109].

4.6. Supplemented Foods

Foods are not only a source of nutrients; their nutritional content can be further enhanced by the addition of extraneous compounds. In Canada, there exists a separate category of supplemented foods, including energy bars and energy drinks that contain added levels of nutrients (e.g., vitamins, minerals and choline) [110]. Thus, the potential exists for use of bioactive peptides with well-defined physiological roles to be incorporated into commercially available foods and drinks under this regulatory measure. However, this may require robust evidence of biological effect (as demonstrated by studies in human subjects, for example) and consistency before becoming a routine practice. The lack of consistency in natural products like peptides and hydrolysates has long been a limiting factor in better ascertaining their specific roles [111].

4.7. Natural Health Products

Not all bioactive peptides are meant to be foods. Many are better suited for use as health products, which can be addressed under the "natural product" category. The growing interest in non-pharmaceutical drugs is a multibillion-dollar industry worldwide, and many bioactive peptides could find successful applications under its umbrella. One of the favorite terms used by both researchers and industry has been "nutraceutical". A recent search on PubMed for "nutraceutical" had over 3000 hits, with barely 300 for "natural health product" (personal observation, May 2018). However, despite its apparent popularity, the term "nutraceutical" remains poorly defined, with various interpretations and minimal legal/regulatory value [112,113]. From a regulatory perspective, Health Canada uses the term "natural health product" (NHP) and regulates manufacture and sale of such products through the NHP regulations made under the F&D Act [113]. In the United States, the Food and Drug Administration (US FDA) has a similar category of "dietary supplements" [114].

To date, a number of bioactive peptides have been cleared for use under these regulatory systems. The Canadian NHP database already includes "medicinal" ingredients such as casein phosphopeptides, glutamine peptides, and LKPNM (a pentapeptide derived from bonito protein), as well as the hydrolysates of fish protein, lupine, collagen, casein, and shrimp, to name a few [115]. Similarly, the US FDA maintains a list of new dietary ingredients that includes peptides derived from fish, shrimp, sesame, and silk fibroin protein, as well as hydrolysates of egg albumin and milk protein [116]. Given the beneficial roles of bioactive peptides on various physiological systems, this category is likely to be the preferred non-food option for future commercialization.

Interestingly, Schedule 1 of the Canadian NHP regulations specifically mentions (free) amino acids [117]; hence, it could be extrapolated to include synthetic short (2–10 amino acids) peptides in addition. Indeed, non-natural synthesized peptides such as anidulafungin (anti-fungal) and palmitoyl tetrapeptide-7 (skin conditioning agent) are listed in the Canadian NHP database under a separate category [115]. This is a novel option that merits further examination and may become a global model for regulatory approval of synthetic peptides with health benefits.

4.8. Pharmaceuticals

Finally, the most stringent regulatory requirements are reserved for the pharmaceuticals. Unlike food and supplements, pharmaceuticals can be used in invasive routes (e.g., intravenous and subcutaneous) or can be prescribed for specific diseases. However, given the variability in many "natural" products, limited opportunities for patent protection, and the lack of human clinical trials, the pharmaceutical route remains virtually inaccessible to most bioactive peptide formulations [111,118–120]. While the potential exists for a handful of synthetic peptides with high potency to break into this field, it would only be realized upon the completion of prohibitively expensive and time-consuming clinical trials, and only for those with robust and unequivocal effects on disease processes. With the legal, financial, and ethical challenges involved, this is unlikely to be a common option in the foreseeable future.

In summary, an understanding of the prevalent and evolving regulatory environment is critical for the success in translating basic discoveries in this field to viable products for improving human health. Given the range of options available, it is advisable to move beyond imprecise and overly broad terminology, and focus on placing novel formulations of bioactive peptides on their appropriate place along the food-drug continuum. Food derived bioactive peptides offer much promise in improving human health, while providing a valuable resource for food producers to prepare value-added products and better utilize the often-wasted by-products. A better understanding of manufacturing, consumer-related, and regulatory aspects would enable broader acceptance and faster utilization of their potential.

5. Conclusions

Further studies are required for the future use of food-derived bioactive peptides for the prevention and management of chronic diseases. As there are many factors that may influence the production of bioactive peptides, there is still a need to develop a more scalable, affordable, and consistent production technique. The major challenges and future research opportunities associated with the food-derived bioactive peptides are illustrated through a simple line diagram (Figure 1). It is also important to investigate the impact of the co-existing food matrix on absorption of these bioactive peptides. Finally, further research is also required to evaluate the physiological efficacy of these food-derived peptides in human clinical studies. Such scientific knowledge will be helpful for the regulatory bodies to categorize these products, which would facilitate their commercial use to improve human health and wellness.

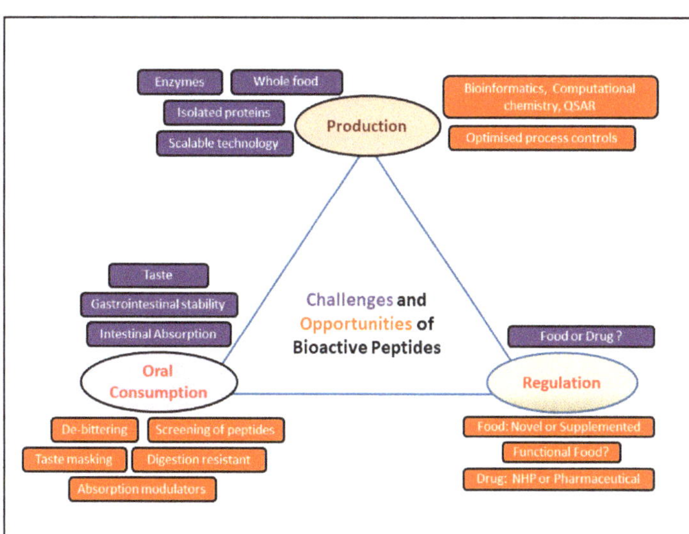

Figure 1. Challenges and potential solutions to utilization of bioactive peptides in human health. The three major aspects attached with the utilizations of food-derived bioactive peptides are (1) production; (2) oral consumption; and (3) regulation. The figure highlights the challenges and future opportunities those are associated with each of the aspects.

Acknowledgments: The research program in Majumder's laboratory is supported by grants from National Institute of Health to Nebraska Center for the Prevention of Obesity Diseases through Dietary Molecules (P20GM104320), the Nebraska Department of Agriculture, Nebraska Dry Bean Commission, University of Nebraska Collaboration Initiative, and Frank E. Mussehl and Inez L. Mussehl Poultry Research Fund.

Conflicts of Interest: The authors declare no conflicts of interest.

References

1. Daliri, E.B.M.; Oh, D.H.; Lee, B.H. Bioactive Peptides. *Foods* **2017**, *6*, 32. [CrossRef] [PubMed]
2. Korhonen, H.; Pihlanto, A. Bioactive peptides: Production and functionality. *Int. Dairy J.* **2006**, *16*, 945–960. [CrossRef]
3. Kitts, D.D.; Weiler, K. Bioactive proteins and peptides from food sources. Applications of bioprocesses used in isolation and recovery. *Curr. Pharm. Des.* **2003**, *9*, 1309–1323. [CrossRef] [PubMed]
4. Sánchez, A.; Vázquez, A. Bioactive peptides: A review. *FQS* **2017**, *1*, 29–46. [CrossRef]
5. Chakrabarti, S.; Jahandideh, F.; Wu, J. Food-derived bioactive peptides on inflammation and oxidative stress. *Biomed. Res. Int.* **2014**, 608979. [CrossRef] [PubMed]
6. Soory, M. Nutritional antioxidants and their applications in cardiometabolic diseases. *Infect. Disord. Drug Targets* **2012**, *12*, 388–401. [CrossRef] [PubMed]
7. Rutherfurd-Markwick, K.J. Food proteins as a source of bioactive peptides with diverse functions. *Br. J. Nutr.* **2012**, *108*, S149–S157. [CrossRef] [PubMed]
8. Fields, K.; Falla, T.J.; Rodan, K.; Bush, L. Bioactive peptides: Signaling the future. *J. Cosmet. Dermatol.* **2009**, *8*, 8–13. [CrossRef] [PubMed]
9. Moller, N.P.; Scholz-Ahrens, K.E.; Roos, N.; Schrezenmeir, J. Bioactive peptides and proteins from foods: Indication for health effects. *Eur. J. Nutr.* **2008**, *47*, 171–182. [CrossRef] [PubMed]
10. Moldes, A.B.; Vecino, X.; Cruz, J.M. Nutraceuticals and Food Additives. In *Current Developments in Biotechnology and Bioengineering: Food and Beverages Industry*, 1st ed.; Pandey, A., Sanromán, M.A., Du, G., Soccol, C.R., Dussap, C.G., Eds.; Elsevier: Amsterdam, The Netherlands, 2016; pp. 143–164. ISBN 9780444636775.
11. Haque, E.; Chand, R.; Kapila, S. Biofunctional properties of bioactive peptides of milk origin. *Food Rev. Int.* **2009**, *25*, 28–43. [CrossRef]
12. Fu, Y.; Therkildsen, M.; Aluko, R.E.; Lametsch, R. Exploration of collagen recovered from animal by-products as a precursor of bioactive peptides: Successes and challenges. *Crit. Rev. Food Sci. Nutr.* **2018**, 1–17. [CrossRef] [PubMed]
13. Przybylski, R.; Firdaous, L.; Châtaigné, G.; Dhulster, P.; Nedjar, N. Production of an antimicrobial peptide derived from slaughterhouse by-product and its potential application on meat as preservative. *Food Chem.* **2016**. [CrossRef] [PubMed]
14. Gu, Y.; Majumder, K.; Wu, J. QSAR-aided in silico approach in evaluation of food proteins as precursors of ACE inhibitory peptides. *Food Res. Int.* **2011**, *44*, 2465–2474. [CrossRef]
15. Perez Espitia, P.J.; de Fátima Ferreira Soares, N.; dos Reis Coimbra, J.S.; de Andrade, N.J.; Souza Cruz, R.; Alves Medeiros, E.A. Bioactive Peptides: Synthesis, Properties, and Applications in the Packaging and Preservation of Food. *Compr. Rev. Food Sci. Food Saf.* **2012**, *11*, 187–204. [CrossRef]
16. Gobbetti, M.; Ferranti, P.; Smacchi, E.; Goffredi, F.; Addeo, F. Production of Angiotensin-I-Converting-Enzyme-Inhibitory Peptides in Fermented Milks Started by Lactobacillus delbrueckii subsp. bulgaricus SS1 and Lactococcus lactis subsp. cremoris FT4. *Appl. Environ. Microbiol.* **2000**, *66*, 3898–3904. [CrossRef] [PubMed]
17. El-Fattah, A.M.A.; Sakr, S.S.; El-Dieb, S.M.; Elkashef, H.A.S. Bioactive peptides with ACE-I and antioxidant activity produced from milk proteolysis. *Int. J. Food Prop.* **2017**, *20*, 3033–3042. [CrossRef]
18. Ferri, M.; Graen-Heedfeld, J.; Bretz, K.; Guillon, F.; Michelini, E.; Calabretta, M.M.; Lamborghini, M.; Gruarin, N.; Roda, A.; Kraft, A.; et al. Peptide fractions obtained from rice by-products by means of an environment-friendly process show in vitro health-related bioactivities. *PLoS ONE* **2017**, *12*, e0170954. [CrossRef] [PubMed]
19. Fu, Y.; Liu, J.; Hansen, E.T.; Bredie, W.L.P.; Lametsch, R. Structural characteristics of low bitter and high umami protein hydrolysates prepared from bovine muscle and porcine plasma. *Food Chem.* **2018**, *257*, 163–171. [CrossRef] [PubMed]

20. Mora, L.; Bolumar, T.; Heres, A.; Toldrá, F. Effect of cooking and simulated gastrointestinal digestion on the activity of generated bioactive peptides in aged beef meat. *Food Funct.* **2017**, *8*, 4347–4355. [CrossRef] [PubMed]
21. Aspri, M.; Leni, G.; Galaverna, G.; Papademas, P. Bioactive properties of fermented donkey milk, before and after in vitro simulated gastrointestinal digestion. *Food Chem.* **2018**, *268*, 476–484. [CrossRef] [PubMed]
22. Vieira, E.F.; das Neves, J.; Vitorino, R.; Dias da Silva, D.; Carmo, H.; Ferreira, I.M. Impact of in vitro Gastrointestinal Digestion and Transepithelial Transport on Antioxidant and ACE-Inhibitory Activities of Brewer's Spent Yeast Autolysate. *J. Agric. Food Chem.* **2016**, *64*, 7335–7341. [CrossRef] [PubMed]
23. Picariello, G.; Miralles, B.; Mamone, G.; Sánchez-Rivera, L.; Recio, I.; Addeo, F.; Ferranti, P. Role of intestinal brush border peptidases in the simulated digestion of milk proteins. *Mol. Nutr. Food Res.* **2015**, *59*, 948–956. [CrossRef] [PubMed]
24. Rizzello, C.G.; Lorusso, A.; Russo, V.; Pinto, D.; Marzani, B.; Gobbetti, M. Improving the antioxidant properties of quinoa flour through fermentation with selected autochthonous lactic acid bacteria. *Int. J. Food Microbiol.* **2017**, *241*, 252–261. [CrossRef] [PubMed]
25. Aguilar-Toalá, J.E.; Santiago-López, L.; Peres, C.M.; Peres, C.; Garcia, H.S.; Vallejo-Cordoba, B.; González-Córdova, A.F.; Hernández-Mendoza, A. Assessment of multifunctional activity of bioactive peptides derived from fermented milk by specific Lactobacillus plantarum strains. *J. Dairy Sci.* **2017**, *100*, 65–75. [CrossRef] [PubMed]
26. Ahn, J.E.; Park, S.Y.; Atwal, A.; Gibbs, B.F.; Lee, B.H. Angiotensin I-Converting Enzyme (Ace) Inhibitory Peptides From Whey Fermented By Lactobacillus Species. *J. Food Biochem.* **2009**, *33*, 587–602. [CrossRef]
27. Sanjukta, S.; Rai, A.K.; Muhammed, A.; Jeyaram, K.; Talukdar, N.C. Enhancement of antioxidant properties of two soybean varieties of Sikkim Himalayan region by proteolytic Bacillus subtilis fermentation. *J. Funct. Foods* **2015**, *14*, 650–658. [CrossRef]
28. Chaudhury, A.; Duvoor, C.; Reddy Dendi, V.S.; Kraleti, S.; Chada, A.; Ravilla, R.; Marco, A.; Shekhawat, N.S.; Montales, M.T.; Kuriakose, K.; et al. Clinical review of antidiabetic drugs: Implications for type 2 diabetes mellitus management. *Front. Endocrinol.* **2017**, *8*, 6. [CrossRef] [PubMed]
29. Li-Chan, E.C.Y. Bioactive peptides and protein hydrolysates: Research trends and challenges for application as nutraceuticals and functional food ingredients. *Curr. Opin. Food Sci.* **2015**, *1*, 28–37. [CrossRef]
30. Hanke, A.T.; Ottens, M. Purifying biopharmaceuticals: Knowledge-based chromatographic process development. *Trends Biotechnol.* **2014**, *32*, 210–220. [CrossRef] [PubMed]
31. Cheung, I.W.Y.; Li-Chan, E.C.Y. Angiotensin-I-converting enzyme inhibitory activity and bitterness of enzymatically-produced hydrolysates of shrimp (Pandalopsis dispar) processing byproducts investigated by Taguchi design. *Food Chem.* **2010**, *122*, 1003–1012. [CrossRef]
32. Kopf-Bolanz, K.A.; Schwander, F.; Gijs, M.; Vergères, G.; Portmann, R.; Egger, L. Impact of milk processing on the generation of peptides during digestion. *Int. Dairy J.* **2014**, *35*, 130–138. [CrossRef]
33. Kamdem, J.P.; Tsopmo, A. Reactivity of peptides within the food matrix. *J. Food Biochem.* **2017**, e12489. [CrossRef]
34. Jakubczyk, A.; Baraniak, B. Angiotensin I Converting Enzyme Inhibitory Peptides Obtained after in vitro Hydrolysis of Pea (*Pisum sativum* var. Bajka) Globulins. *Biomed. Res. Int.* **2014**, 438459. [CrossRef]
35. Yousr, M.; Howell, N. Antioxidant and ACE Inhibitory Bioactive Peptides Purified from Egg Yolk Proteins. *Int. J. Mol Sci.* **2015**, *16*, 29161–29178. [CrossRef] [PubMed]
36. Holton, T.A.; Vijayakumar, V.; Khaldi, N. Bioinformatics: Current perspectives and future directions for food and nutritional research facilitated by a Food-Wiki database. *Trends Food Sci. Technol.* **2013**, *34*, 5–17. [CrossRef]
37. Minkiewicz, P.; Dziuba, J.; Iwaniak, A.; Dziuba, M.; Darewicz, M. BIOPEP database and other programs for processing bioactive peptide sequences. *J. AOAC Int.* **2008**, *91*, 965–980. [PubMed]
38. Rawlings, N.D.; Barrett, A.J.; Finn, R. MEROPS:the database of proteolytic enzymes, their substrates and inhibitors. *Nucleic Acids Res.* **2016**, *44*, D343–D350. [CrossRef] [PubMed]
39. Zelazko, M.; Chrzanowska, J.; Polanowski, A. Pancreatic proteinases—Species diversity and the appending feeding and biotechnological implications. *Biotechnologia* **2007**, *76*, 107–120.
40. Agyei, D.; Danquah, M.K. Industrial-scale manufacturing of pharmaceutical-grade bioactive peptides. *Biotechnol. Adv.* **2011**, *29*, 272–277. [CrossRef] [PubMed]

41. Erdmann, K.; Cheung, B.W.; Schröder, H. The possible roles of food-derived bioactive peptides in reducing the risk of cardiovascular disease. *J. Nutr. Biochem.* **2008**, *19*, 643–654. [CrossRef] [PubMed]
42. Meyerhof, W. Elucidation of mammalian bitter taste. *Rev. Physiol. Biochem. Pharmacol.* **2005**, *154*, 37–72. [CrossRef] [PubMed]
43. Bumberger, E.; Belitz, H.D. Bitter taste of enzymic hydrolysates of casein—I. Isolation, structural and sensorial analysis of peptides from tryptic hydrolysates of β-casein. *Z. Lebensm. Unters. Forsch.* **1993**, *197*, 14–19. [CrossRef] [PubMed]
44. Maehashi, K.; Huang, L. Bitter peptides and bitter taste receptors. *Cell. Mol. Life Sci.* **2009**, *66*, 1661–1671. [CrossRef] [PubMed]
45. Kim, H.-O.; Li-Chan, E.C.Y. Quantitative Structure−Activity Relationship Study of Bitter Peptides. *J. Agric. Food Chem.* **2006**, *54*, 10102–10111. [CrossRef] [PubMed]
46. Li, L.; Yang, Z.Y.; Yang, X.Q.; Zhang, G.H.; Tang, S.Z.; Chen, F. Debittering effect of Actinomucor elegans peptidases on soybean protein hydrolysates. *J. Ind. Microbiol. Biotechnol.* **2008**, *35*, 41–47. [CrossRef] [PubMed]
47. Huang, W.Q.; Zhong, L.F.; Meng, Z.Z.; You, Z.J.; Li, J.Z.; Luo, X.C. The Structure and Enzyme Characteristics of a Recombinant Leucine Aminopeptidase rLap1 from Aspergillus sojae and Its Application in Debittering. *Appl. Biochem. Biotechnol.* **2015**, *177*, 190–206. [CrossRef] [PubMed]
48. Fu, J.; Li, L.; Yang, X.Q. Specificity of carboxypeptidases from actinomucor elegans and their debittering effect on soybean protein hydrolysates. *Appl. Biochem. Biotechnol.* **2011**, *165*, 1201–1210. [CrossRef] [PubMed]
49. Saha, B.C.; Hayashi, K. Debittering of protein hydrolyzates. *Biotechnol. Adv.* **2001**, *19*, 355–370. [CrossRef]
50. Leksrisompong, P.; Gerard, P.; Lopetcharat, K.; Drake, M. Bitter Taste Inhibiting Agents for Whey Protein Hydrolysate and Whey Protein Hydrolysate Beverages. *J. Food Sci.* **2012**, *77*, S282–S287. [CrossRef] [PubMed]
51. Liu, B.Y.; Zhu, K.X.; Guo, X.N.; Peng, W.; Zhou, H.M. Effect of deamidation-induced modification on umami and bitter taste of wheat gluten hydrolysates. *J. Sci. Food Agric.* **2017**, *97*, 3181–3188. [CrossRef] [PubMed]
52. Zhang, C.; Alashi, A.M.; Singh, N.; Liu, K.; Chelikani, P.; Aluko, R.E. Beef Protein-Derived Peptides as Bitter Taste Receptor T2R4 Blockers. *J. Agric. Food Chem.* **2018**, *66*, 4902–4912. [CrossRef] [PubMed]
53. Hartmann, R.; Meisel, H. Food-derived peptides with biological activity: From research to food applications. *Curr. Opin. Biotechnol.* **2007**, *18*, 163–169. [CrossRef] [PubMed]
54. Majumder, K.; Wu, J. Purification and characterisation of angiotensin i converting enzyme (ACE) inhibitory peptides derived from enzymatic hydrolysate of ovotransferrin. *Food Chem.* **2011**, *126*, 1614–1619. [CrossRef] [PubMed]
55. Fujita, H.; Yoshikawa, M. LKPNM: A prodrug-type ACE-inhibitory peptide derived from fish protein. *Immunopharmacology* **1999**, *44*, 123–127. [CrossRef]
56. Offengenden, M.; Chakrabarti, S.; Wu, J. Chicken Collagen Hydrolysates Differentially Mediate Anti-inflammatory Activity and Type I Collagen Synthesis on Human Dermal Fibroblasts. *Food Sci. Hum. Wellness* **2018**, *7*, 138–147. [CrossRef]
57. Chang, C.; Lahti, T.; Tanaka, T.; Nickerson, M.T. Egg proteins: Fractionation, bioactive peptides and allergenicity. *J. Sci. Food Agric.* **2018**, *98*, 5547–5558. [CrossRef] [PubMed]
58. Nongonierma, A.B.; FitzGerald, R.J. Enhancing bioactive peptide release and identification using targeted enzymatic hydrolysis of milk proteins. *Anal. Bioanal. Chem.* **2018**, *410*, 3407–3423. [CrossRef] [PubMed]
59. Jahandideh, F.; Majumder, K.; Chakrabarti, S.; Morton, J.S.; Panahi, S.; Kaufman, S.; Davidge, S.T.; Wu, J. Beneficial Effects of Simulated Gastro-Intestinal Digests of Fried Egg and Its Fractions on Blood Pressure, Plasma Lipids and Oxidative Stress in Spontaneously Hypertensive Rats. *PLoS ONE* **2014**, *9*, e115006. [CrossRef] [PubMed]
60. Wada, Y.; Lönnerdal, B. Bioactive peptides released by in vitro digestion of standard and hydrolyzed infant formulas. *Peptides* **2015**, *73*, 101–105. [CrossRef] [PubMed]
61. Ng, D.H.C.; Embleton, N.D.; McGuire, W. Hydrolyzed formula compared with standard formula for preterm infants. *JAMA* **2018**, *319*, 1717–1718. [CrossRef] [PubMed]
62. Muheem, A.; Shakeel, F.; Jahangir, M.A.; Anwar, M.; Mallick, N.; Jain, G.K.; Warsi, M.H.; Ahmad, F.J. A review on the strategies for oral delivery of proteins and peptides and their clinical perspectives. *Saudi Pharm. J.* **2016**, *24*, 413–428. [CrossRef] [PubMed]
63. Lundquist, P.; Artursson, P. Oral absorption of peptides and nanoparticles across the human intestine: Opportunities, limitations and studies in human tissues. *Adv. Drug Deliv. Rev.* **2016**, *106*, 256–276. [CrossRef] [PubMed]

64. Artursson, P.; Knight, S.D. Breaking the intestinal barrier to deliver drugs. *Science* **2015**, *347*, 716–717. [CrossRef] [PubMed]
65. Lindmark, T.; Kimura, Y.; Artursson, P. Absorption enhancement through intracellular regulation of tight junction permeability by medium chain fatty acids in Caco-2 cells. *J. Pharmacol. Exp. Ther.* **1998**, *284*, 362–369. [PubMed]
66. Lindmark, T.; Schipper, N.; Lazorová, L.; De Boer, A.G.; Artursson, P. Absorption enhancement in intestinal epithelial Caco-2 monolayers by sodium caprate: Assessment of molecular weight dependence and demonstration of transport routes. *J. Drug Target.* **1998**, *5*, 215–223. [CrossRef] [PubMed]
67. Maher, S.; Kennelly, R.; Bzik, V.A.; Baird, A.W.; Wang, X.; Winter, D.; Brayden, D.J. Evaluation of intestinal absorption enhancement and local mucosal toxicity of two promoters. I. Studies in isolated rat and human colonic mucosae. *Eur. J. Pharm. Sci.* **2009**, *38*, 291–300. [CrossRef] [PubMed]
68. Jin, Y.; Blikslager, A.T. Myosin light chain kinase mediates intestinal barrier dysfunction via occludin endocytosis during anoxia/reoxygenation injury. *Am. J. Physiol. Cell Physiol.* **2016**, *311*, C996–C1004. [CrossRef] [PubMed]
69. Murthy, K.S.; Zhou, H.; Grider, J.R.; Brautigan, D.L.; Eto, M.; Makhlouf, G.M. Differential signalling by muscarinic receptors in smooth muscle: m2-mediated inactivation of myosin light chain kinase via Gi3, Cdc42/Rac1 and p21-activated kinase 1 pathway, and m3-mediated MLC20 (20 kDa regulatory light chain of myosin II) phosphorylat. *Biochem. J.* **2003**, *374*, 145. [CrossRef] [PubMed]
70. Pooga, M.; Langel, Ü. Classes of cell-penetrating peptides. In *Cell-Penetrating Peptides: Methods and Protocols*; Humana Press: New York, NY, USA, 2015; Volume 1324, pp. 3–28, ISBN 9781493928064.
71. Dupont, E.; Prochiantz, A.; Joliot, A. Penetratin story: An overview. In *Cell-Penetrating Peptides: Methods and Protocols*; Humana Press: New York, NY, USA, 2015; Volume 1324, pp. 29–37, ISBN 9781493928064.
72. Vives, E. Present and future of cell-penetrating peptide mediated delivery systems: "Is the Trojan horse too wild to go only to Troy?". *J. Control. Release* **2005**, *109*, 77–85. [CrossRef] [PubMed]
73. Koren, E.; Torchilin, V.P. Cell-penetrating peptides: Breaking through to the other side. *Trends Mol. Med.* **2012**, *18*, 385–393. [CrossRef] [PubMed]
74. Thuenauer, R.; Müller, S.K.; Römer, W. Pathways of protein and lipid receptor-mediated transcytosis in drug delivery. *Expert Opin. Drug Deliv.* **2017**, *14*, 341–351. [CrossRef] [PubMed]
75. Kohli, N.; Westerveld, D.R.; Ayache, A.C.; Verma, A.; Shil, P.; Prasad, T.; Zhu, P.; Chan, S.L.; Li, Q.; Daniell, H. Oral delivery of bioencapsulated proteins across blood-brain and blood-retinal barriers. *Mol. Ther.* **2014**, *22*, 535–546. [CrossRef] [PubMed]
76. Chen, J.; Liu, C.; Shan, W.; Xiao, Z.; Guo, H.; Huang, Y. Enhanced stability of oral insulin in targeted peptide ligand trimethyl chitosan nanoparticles against trypsin. *J. Microencapsul.* **2015**, *32*, 632–641. [CrossRef] [PubMed]
77. Pridgen, E.M.; Alexis, F.; Kuo, T.T.; Levy-Nissenbaum, E.; Karnik, R.; Blumberg, R.S.; Langer, R.; Farokhzad, O.C. Transepithelial transport of Fc-targeted nanoparticles by the neonatal fc receptor for oral delivery. *Sci. Transl. Med.* **2013**, *5*, 213ra167. [CrossRef] [PubMed]
78. Harokopakis, E.; Hajishengallis, G.; Michalek, S.M. Effectiveness of liposomes possessing surface-linked recombinant B subunit of cholera toxin as an oral antigen delivery system. *Infect. Immun.* **1998**, *66*, 4299–4304. [PubMed]
79. Geissler, S.; Zwarg, M.; Knütter, I.; Markwardt, F.; Brandsch, M. The bioactive dipeptide anserine is transported by human proton-coupled peptide transporters. *FEBS J.* **2010**, *277*, 790–795. [CrossRef] [PubMed]
80. Satake, M.; Enjoh, M.; Nakamura, Y.; Takano, T.; Kawamura, Y.; Arai, S.; Shimizu, M. Transepithelial Transport of the Bioactive Tripeptide, Val-Pro-Pro, in Human Intestinal Caco-2 Cell Monolayers. *Biosci. Biotechnol. Biochem.* **2002**, *66*, 378–384. [CrossRef] [PubMed]
81. Bejjani, S.; Wu, J. Transport of IRW, an Ovotransferrin Derived Antihypertensive Peptide, in Human Intestinal Epithelial Caco-2 cells. *J. Agric. Food Chem.* **2013**, *61*, 1487–1492. [CrossRef] [PubMed]
82. Miner-Williams, W.M.; Stevens, B.R.; Moughan, P.J. Are intact peptides absorbed from the healthy gut in the adult human? *Nutr. Res. Rev.* **2014**, *27*, 308–329. [CrossRef] [PubMed]
83. Santiago-Lopez, L.; F. Gonzalez-Cordova, A.; Hernandez-Mendoza, A.; Vallejo-Cordoba, B. Potential Use of Food Protein-Derived Peptides in the Treatment of Inflammatory Diseases. *Protein Pept. Lett.* **2017**, *24*, 137–145. [CrossRef] [PubMed]
84. Wang, C.Y.; Liu, S.; Xie, X.-N.; Tan, Z.R. Regulation profile of the intestinal peptide transporter 1 (PepT1). *Drug Des. Dev. Ther.* **2017**, *11*, 3511–3517. [CrossRef] [PubMed]

85. Zhang, H.; Hu, C.-A.A.; Kovacs-Nolan, J.; Mine, Y. Bioactive dietary peptides and amino acids in inflammatory bowel disease. *Amino Acids* **2015**, *47*, 2127–2141. [CrossRef] [PubMed]
86. De Medina, F.S.; Daddaoua, A.; Requena, P.; Capitán-Cañadas, F.; Zarzuelo, A.; Dolores Suárez, M.; Martínez-Augustin, O. New insights into the immunological effects of food bioactive peptides in animal models of intestinal inflammation. *Proc. Nutr. Soc.* **2010**, *69*, 454–462. [CrossRef] [PubMed]
87. Mandigers, P.J.J.; Biourge, V.; German, A.J. Efficacy of a commercial hydrolysate diet in eight cats suffering from inflammatory bowel disease or adverse reaction to food. *Tijdschr. Diergeneeskd.* **2010**, *135*, 668–672. [PubMed]
88. Shi, Y.; Rupa, P.; Jiang, B.; Mine, Y. Hydrolysate from eggshell membrane ameliorates intestinal inflammation in mice. *Int. J. Mol. Sci.* **2014**, *15*, 22728–22742. [CrossRef] [PubMed]
89. Epstein, J.; Seitz, R.; Dhingra, N.; Ganz, P.R.; Gharehbaghian, A.; Spindel, R.; Teo, D.; Reddy, R. Role of regulatory agencies. *Biol. J. Int. Assoc. Biol. Stand.* **2009**, *37*, 94–102. [CrossRef] [PubMed]
90. L'abbé, M.R.; Dumais, L.; Chao, E.; Junkins, B. Health claims on foods in Canada. *J. Nutr.* **2008**, *138*, 1221S–1227S. [CrossRef] [PubMed]
91. Ellwood, K.C.; Trumbo, P.R.; Kavanaugh, C.J. How the US Food and Drug Administration evaluates the scientific evidence for health claims. *Nutr. Rev.* **2010**, *68*, 114–121. [CrossRef] [PubMed]
92. Tapsell, L.C. Evidence for health claims: A perspective from the Australia-New Zealand region. *J. Nutr.* **2008**, *138*, 1206S–1209S. [CrossRef] [PubMed]
93. Government of Canada. Food and Drugs Act (R.S.c., 1985, c. F-27). Available online: http://laws-lois.justice.gc.ca/eng/acts/F-27/FullText.html (accessed on 9 August 2018).
94. Coppens, P.; da Silva, M.F.; Pettman, S. European regulations on nutraceuticals, dietary supplements and functional foods: A framework based on safety. *Toxicology* **2006**, *221*, 59–74. [CrossRef] [PubMed]
95. Leroy, F.; De Vuyst, L. Fermented food in the context of a healthy diet: How to produce novel functional foods? *Curr. Opin. Clin. Nutr. Metab. Care* **2014**, *17*, 574–581. [CrossRef] [PubMed]
96. Frias, J.; Martinez-Villaluenga, C.; Peñas, E. *Fermented Foods in Health and Disease Prevention*, 1st ed.; Frias, J., Martinez-Villaluenga, C., Peñas, E., Eds.; Academic Press: Cambridge, MA, USA, 2017; ISBN 9780128023099.
97. Government of Canada. Justice Laws Website. Food and Drug Regulations (CRC C.870). Available online: http://laws-lois.justice.gc.ca/eng/regulations/C.R.C.%2C_c._870/page-102.html#h-142 (accessed on 9 August 2018).
98. Paul, R.H.; Frestedt, J.; Magurany, K. GRAS from the ground up: Review of the Interim Pilot Program for GRAS notification. *Food Chem. Toxicol.* **2017**, *105*, 140–150. [CrossRef] [PubMed]
99. U.S. Food & Drug Administration. Food. Generally Recognized as Safe (GRAS). Available online: https://www.fda.gov/Food/IngredientsPackagingLabeling/GRAS/default.htm (accessed on 9 August 2018).
100. Hunter, P.M.; Hegele, R.A. Functional foods and dietary supplements for the management of dyslipidaemia. *Nat. Rev. Endocrinol.* **2017**, *13*, 278–288. [CrossRef] [PubMed]
101. Matos, J.; Cardoso, C.; Bandarra, N.M.; Afonso, C. Microalgae as healthy ingredients for functional food: A review. *Food Funct.* **2017**, *8*, 2672–2685. [CrossRef] [PubMed]
102. Hobbs, J.E.; Malla, S.; Sogah, E.K. Regulatory Frameworks for Functional Food and Supplements. *Can. J. Agric. Econ.* **2014**, *62*, 569–594. [CrossRef]
103. Patel, D.; Dufour, Y.; Domigan, N. Functional food and nutraceutical registration processes in Japan and China: A diffusion of innovation perspective. *J. Pharm. Pharm. Sci.* **2008**, *11*, 1–11. [CrossRef] [PubMed]
104. Govt of Japan Ministry of Health, Labour and Welfare: Food with Health Claims, Food for Special Dietary Uses, and Nutrition Labeling. Available online: https://www.mhlw.go.jp/english/topics/foodsafety/fhc/02.html (accessed on 9 August 2018).
105. Joint Food & Agriculture Organization (FAO)/World Health Organization (WHO). *Codex Alimentarius* Commission. CODEX STAN 72-1981 Standard for Infant Formula and Formulas for Special Medical Purposes Intended for Infants Sections A&B Revision 2007. Amended 2016. Available online: http://www.fao.org/fao-who-codexalimentarius/sh-proxy/fr/?lnk=1&url=https%253A%252F%252Fworkspace.fao.org%252Fsites%252Fcodex%252FStandards%252FCODEX%2BSTAN%2B72-1981%252FCXS_072e.pdf (accessed on 9 August 2018).
106. Institute of Medicine (US) Committee on the Evaluation of the Addition of Ingredients New to Infant Formula. *Infant Formula: Evaluating the Safety of New Ingredients*; National Academies Press: Washington, DC, USA, 2004; ISBN 978-0-309-09150-3.

107. Vandenplas, Y. Prevention and Management of Cow's Milk Allergy in Non-Exclusively Breastfed Infants. *Nutrients* **2017**, *9*, 731. [CrossRef] [PubMed]
108. von Berg, A. Modified proteins in allergy prevention. *Nestle Nutr. Workshop Ser. Pediatr. Program* **2009**, *64*, 239–247, discussion 247–257. [CrossRef] [PubMed]
109. Salvatore, S.; Vandenplas, Y. Hydrolyzed Proteins in Allergy. *Nestle Nutr. Workshop Ser. Pediatr. Program* **2016**, *86*, 11–27. [CrossRef]
110. Government of Canada. Category Specific Guidance for Temporary Marketing Authorization: Supplemented Food. Available online: https://www.canada.ca/en/health-canada/services/food-nutrition/legislation-guidelines/guidance-documents/category-specific-guidance-temporary-marketing-authorization-supplemented-food.html (accessed on 9 August 2018).
111. Gilani, G.S.; Xiao, C.; Lee, N. Need for accurate and standardized determination of amino acids and bioactive peptides for evaluating protein quality and potential health effects of foods and dietary supplements. *J. AOAC Int.* **2008**, *91*, 894–900. [PubMed]
112. Santini, A.; Cammarata, S.M.; Capone, G.; Ianaro, A.; Tenore, G.C.; Pani, L.; Novellino, E. Nutraceuticals: Opening the debate for a regulatory framework. *Br. J. Clin. Pharmacol.* **2018**, *84*, 659–672. [CrossRef] [PubMed]
113. Aronson, J.K. Defining "nutraceuticals": Neither nutritious nor pharmaceutical. *Br. J. Clin. Pharmacol.* **2017**, *83*, 8–19. [CrossRef] [PubMed]
114. U.S. Food & Drug Administration. Dietary Supplements. Available online: https://www.fda.gov/Food/DietarySupplements/ (accessed on 9 August 2018).
115. Health Canada, Natural Health Products Ingredients Database. Available online: http://webprod.hc-sc.gc.ca/nhpid-bdipsn/search-rechercheReq.do (accessed on 9 August 2018).
116. U.S. Food & Drug Administration. New Dietary Ingredients Notification Process—Submitted 75-Day Premarket Notifications for New Dietary Ingredients. Available online: https://www.fda.gov/Food/DietarySupplements/NewDietaryIngredientsNotificationProcess/ucm534510.htm (accessed on 9 August 2018).
117. Government of Canada. Natural Health Products Regulations. Available online: http://laws-lois.justice.gc.ca/eng/regulations/SOR-2003-196/page-1.html (accessed on 9 August 2018).
118. Parveen, A.; Parveen, B.; Parveen, R.; Ahmad, S. Challenges and guidelines for clinical trial of herbal drugs. *J. Pharm. Bioallied Sci.* **2015**, *7*, 329–333. [CrossRef] [PubMed]
119. Paller, C.J.; Denmeade, S.R.; Carducci, M.A. Challenges of conducting clinical trials of natural products to combat cancer. *Clin. Adv. Hematol. Oncol.* **2016**, *14*, 447–455. [PubMed]
120. Dwyer, J.T.; Coates, P.M.; Smith, M.J. Dietary Supplements: Regulatory Challenges and Research Resources. *Nutrients* **2018**, *10*, 41. [CrossRef] [PubMed]

nutrients

MDPI

Review

The Use of Glycomacropeptide in Patients with Phenylketonuria: A Systematic Review and Meta-Analysis

Maria João Pena [1,*], Alex Pinto [2,3], Anne Daly [2], Anita MacDonald [2], Luís Azevedo [4,5,6], Júlio César Rocha [6,7,8] and Nuno Borges [6,9]

1 Departamento de Biomedicina, Unidade de Bioquímica, Faculdade de Medicina, Universidade do Porto, 4200-319 Porto, Portugal
2 Department of Dietetics, Birmingham Children's Hospital, Birmingham B4 6NH, UK; alex.pinto@nhs.net (A.P.); a.daly3@nhs.net (A.D.); anita.macdonald@nhs.net (A.M.)
3 Faculty of Health & Human Sciences, University of Plymouth, Plymouth PL6 8BH, UK
4 Faculdade de Medicina, Universidade do Porto, 4200-319 Porto, Portugal; lazevedo@med.up.pt
5 Department of Community Medicine, Information and Health Decision Sciences (MEDCIDS), 4200-450 Porto, Portugal
6 Center for Health Technology and Services Research (CINTESIS), 4200-450 Porto, Portugal; julio.rocha@chporto.min-saude.pt (J.C.R.); nunoborges@fcna.up.pt (N.B.)
7 Centro de Genética Médica Dr Jacinto de Magalhães, Centro Hospitalar Universitário do Porto, 4099-028 Porto, Portugal
8 Centro de Referência na área das Doenças Hereditárias do Metabolismo, Centro Hospitalar Universitário do Porto—CHP EPE, 4099-001 Porto, Portugal
9 Faculdade de Ciências da Nutrição e Alimentação, Universidade do Porto, 4200-465 Porto, Portugal
* Correspondence: mmom12006@med.up.pt; Tel.: +35-122-042-6659

Received: 9 October 2018; Accepted: 12 November 2018; Published: 18 November 2018

Abstract: In phenylketonuria (PKU), synthetic protein derived from L-amino acids (AAs) is essential in a low-phenylalanine (Phe) diet. Glycomacropeptide (GMP), an intact protein, is very low in Phe in its native form. It has been modified and adapted for PKU to provide an alternative protein source through supplementation with rate-limiting amino acids (GMP-AAs), although it still contains residual Phe. This review aims to systematically evaluate published intervention studies on the use of GMP-AAs in PKU by considering its impact on blood Phe control (primary aim) and changes in tyrosine control, nutritional biomarkers, and patient acceptability or palatability (secondary aims). Four electronic databases were searched for articles published from 2007 to June 2018. Of the 274 studies identified, only eight were included. Bias risk was assessed and a quality appraisal of the body of evidence was completed. A meta-analysis was performed with two studies with adequate comparable methodology which showed no differences between GMP-AAs and AAs for any of the interventions analysed. This work underlines the scarcity and nature of studies with GMP-AAs interventions. All were short-term with small sample sizes. There is a need for better-designed studies to provide the best evidence-based recommendations.

Keywords: phenylketonuria; glycomacropeptide; amino acids; phenylalanine; metabolic control; nutritional biomarkers; acceptability

1. Introduction

Phenylketonuria (PKU, OMIM # 261200) is the most common inborn error of amino acid metabolism and is caused by a defect in phenylalanine (Phe) hydroxylase (PAH; EC 1.14.16.1) or in its cofactor, tetrahydrobiopterin (BH_4). The resulting accumulation of Phe in blood and brain causes irreversible neurological impairment [1].

The low-Phe diet introduced in the 1950s by Dr. Horst Bickel was a milestone that allowed avoidance of severe complications for patients with PKU [2]. Untreated PKU may lead to irreversible intellectual disability, microcephaly, motor deficits, eczematous rash, autism, seizures, developmental problems, aberrant behaviour, and psychiatric symptoms [3]. Dietary treatment requires natural protein and Phe restrictions, together with synthetic protein substitutes that provide most of the nitrogen in the diet [4]. The availability of protein substitutes in Europe as well as the nutritional profile of protein substitutes available in Portugal were previously reported. Differences in the availability across European countries and nutritional inconsistencies were found [5].

Following Kure's first description of the impact of BH_4 in PKU in 1999 [6], pharmacological treatment with sapropterin has allowed a relaxation of dietary restrictions in a subgroup of patients, mainly those with mild or moderate PKU. This compound acts as a pharmaceutical chaperone [3], but almost all patients require a low-Phe diet supplemented with a synthetic protein derived from L-amino acids (AAs) [3]. PKU requires lifelong treatment in order to keep blood Phe control within acceptable target ranges, but dietary adherence is challenging, especially in adolescence and adulthood [7].

In the last decade, glycomacropeptide (GMP), a whey-based natural protein derived from the cheese manufacturing process, has been introduced for PKU [8]. It contains only residual amounts of Phe, tyrosine (Tyr), and tryptophan [9], and has many functional and physiological properties. It acts as a prebiotic, and has anti-inflammatory and nutraceutical properties, creating an attractive peptide for patients with inherited metabolic disorders as an alternative protein replacement for AAs [10]. GMP is an incomplete intact protein, but in PKU it is supplemented with any deficient amino acids (GMP-AAs) to offer a more nutritionally complete product [11].

In a preclinical study, wild-type and PKU mice were fed diets consisting of 20% protein from casein, AAs, or GMP-AAs. In this study, the GMP-AAs group showed similar growth and significantly reduced concentrations of Phe in plasma and brain compared to those fed by conventional sources [12]. Another study sought to evaluate the effect of three diets (GMP-AAs, AAs, and casein) on plasma amino acids, cytokines, fat and lean mass, and acute energy balance in PKU and wild-type mice. The PKU mice had growth and lean mass similar to the wild-type mice fed GMP-AAs or AAs. However, the GMP-AAs significantly reduced energy expenditure, food intake and plasma Phe concentrations in PKU mice, whereas AAs and casein induced metabolic stress [13]. Neurotransmitter concentrations and behavioural phenotype were found to be similar in PKU mice fed with either GMP-AAs or AAs [14]. In a further animal study, GMP-AAs showed prebiotic properties by positively modulating the gut microbiota, increasing short-chain fatty acids, and reducing inflammatory markers [15]. A study by Solverson et al. [16] reported potential long-term benefits for bone health using GMP-AAs.

Overall, the studies in PKU mice showed a positive influence of GMP-AAs. However, scientific evidence from clinical studies that support the use of GMP-AAs as a major source of protein in PKU patients is less robust. Doubts still persist regarding the potential effect on patients of the residual Phe provided by GMP-AAs as well as how the nutritional biomarkers are influenced by GMP-AAs intake [10,17–27].

The primary aim was to systematically review the existing literature relating to the influence of residual Phe in GMP-AAs on blood Phe control. The secondary aims were to evaluate the impact on blood Tyr metabolic control, changes in nutritional biomarkers, and the acceptability or palatability of GMP products.

2. Materials and Methods

2.1. Review Question

A systematic literature search was performed according to the Preferred Reporting Items for Systematic Reviews and Meta-Analysis (PRISMA) guidelines [28]. The protocol is registered with the "International prospective register of systematic reviews" (PROSPERO) with systematic review number CRD42018098873.

Inclusion criteria included articles reporting observational or interventional studies. Articles of preclinical studies (defined as not providing clinical outcome data) or abstracts were excluded. Based on the Patients, Intervention, Comparator, Outcomes (PICO) approach, the patients/populations under study included male and female subjects diagnosed with PKU, with ages ranging from infancy to adulthood, under treatment with diet only or diet plus sapropterin, and who were willing to take GMP-AAs or AAs as their primary nitrogen source or cheese made of GMP. Exclusion criteria for patients/populations were pregnancy and no dietary treatment.

2.2. Search Strategy

Eligible literature published from 2007 to June 2018 was obtained from PubMed, CENTRAL Cochrane Library, Scopus and Web of Science. Studies were sought with the following terms: PubMed query—("Phenylketonuria" [All fields] OR "Phenylketonuria" [MeSH TERM] OR "PKU" [All fields]) AND ("Glycomacropeptide" [All fields] OR "kappa-casein glycomacropeptide" [Supplementary Concept] OR "caseinomacropeptide" [Supplementary Concept] OR GMP [All fields]); CENTRAL Cochrane Library query—#1. "phenylketonuria": ti,ab,kw, #2. MeSH descriptor: [Phenylketonurias] explode all trees, #3. "PKU", #4. #1 or #2 or #3, #5. "glycomacropeptide", #6. #4 and #5; Scopus query—("Phenylketonuria" OR "PKU") AND "Glycomacropeptide"; Web of Science query—#1. TS = Phenylketonuria, #2. TS = PKU, #3. TS = Glycomacropeptide, #4. #1 OR #2, #5. #3 AND #4.

2.3. Study Selection

The first stage in the process was to review the titles and abstracts of the studies. These were screened independently by two investigators (M.J.P. and A.P.) based on the inclusion and exclusion criteria. Articles of overlapping participants were also screened and considered independent of the "parent" study. A record number was assigned to each included study. Any disagreements were overcome by consensus. When a research study was considered eligible, it was selected for full text review. Of the 274 studies identified, eight were eligible for inclusion.

2.4. Data Extraction

Data was extracted by two independent investigators (M.J.P. and A.P.): author and year, country, study design, length of intervention, sample size, patients' characteristics, intervention features, comparator features, and outcomes (blood Phe levels, blood Tyr levels, blood urea nitrogen (BUN), glucose levels and acceptability/palatability). For all included studies, mean $\pm$ standard deviation (SD) or standard error of mean (SEM) or median and interquartile range (IQR) were used for data extracted.

2.5. Quality Appraisal

The quality of all included studies was assessed using the Grading of Recommendations Assessment, Development and Evaluation (GRADE) system [29]. The GRADE ranks as follows: not serious, serious and very serious. The GRADE level of evidence was determined independently by two authors (M.J.P. and L.A.), and consensus was achieved by discussion.

2.6. Assessment of Risk of Bias

The Cochrane Collaboration's domain-based evaluation tool as described in Chapter 8, Section 8.5, in the Cochrane Handbook for Systematic Reviews of Interventions was used to assess risk of bias of randomised clinical trials (RCTs) [30]. This tool comprises six domains: random sequence generation (selection bias); allocation concealment (selection bias); blinding of participants and personnel (performance bias); blinding of outcome assessment (detection bias); incomplete outcome data (attrition bias), and selective reporting (reporting bias). Each RCT was rated as low risk, unclear risk or high risk of bias.

The Risk of Bias in Non-Randomised Studies of Interventions (ROBINS-I) assessment tool was used for non-randomised studies (observational studies). This tool includes seven specific bias domains, pre-intervention and post-intervention [31]. The domains are: (1) confounding; (2) selection of participants; (3) classification of intervention; (4) deviation from interventions; (5) missing outcome data; (6) measurement of outcomes; and (7) selection of reported result overall. Risk of bias was rated as 0—no information; 1—low risk; 2—moderate risk; 3—serious risk; and 4—critical risk.

Two authors independently assessed risk of bias (M.J.P. and L.A.) of the included articles. Disagreements were managed by consensus.

2.7. *Data Analysis*

Meta-analysis was performed using Review Manager Version 5.3 (The Nordic Cochrane Centre, The Cochrane Collaboration 2014, Portland, OR, USA).

Our primary question was about the effect of GMP intervention on altering blood Phe concentrations in PKU. Due to absence of statistical information and assuming that randomisation was well conducted, we compared the final values of blood Phe. The same approach was applied to the secondary outcomes (blood Tyr, BUN, glucose). The secondary outcome acceptability/palatability was compiled in a table.

In two RCTs with sufficient methodological similarity [18,22], a meta-analysis was carried out. The study of Ahring et al. [18] tested four drink mixtures (DMs 1–4), consisting of GMP or AAs or a combination. For the purposes of analysis, we only considered DM3 and DM4. In the same study, the values of BUN and glucose were available in mmol/L which were converted to mg/dL. In these two studies, GMP-AAs provided 1.8 mg Phe/g of protein equivalent. A forest plot was generated and calculated the mean difference (MD) as the effect measure. We combined the MD with the use of the random-effects model. The degree of statistical heterogeneity between studies was assessed with the use of the I^2 statistic. We reported statistical heterogeneity as important if the I^2 statistic was $\geq$40%, according to the Cochrane guidelines. Significance was set at the level of P-value less than 0.05.

3. Results

3.1. *Study Selection*

Figure 1 describes the process of study selection according to PRISMA. The first literature search identified 274 articles. Initial screening identified 12 papers for full text review. From this, 4 were eliminated as they failed to meet the exclusion criteria. Eight studies were eligible for the systematic review and meta-analysis was performed for only two studies.

3.2. *Study Characteristics*

Table 1 summarizes the main characteristics of all included articles. Only two studies were considered RCTs with crossover according to the Consolidated Standards of Reporting Trials (CONSORT) guidelines [32] and the remaining six studies were as follows: two crossover clinical studies, two clinical studies, one retrospective study, and one cross-sectional study. Four studies were conducted in the United States at the University of Wisconsin–Madison. The remaining four studies were performed in the United Kingdom, Portugal, Denmark, and Egypt. Studies were published between 2007 and 2018, with the vast majority published since 2010.

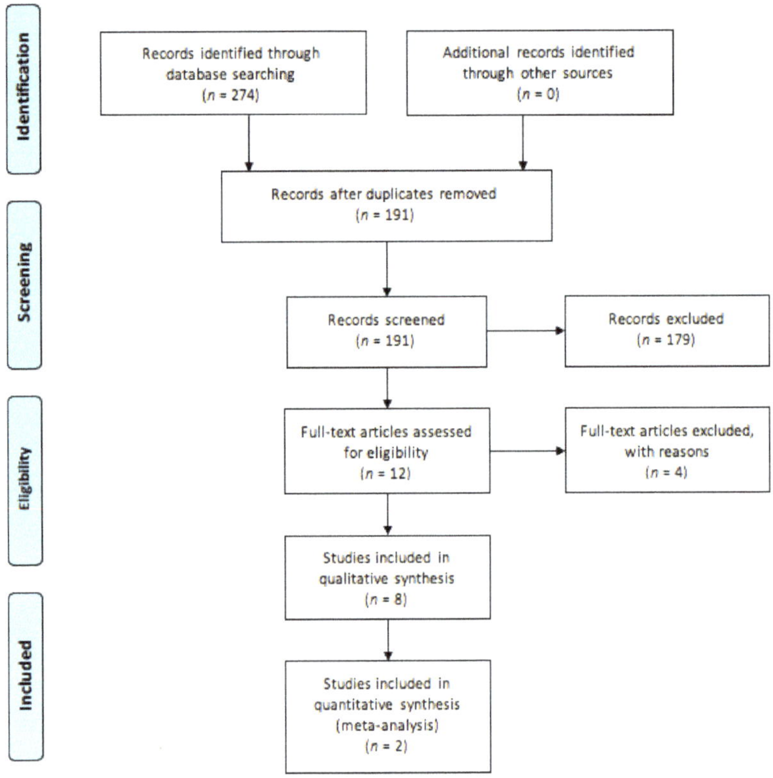

Figure 1. Preferred Reporting Items for Systematic Reviews and Meta-Analysis (PRISMA) study flow diagram describing process of study selection. Reviews or preclinical studies (defined as not providing clinical outcome data) and abstracts were excluded. Full-text articles that provided no outcome of interest were also excluded.

Table 1. Characteristics of studies included in the systematic review.

Author, Year (Ref.)	Country	Study Design	Sample Size (*N*)	Age (Range)—Years	Gender	PKU Phenotype
Lim et al. 2007 [10]	United States	Cross-sectional study	49	12–42	N/A	N/A
van Calcar et al. 2009 [17]	United States	Crossover clinical study	11	23 ± 7 (11–31)	4 F; 7 M	10 classical; 1 variant form
MacLeod et al. 2010 [20]	United States	Crossover clinical study	11	23 ± 7 (11–31)	4 F; 7 M	11 classical
Zaki et al. 2016 [21]	Egypt	Clinical study	10	6.73 [5.02; 11.79]	4 F; 6 M	10 classical
Ney et al. 2016 [22]	United States	Randomised crossover clinical trial	30	15–49	18 F; 12 M	20 classical; 10 variant form
Daly et al. 2017 [23]	United Kingdom	Clinical study	22	11 (6–16)	9 F; 13 M	N/A
Pinto et al. 2017 [24]	Portugal	Retrospective, longitudinal study	11	27 ± 10 (13–42)	8 F; 3 M	6 classical; 4 mild; 1 HPA
Ahring et al. 2018 [18]	Denmark	Randomised crossover clinical trial	8 [1]	33.25 ± 11.21 (15–48)	7 F; 1 M	8 classical

F: female; HPA: hyperphenylalaninemia; M: male; N/A: not available; PKU: phenylketonuria. Data are presented as mean ± standard deviation or median [interquartile range]. [1] Initial sample size was of eight patients but only six patients completed the study.

The total sample size of the included articles was 139 participants, since the participants of the study of MacLeod et al. [20] were recruited from the "parent" study of van Calcar et al. [17]. The largest trial conducted in patients with PKU taking GMP-AAs was the study by Ney et al. [22], with a total of 30 participants. The participants in most of the studies were adults, with the exception of the articles from Zaki et al. [21] and Daly et al. [23], that recruited children with PKU. Regarding the PKU phenotype, the predominant form was classical PKU.

3.3. *Treatment and Outcome Measures*

Table 2 illustrates the characteristics of treatment and outcome measures. The length of intervention is quite variable across studies, ranging from eight days to twenty months. In the studies of van Calcar et al. [17] and MacLeod et al. [20], subjects consumed the AAs diet or the GMP-AAs diet for four days. In the work performed by Zaki et al. [21], the study was divided into two periods, each lasting nine weeks each. In one of the periods, children were given 50% of their total protein substitute as GMP made with cheese and the remaining 50% was given in the form of AAs. In the other period, the total protein substitute was taken in the form of AAs. In the study of Ney et al. [22], subjects consumed for three weeks each, in a random order, AAs or GMP-AAs, separated by a washout period of three weeks with AAs. In the work of Daly et al. [23], 12 children received GMP-AAs (partially or fully to replace AAs but individually titrated according to their blood Phe control) and 9 subjects received AAs as their protein substitute. In the retrospective study conducted by Pinto et al. [24] with 11 subjects, GMP-AAs partially or fully substituted AAs. In the study performed by Ahring et al. [18], subjects tested four DMs (1–4) in a random order at each visit (DM1 = GMP; DM2 = AAs (equivalent amino acid profile to DM1); DM3 = GMP + AAs; DM4 = AAs (equivalent amino acid profile to DM3 but without Phe).

Table 2. Characteristics of treatment and outcome measures of the included studies.

Author, Year (Ref.)	Length of Intervention	Intervention	Comparator	Primary Outcome	Secondary Outcomes
Lim et al. 2007 [10]	N/A	GMP-AAs	AAs	N/A	Acceptability *
van Calcar et al. 2009 [17]	Two treatments for four days each: AAs (days 1–4) and GMP-AAs (days 5–8)	Period I—0% GMP-AAs; Period II—100% GMP-AAs; 11 patients	Period I—100% AAs; Period II—0% AAs; 11 patients	Blood Phe	Blood Tyr BUN Glucose Acceptability *
MacLeod et al. 2010 [20]	Two treatments for four days each: AAs (days 1–4) and GMP-AAs (days 5–8)	Period I—0% GMP-AAs; Period II—100% GMP-AAs; 11 patients	Period I—100% AAs; Period II—0% AAs; 11 patients	Blood Phe	Blood Tyr Acceptability *
Zaki et al. 2016 [21]	Eighteen weeks	Period I—50% GMP; Period II—0% GMP; 10 patients	Period I—50% AAs; Period II—100% AAs; 10 patients	Blood Phe	Urea/BUN Acceptability *
Ney et al. 2016 [22]	Eleven weeks	Three weeks each of GMP-AAs or AAs; 15 patients in each arm	Three weeks each of GMP-AAs or AAs; 15 patients in each arm	Blood Phe	Blood Tyr BUN Glucose Acceptability *
Daly et al. 2017 [23]	Twenty-six weeks	12 patients—GMP-AAs	9 patients—AAs	Blood Phe	Blood Tyr Acceptability *
Pinto et al. 2017 [24]	Twenty months	11 patients—GMP-AAs	11 patients—AAs	Blood Phe	Blood Tyr Urea/BUN Glucose
Ahring et al. 2018 [18]	Four visits, analysis at five timepoints (0, 15, 30, 60, 120 and 240 min)	6 patients tested the four DMs (DM1 = GMP; DM3 = GMP + AAs)	6 patients tested the four DMs [DM2 = AAs (equivalent amino acid profile to DM1); DM4 = AAs (equivalent amino acid profile to DM3 but without Phe)]	Blood Phe	Blood Tyr BUN Glucose Acceptability *

AAs: synthetic protein derived from L-amino acids; BUN: blood urea nitrogen; DM: drink mixture; GMP: glycomacropeptide; GMP-AA: glycomacropeptide supplemented with amino acids; N/A: not available; Phe: phenylalanine; PKU: phenylketonuria; Tyr: tyrosine. * The results of acceptability are shown in Table 3.

Table 3. Acceptability of GMP products versus AAs.

Author, Year (Ref.)	Method	Number of Items Evaluated	Type of Items Evaluated	Main Findings
Lim et al. 2007 [10]	Five-point hedonic scale [1]	Seven products (five GMP-AAs and two AAs)	GMP-AAs (strawberry pudding, strawberry fruit leather, chocolate beverage, snack crackers, orange sports beverage) and AAs (crackers, chocolate beverage)	Decreasing order of overall acceptability—strawberry pudding (4.2 ± 0.9), snack cracker (3.6 ± 1.4), strawberry fruit leather (3.4 ± 1.0), chocolate beverage (3.3 ± 1.0), orange sports beverage (3.3 ± 1.1), AAs in crackers (2.9 ± 1.3), AAs in a chocolate beverage (2.5 ± 1.4)
van Calcar et al. 2009 [17]	No methodology described	Six GMP-AAs and subject's usual AAs	GMP-AAs (orange-flavoured sports beverage, chocolate-flavoured or caramel-flavoured beverage, chocolate or strawberry pudding, cinnamon crunch bar) and subject's usual AAs	After consuming the GMP-AAs diet for four days, 10 of 11 subjects claimed that the GMP-AAs products were superior in sensory qualities to their usual AAs. Moreover, at the end of the study, 6 of 7 adults expressed a strong preference to consume GMP-AAs products rather than their usual AAs
MacLeod et al. 2010 [20]	Four questions, motivation-to-eat VAS questionnaires	Six GMP-AAs and subject's usual AAs	GMP-AAs (orange-flavoured sports beverage, chocolate-flavoured or caramel-flavoured beverage, chocolate or strawberry pudding, cinnamon crunch bar) and subject's usual AAs	The motivation-to-eat VAS profiles were not significantly different at any timepoint between the AAs (day 4) and GMP-AAs (day 8)
Zaki et al. 2016 [21]	Questionnaire	N/A	N/A	Throughout the study, all patients preferred the diet supplemented with GMP over the classical AAs due to better taste and satiety
Ney et al., 2016 [22]	Six-question survey and six-point scale [2]	Fifteen AAs and N/A the exact number of GMP-AAs	N/A	AAs vs GMP-AAs (1) 3.97 ± 0.24 vs 4.90 ± 0.18, $P = 0.001$ (2) 4.79 ± 0.22 vs 5.07 ± 0.16, $P = 0.366$ (3) 4.50 ± 0.25 vs 4.86 ± 0.19, $P = 0.172$ (4) 4.19 ± 0.18 vs 4.69 ± 0.16, $P = 0.019$ (5) 3.83 ± 0.26 vs 4.72 ± 0.27, $P = 0.003$ (6) 3.34 ± 0.31 vs 4.47 ± 0.23, $P = 0.001$
Daly et al., 2017 [23]	Acceptability questionnaires (taste, smell, texture, mouthfeel and overall acceptability)	N/A	In the GMP-AAs group, subjects took a berry flavoured GMP-AAs powder (35 g sachet = 20 g protein equivalent) which subjects prepared with water or low-protein milk	All of the subjects in the GMP-AAs group described the protein substitute as acceptable, with improved taste, mouth feel, texture, and smell compared to their conventional AAs
Pinto et al., 2017 [24]	N/A	N/A	N/A	N/A
Ahring et al., 2018 [18]	Two questions—VAS [3]	Four DMs	DM1 = GMP; DM2 = AAs (equivalent amino acid profile as DM1); DM3 = GMP + AAs (0.16 g Phe/100 g amino acids present in GMP); DM4 = AAs (equivalent amino acid profile as DM3 but without Phe)	1) DM1: 36 ± 18, DM2: 41 ± 16, DM3: 28 ± 27, DM4: 35 ± 30); 2) DM1: 34 ± 31, DM2: 44 ± 22, DM3: 36 ± 28, DM4: 26 ± 22); all comparisons (DM1 and DM2, DM3 and DM4, DM3 to DM1 and DM2, respectively) were statistically insignificant

AAs: synthetic protein derived from L-amino acids; DM: drink mixture; GMP: glycomacropeptide; GMP-AAs: glycomacropeptide supplemented with amino acids; N/A: not available; VAS: visual analogue scale. Data are presented as mean ± standard deviation or mean ± SEs (in the case of Ney et al., 2016). [1] Five sensory categories—appearance, odour, taste, texture and overall acceptability (1 = dislike very much; 2 = dislike; 3 = neither like nor dislike; 4 = like; 5 = like very much). [2] Six questions: (1) How much do you like your AAs/GMP-AAs?; (2) How easy is it to prepare your AAs/GMP-AAs?; (3) How willing are you to take AAs/GMP-AAs three times a day?; (4) How easy is it to stay on your phenylketonuria diet when you are using AAs/GMP-AAs?; (5) How comfortable are you eating AAs/GMP-AAs in social situations?; (6) Overall, how convenient is it to take and consume AAs/GMP-AAs away from home? (1 = dislike extremely; 2 = dislike; 3 = somewhat dislike; 4 = somewhat like; 5 = like; 6 = like extremely). [3] Two questions: (1) How satisfied are you? and (2) How does the DM taste? This was presented to patients as a horizontal line, ranking from 0 = very hungry to 100 = very satisfied and from 0 = bad taste to 100 = good taste.

Considering the outcome measures, only the study by Lim et al. [10] evaluated acceptability. The remaining studies used blood Phe as a primary outcome measure. Blood Tyr was measured in all studies, with exception of the studies of Lim et al. [10] and Zaki et al. [21]. BUN was measured in the studies of van Calcar et al. [17], Ney et al. [22], and Ahring et al. [18]. In the studies of Zaki et al. [21] and Pinto et al. [24], only the values of urea were available. Glucose was measured in the studies of van Calcar et al. [17], Ney et al. [22], Pinto et al. [24], and Ahring et al. [18]. Acceptability was assessed by all apart from Pinto et al. [24].

3.4. Acceptability/Palatability of GMP Products

Acceptability is a hedonic response affected by the organoleptic properties of products, among others. Measuring acceptability is both subjective and complex, with many different methodologies available. Acceptability of GMP products was determined based on different methodologies as illustrated in Table 3. The included studies showed that GMP products were well accepted by patients. There is evidence suggesting that GMP products based on natural protein source are more palatable than protein substitutes based on mono amino acids. However, it is important to highlight the lack of uniformity in the methods used to evaluate this parameter. The presentation form of the products was also variable, some studies used solid food whereas other studies used only drinks.

3.5. Quality Appraisal

Using the GRADE system, inconsistency and imprecision were the most common reasons for downgrading (Table 4).

Table 4. Quality of all included studies according to Grading of Recommendations Assessment, Development and Evaluation (GRADE) system.

Outcomes	Number of Studies	Study Design	Risk of Bias	Inconsistency	Indirectness	Imprecision
Blood Phe	2	Randomised trials	Not serious	Serious	Not serious	Very serious
	5	Observational studies	Not serious	Serious	Not serious	Very serious
Blood Tyr	2	Randomised trials	Not serious	Serious	Not serious	Very serious
	4	Observational studies	Not serious	Serious	Not serious	Very serious
BUN	2	Randomised trials	Not serious	Serious	Not serious	Very serious
	3	Observational studies	Not serious	Serious	Not serious	Very serious
Glucose	2	Randomised trials	Not serious	Serious	Not serious	Very serious
	4	Observational studies	Not serious	Serious	Not serious	Very serious
Acceptability	2	Randomised trials	Not serious	Serious	Not serious	Very serious
	5	Observational studies	Not serious	Serious	Not serious	Very serious

BUN: blood urea nitrogen; Phe: phenylalanine; Tyr: tyrosine. The GRADE ranks as follows: not serious, serious, and very serious.

3.6. Assessment of Risk of Bias

Risk of bias for RCTs was evaluated according to the Cochrane guidelines (Figures 2 and 3). Only two out of eight studies were considered RCTs. For the domain random sequence generation (selection of bias), 1/2 rated as unclear and 1/2 rated as low; for the domain allocation concealment (selection bias), 2/2 rated as high; for the domain blinding of participants and personnel (performance bias), 1/2 rated as low and 1/2 rated as high; for the domain blinding of outcome assessment (detection bias), 2/2 rated as unclear; for the domain incomplete outcome data (attrition bias), 1/2 rated as unclear and 1/2 rated as low; for the domain selective reporting (reporting bias), 2/2 rated as low.

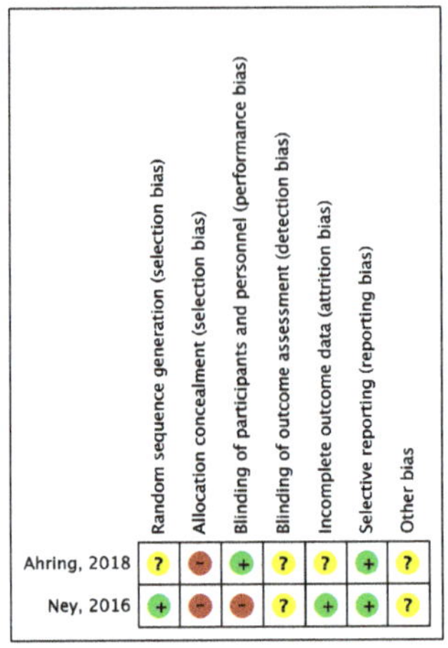

Figure 2. Risk of bias summary across randomised controlled trials. Low risk of bias: green "+"; Unclear risk of bias: yellow "?"; High risk of bias: red "−".

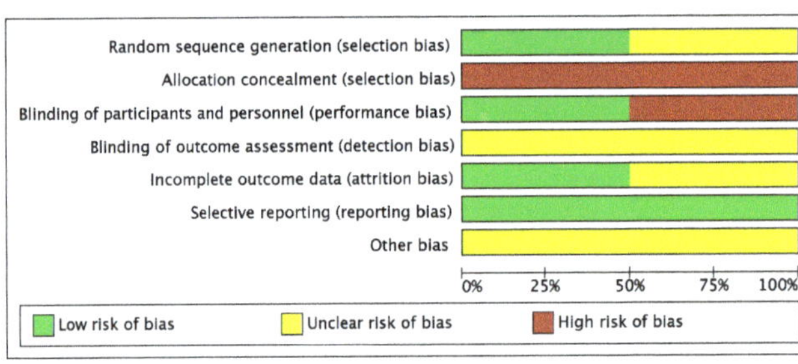

Figure 3. Risk of bias graph across randomised controlled trials. Low risk of bias: green; Unclear risk of bias: yellow; High risk of bias: red.

Risk of bias for observational studies was evaluated using ROBINS-I tool (Table 5). In domains 1 and 2, 5/5 were rated as serious; in domains 3, 4 and 5, 5/5 rated as low; in domains 6 and 7, 4/5 were rated as low and 1/5 rated as serious; and overall, 5 of 5 were rated as moderate risk of bias. All studies provided sound evidence for non-randomised studies but cannot be considered comparable to well-performed randomised trials.

Table 5. Risk of bias in non-randomised studies according to the Risk of Bias in Non-Randomised Studies of Interventions (ROBINS-I) tool.

Author, year (Ref.)	Domain 1	Domain 2	Domain 3	Domain 4	Domain 5	Domain 6	Domain 7	Overall
Lim et al. 2007 * [10]	N/A	N/A	N/A	N/A	N/A	N/A	N/A	N/A
van Calcar et al. 2009 [17]	3	3	1	1	1	1	1	2—Moderate
MacLeod et al. 2010 [20]	3	3	1	1	1	1	1	2—Moderate
Zaki et al. 2016 [21]	3	3	1	1	1	3	3	2—Moderate
Daly et al. 2017 [23]	3	3	1	1	1	1	1	2—Moderate
Pinto et al. 2017 [24]	3	3	1	1	1	1	1	2—Moderate

N/A. not applicable; Domain 1: confounding; Domain 2: selection of participants; Domain 3: classification of intervention; Domain 4: deviation from interventions; Domain 5: missing outcome data; Domain 6: measurement of outcomes; Domain 7: selection of reported result; Overall. Risk of bias assessment: 0—No information; 1—Low; 2—Moderate; 3—Serious; 4—Critical. * Non-comparative study only acceptability of GMP products is evaluated, therefore this tool is not applicable in this case.

3.7. Meta-Analysis

Focusing on the primary outcome (blood Phe levels), the meta-analysis showed no significant differences between GMP-AAs and AAs (MD = 123.36 μmol/L (−35.18, 281.89); I^2 = 0%; P = 0.13; two studies; N = 72 participants; Figure 4), although a tendency to lower Phe concentrations in patients treated with AAs was observed.

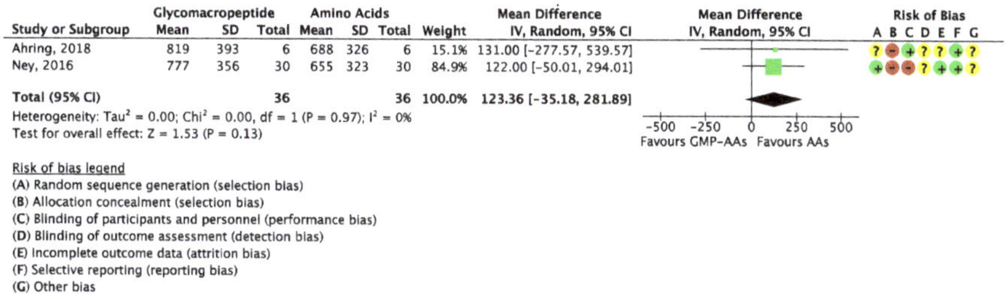

Figure 4. Forest plot of studies with data on the effect of glycomacropeptide interventions on blood phenylalanine levels. The analysis included data from two studies with a total of 72 participants. AAs: synthetic protein derived from L-amino acids; CI: confidence interval; df: degrees of freedom; GMP-AAs: glycomacropeptide supplemented with amino acids; IV: intravitreal; SD: standard deviation.

The overall treatment effect on blood Tyr levels was not statistically significant (MD = −3.91 μmol/L (−8.12, 0.31); I^2 = 0%; P = 0.07; two studies; N = 72 participants; Figure 5) and patients treated with AAs tended to have higher levels of Tyr.

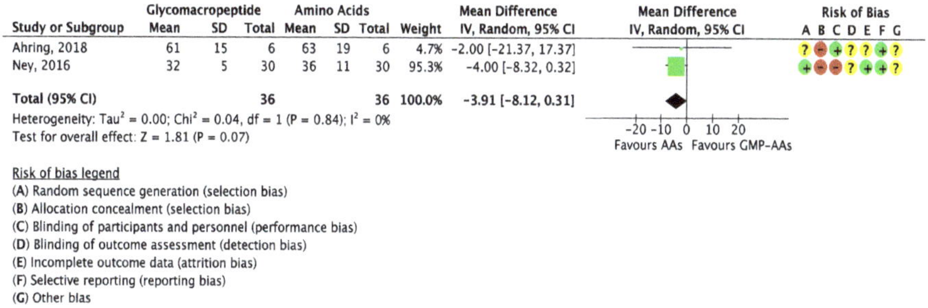

Figure 5. Forest plot of studies with data on glycomacropeptide interventions on blood tyrosine levels. The analysis included data from two studies with a total of 72 participants.AAs: synthetic protein derived from L-amino acids; CI: confidence interval; df: degrees of freedom; GMP-AAs: glycomacropeptide supplemented with amino acids; IV: intravitreal; SD: standard deviation.

The meta-analysis for BUN reported no significant differences between GMP-AAs and AAs (MD = −0.22 mg/dL (−1.49, 1.04); I^2 = 0%; P = 0.73; two studies; N = 72 participants; Figure 6); nor did the meta-analysis for glucose levels (MD = −1.33 mg/dL (−7.51, 4.85); I^2 = 57%; P = 0.67; two studies; N = 72 participants; Figure 7).

When analysing BUN, the value of SD of DM4 was imputed since no value was reported. It was calculated from the arithmetic mean of SD of DM2 from baseline and final and DM4 from baseline.

The studies included in this meta-analysis were quite consistent in all outcomes as a result of I^2 values, a measure of heterogeneity. Nevertheless, the length of study was different between studies, and in the study of Ahring et al. [18], patients had high blood Phe levels at the start of the study and this aspect could have masked the results.

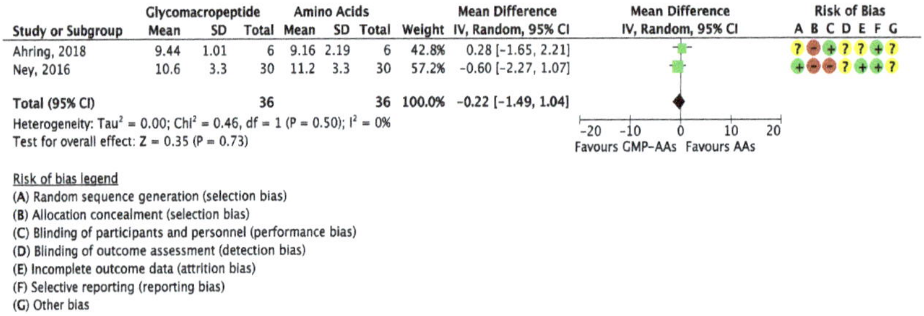

Figure 6. Forest plot of studies with data on the effect of glycomacropeptide interventions on blood urea nitrogen. The analysis included data from two studies with a total of 72 participants.AAs: synthetic protein derived from L-amino acids; CI: confidence interval; df: degrees of freedom; GMP-AAs: glycomacropeptide supplemented with amino acids; IV: intravitreal; SD: standard deviation.

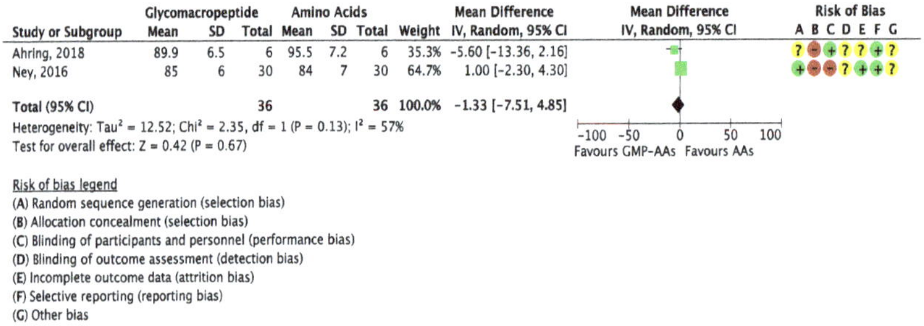

Figure 7. Forest plot of studies with data on the effect of glycomacropeptide interventions on glucose levels. The analysis included data from two studies with a total of 72 participants. AAs: synthetic protein derived from L-amino acids; CI: confidence interval; df: degrees of freedom; GMP-AAs: glycomacropeptide supplemented with amino acids; IV: intravitreal; SD: standard deviation.

4. Discussion

This is the first systematic review and meta-analysis addressing the use of GMP in the nutritional management of PKU. This study was designed with the aim of reviewing the current literature on the use of GMP in PKU and the effect of residual Phe in GMP on blood Phe control, biochemical status, and palatability.

Overall, pooled results based on two RCTs reported no significant effect for all outcome measures. For blood Phe control, in the adult studies, meta-analysis showed a tendency in favour of AAs despite no clinical significance. AAs have no added Phe and the effect of the extra Phe provided by the GMP-AAs may have been masked as adult subjects started with higher baseline blood Phe [18]. Children maintain lower blood Phe target concentrations so may have less tolerance with additional Phe sources. In addition, fever and recurrent infections are more likely to impact on blood Phe control in children [33]. It is well known that administration of AAs during any acute phases suppresses Phe levels, improving metabolic control [3]. So far, it remains undocumented if GMP-AAs intake can suppress the rise in Phe levels in a similar way to AAs, as little is known about the kinetics of GMP-AAs in PKU. Additionally, the impact of GMP-AAs on glucose metabolism and anabolic pathways remains to be studied, and ultimately an influence on Phe levels cannot be dismissed. The studies by Zaki et al. [21] and Daly et al. [23], investigated the effect on blood Phe control using two different formulations of GMP in 10 and 22 children with PKU, respectively. The different interventions in these two studies prevented subgroup analysis, which would have enabled a better understanding of the impact of GMP in the paediatric population versus adulthood. So far, the research about the effects of GMP in children is still insufficient to advocate its use as a safe alternative to the traditional treatment. A systematic review with three trials evaluating the use of protein substitutes in PKU concluded that the current evidence is scarce and until robust evidence from RCTs is obtained, the use of all protein substitutes should be monitored carefully [34]. Nevertheless, the clinical use of AAs for several decades counterweighs the scarcity of scientific evidence emerging from RCTs [3].

When we performed meta-analysis on the effect of GMP-AAs versus AAs on blood Tyr levels, patients treated with AAs tended to have higher levels of Tyr. Tyr is considered a conditionally essential amino acid in PKU since it is produced from Phe and without treatment with a Tyr-supplemented protein substitute, Tyr deficiency is seen. The study of Ney et al. [22] reported that despite significantly higher intakes of Tyr in patients consuming a low-Phe diet in combination with AAs when compared to GMP-AAs, fasting plasma levels of Tyr were not statistically different. Moreover, the study of Pinto et al. [24] showed an increase in blood Tyr (even when dietary Tyr intake was lower) when patients consumed GMP-AAs.

A study performed in PKU mice showed that GMP-AAs acted as a prebiotic [15], shaping the gut microbiota. The GMP-AAs effects on gut microbiota may influence Tyr bioavailability [26]. Tyr is one of the amino acids with the lowest solubility [35], which can interfere with gut absorption [26].

For BUN and glucose levels, no conclusions can be reached. Subjects in the studies had similar protein intakes, irrespective of taking GMP-AAs or AAs. BUN is an indicator of the relationship between nutritional status and protein metabolism of patients [36]. In the study by van Calcar et al. [17], performed with 11 subjects, BUN was significantly lower and plasma insulin was higher when measured 2.5 h after eating a breakfast containing GMP-AAs. Glycaemia is known to be influenced by amino acid intake [37].

A further objective was to evaluate the acceptability/palatability of GMP products. Despite the different approaches used to measure acceptability in the included studies [10,17,18,20–23], GMP products were well accepted by patients. A very recent study from Proserpio et al. [38] published after our literature selection sought to explore the liking of low-Phe products (GMP products versus AAs) as well as to obtain a sensory description of them using the check-all-that-apply (CATA) method in 86 subjects with PKU in an ambulatory setting. The CATA questionnaire is a rapid sensory profiling approach to characterize foods based on sensory attributes. This is the first evidence of the sensory properties of GMP products in PKU subjects. The study included eight samples: four GMP products and four AAs flavoured with neutral, chocolate, strawberry, and tomato aromas. GMP products flavoured with chocolate and strawberry aromas were the most appreciated. The CATA method appears as a suitable method to fine-tune organoleptic properties to help improve dietary adherence. Nevertheless, this study does not provide data about the long-term acceptance of GMP products with patients and whilst the palatability of protein substitutes is important it is essential to assess the impact on metabolic control of any formulation that provides a source of Phe in all age groups and categories of patients with PKU.

This systematic review has several strengths and limitations. The main strength is that it provides a compilation of the available evidence of GMP interventions and gives an overview of the current status. This will help in PKU guideline production. This study unveils the main flaws in the design of GMP interventions. First, among the eight studies included in this work, only two were RCTs, studies at the top of the hierarchy of evidence. Although high-quality observational studies can also produce comparable responses, well-conducted RCTs are still the gold-standard of evidence [39]. Secondly, all studies consisted of small sample sizes but in the context of PKU this cannot be undervalued due to the rarity of the disorder. Moreover, the RCT studies were short-term, and the adults did not have good metabolic control at baseline and had variable phenotypic presentations.

The present systematic review and meta-analysis raises important aspects in the scope of PKU research. It would be ideal to create a group with PKU experts to develop standards in planning and designing better-quality studies for protein substitute research. However, it should be acknowledged that RCTs on protein substitutes are difficult to conduct due to food neophobia and poor acceptability of protein substitutes.

5. Conclusions

The two studies that qualified for comparable investigation failed to show any reduction in plasma Phe, despite GMP-AAs providing 1.8 mg Phe/g of protein equivalent. This might be explained by the small number of available studies, small sample sizes, and short lengths of study. Considering that PKU is a chronic disease and requires lifelong treatment, further long-term research is warranted to understand in depth the safety and health benefits of GMP in the context of PKU. In the interim, the use of GMP in children should be carefully managed.

Author Contributions: M.J.P. was involved in all processes of the review; A.P. was involved in study selection and data extraction. A.D. and A.M. provided valuable contributions for the protocol design and also provided important contents for the manuscript. L.A. contributed to GRADE and risk of bias assessment, and to data analysis. J.C.R. and N.B. were involved in all steps of the review. All authors contributed to the development of the study and approved the final version of the manuscript.

Funding: This article was supported by ERDF through the operation POCI-01-0145-FEDER-007746 funded by the Programa Operacional Competitividade e Internacionalização (COMPETE2020), and by national funds through Fundação para a Ciência e a Tecnologia (FCT) within CINTESIS, R&D Unit (reference UID/IC/4255/2013). M.J.P. was partially funded by the project NORTE-08-5369-FSE-000018, supported by Norte Portugal Regional Programme (Norte 2020), under the PORTUGAL 2020 Partnership Agreement, through the European Regional Development Fund (ERDF).

Acknowledgments: M.J.P. was partially funded by the project NORTE-08-5369-FSE-000018, supported by Norte Portugal Regional Programme (Norte 2020), under the PORTUGAL 2020 Partnership Agreement, through the European Regional Development Fund (ERDF).

Conflicts of Interest: Alex Pinto has received an educational grant from Cambrooke Therapeutics and grants from Vitaflo, Nutricia, Merck Serono, and Biomarin to attend scientific meetings. Anne Daly has received grants, lecturing honoraria, consulting fees, and a PhD from Vitaflo Ltd., Nutricia Ltd., Firstplay dietary foods, and Mevalia. Anita MacDonald has received research funding and honoraria from Nutricia, Vitaflo International, Biomarin, Mevalia, and Pharma Galen. She is a member of the European Nutrition Expert Panel (Biomarin), and a member of the following advisory boards: the European PKU Group Board (Biomarin), Element (Danone-Nutricia), Excemed, Arla, and Applied Pharma Research. Júlio César Rocha is member of the European Nutrition Expert Panel (Biomarin) and of the advisory boards of Applied Pharma Research and Nutricia. He has received speaker's fees from Merck Serono, Biomarin, Nutricia, Vitaflo, and Cambrooke.

References

1. Blau, N.; Van Spronsen, F.J.; Levy, H.L. Phenylketonuria. *Lancet* **2010**, *376*, 1417–1427. [CrossRef]
2. Bickel, H.; Gerrard, J.; Hickmans, E.M. Preliminary communication. *Lancet* **1953**, *262*, 812–813. [CrossRef]
3. Van Wegberg, A.M.J.; MacDonald, A.; Ahring, K.; Bélanger-Quintana, A.; Blau, N.; Bosch, A.M.; Burlina, A.; Campistol, J.; Feillet, F.; Giżewska, M.; et al. The complete European guidelines on phenylketonuria: Diagnosis and treatment. *Orphanet J. Rare Dis.* **2017**, *12*, 1–56. [CrossRef] [PubMed]
4. MacDonald, A.; Rocha, J.C.; van Rijn, M.; Feillet, F. Nutrition in phenylketonuria. *Mol. Genet. MeTab.* **2011**, *104*. [CrossRef] [PubMed]
5. Pena, M.J.; De Almeida, M.F.; Van Dam, E.; Ahring, K.; Bélanger-Quintana, A.; Dokoupil, K.; Gokmen-Ozel, H.; Lammardo, A.M.; MacDonald, A.; Robert, M.; et al. Protein substitutes for phenylketonuria in Europe: Access and nutritional composition. *Eur. J. Clin. Nutr.* **2016**, *70*, 785–789. [CrossRef] [PubMed]
6. Kure, S.; Hou, D.; Ohura, T.; Iwamoto, H.; Suzuki, S.; Sugiyama, N.; Sakamoto, O.; Fujii, K.; Matsubara, Y.; Narisawa, K. Tetrahydrobiopterin-responsive phenylalanine hydroxylase deficiency. *J. Pediatr.* **1999**, *135*, 375–378. [CrossRef]
7. MacDonald, A.; Van Rijn, M.; Gokmen-Ozel, H.; Burgard, P. The reality of dietary compliance in the management of phenylketonuria. *J. Inherit. Metab. Dis.* **2010**, *33*, 665–670. [CrossRef] [PubMed]
8. MacLeod, E.L.; Ney, D.M. Nutritional management of phenylketonuria. *Ann. Nestle* **2010**, *68*, 58–69. [CrossRef] [PubMed]
9. LaClair, C.E.; Ney, D.M.; MacLeod, E.L.; Etzel, M.R. Purification and use of glycomacropeptide for nutritional management of phenylketonuria. *J. Food Sci.* **2009**, *74*, 1–19. [CrossRef] [PubMed]

10. Lim, K.; van Calcar, S.C.; Nelson, K.L.; Gleason, S.T.; Ney, D.M. Acceptable low-phenylalanine foods and beverages can be made with glycomacropeptide from cheese whey for individuals with PKU. *Mol. Genet. MeTab.* **2007**, *92*, 176–178. [CrossRef] [PubMed]
11. Ney, D.M.; Etzel, M.R. Designing medical foods for inherited metabolic disorders: Why intact protein is superior to amino acids. *Curr. Opin. Biotechnol.* **2017**, *44*, 39–45. [CrossRef] [PubMed]
12. Ney, D.M.; Hull, A.K.; van Calcar, S.C.; Liu, X.; Etzel, M.R. Dietary glycomacropeptide supports growth and reduces the concentrations of phenylalanine in plasma and brain in a murine model of phenylketonuria. *J. Nutr.* **2008**, *138*, 316–322. [CrossRef] [PubMed]
13. Solverson, P.; Murali, S.G.; Brinkman, A.S.; Nelson, D.W.; Clayton, M.K.; Yen, C.-L.E.; Ney, D.M. Glycomacropeptide, a low-phenylalanine protein isolated from cheese whey, supports growth and attenuates metabolic stress in the murine model of phenylketonuria. *AJP Endocrinol. MeTab.* **2012**, *302*, E885–E895. [CrossRef] [PubMed]
14. Sawin, E.A.; Murali, S.G.; Ney, D.M. Differential effects of low-phenylalanine protein sources on brain neurotransmitters and behavior in C57Bl/6-Pah(enu2) mice. *Mol. Genet. MeTab.* **2014**, *111*, 452–461. [CrossRef] [PubMed]
15. Sawin, E.A.; De Wolfe, T.J.; Aktas, B.; Stroup, B.M.; Murali, S.G.; Steele, J.L.; Ney, D.M. Glycomacropeptide is a prebiotic that reduces *Desulfovibrio* bacteria, increases cecal short-chain fatty acids, and is anti-inflammatory in mice. *Am. J. Physiol. Liver Physiol.* **2015**, *309*, G590–G601. [CrossRef] [PubMed]
16. Solverson, P.; Murali, S.G.; Litscher, S.J.; Blank, R.D.; Ney, D.M. Low bone strength is a manifestation of phenylketonuria in mice and is attenuated by a glycomacropeptide diet. *PLoS ONE* **2012**, *7*, e45165. [CrossRef] [PubMed]
17. Van Calcar, S.C.; MacLeod, E.L.; Gleason, S.T.; Etzel, M.R.; Clayton, M.K.; Wolff, J.A.; Ney, D.M. Improved nutritional management of phenylketonuria by using a diet ontaining glycomacropeptide compared with amino acids. *Am. J. Clin. Nutr.* **2009**, *89*, 1068–1077. [CrossRef] [PubMed]
18. Ahring, K.K.; Lund, A.M.; Jensen, E.; Jensen, T.G.; Brøndum-Nielsen, K.; Pedersen, M.; Bardow, A.; Holst, J.J.; Rehfeld, J.F.; Møller, L.B. Comparison of glycomacropeptide with phenylalanine free-synthetic amino acids in test meals to PKU patients: No significant differences in biomarkers, including plasma phe levels. *J. Nutr. MeTab.* **2018**, *2018*. [CrossRef] [PubMed]
19. Stroup, B.M.; Nair, N.; Murali, S.G.; Broniowska, K.; Rohr, F.; Levy, H.L.; Ney, D.M. Metabolomic markers of essential fatty acids, carnitine, and cholesterol metabolism in adults and adolescents with phenylketonuria. *J. Nutr.* **2018**, *148*, 194–201. [CrossRef] [PubMed]
20. MacLeod, E.L.; Clayton, M.K.; van Calcar, S.C.; Ney, D.M. Breakfast with glycomacropeptide compared with amino acids suppresses plasma ghrelin levels in individuals with phenylketonuria. *Mol. Genet. MeTable* **2010**, *100*, 303–308. [CrossRef] [PubMed]
21. Zaki, O.K.; El-Wakeel, L.; Ebeid, Y.; Ez Elarab, H.S.; Moustafa, A.; Abdulazim, N.; Karara, H.; Elghawaby, A. The use of glycomacropeptide in dietary management of phenylketonuria. *J. Nutr. MeTab.* **2016**, *2016*. [CrossRef] [PubMed]
22. Ney, D.M.; Stroup, B.M.; Clayton, M.K.; Murali, S.G.; Rice, G.M.; Rohr, F.; Levy, H.L. Glycomacropeptide for nutritional management of phenylketonuria: A randomized, controlled, crossover trial. *Am. J. Clin. Nutr.* **2016**, *104*, 334–345. [CrossRef] [PubMed]
23. Daly, A.; Evans, S.; Chahal, S.; Santra, S.; MacDonald, A. Glycomacropeptide in children with phenylketonuria: Does its phenylalanine content affect blood phenylalanine control? *J. Hum. Nutr. Diet.* **2017**, *30*, 515–523. [CrossRef] [PubMed]
24. Pinto, A.; Almeida, M.F.; Ramos, P.C.; Rocha, S.; Guimas, A.; Ribeiro, R.; Martins, E.; Bandeira, A.; MacDonald, A.; Rocha, J.C. Nutritional status in patients with phenylketonuria using glycomacropeptide as their major protein source. *Eur. J. Clin. Nutr.* **2017**, *71*, 1230–1234. [CrossRef] [PubMed]
25. Stroup, B.M.; Sawin, E.A.; Murali, S.G.; Binkley, N.; Hansen, K.E.; Ney, D.M. Amino acid medical foods provide a high dietary acid load and increase urinary excretion of renal net acid, calcium, and magnesium compared with glycomacropeptide medical foods in phenylketonuria. *J. Nutr. MeTab.* **2017**, *2017*. [CrossRef] [PubMed]

26. Ney, D.M.; Murali, S.G.; Stroup, B.M.; Nair, N.; Sawin, E.A.; Rohr, F.; Levy, H.L. Metabolomic changes demonstrate reduced bioavailability of tyrosine and altered metabolism of tryptophan via the kynurenine pathway with ingestion of medical foods in phenylketonuria. *Mol. Genet. MeTab.* **2017**, *121*, 96–103. [CrossRef] [PubMed]
27. Stroup, B.M.; Ney, D.M.; Murali, S.G.; Rohr, F.; Gleason, S.T.; Van Calcar, S.C.; Levy, H.L. Metabolomic insights into the nutritional status of adults and adolescents with phenylketonuria consuming a low-phenylalanine diet in combination with amino acid and glycomacropeptide medical foods. *J. Nutr. MeTab.* **2017**, *2017*. [CrossRef] [PubMed]
28. Moher, D.; Liberati, A.; Tetzlaff, J.; Altman, D.G.; Altman, D.; Antes, G.; Atkins, D.; Barbour, V.; Barrowman, N.; Berlin, J.A.; et al. Preferred reporting items for systematic reviews and meta-analyses: The PRISMA statement. *PLoS Med.* **2009**, *6*. [CrossRef] [PubMed]
29. Guyatt, G.; Oxman, A.D.; Akl, E.A.; Kunz, R.; Vist, G.; Brozek, J.; Norris, S.; Falck-Ytter, Y.; Glasziou, P.; Debeer, H.; et al. GRADE guidelines: 1. Introduction—GRADE evidence profiles and summary of findings tables. *J. Clin. Epidemiol.* **2011**, *64*, 383–394. [CrossRef] [PubMed]
30. O'Connor, D.; Green, S.; Higgins, J.P. Defining the review question and developing criteria for including studies. *Cochrane Handb. Syst. Rev. Interv. Cochrane Book Ser.* **2008**, 81–94. [CrossRef]
31. Sterne, J.A.; Hernán, M.A.; Reeves, B.C.; Savović, J.; Berkman, N.D.; Viswanathan, M.; Henry, D.; Altman, D.G.; Ansari, M.T.; Boutron, I.; et al. ROBINS-I: A tool for assessing risk of bias in non-randomised studies of interventions. *BMJ* **2016**, *355*, 4–10. [CrossRef] [PubMed]
32. Moher, D.; Hopewell, S.; Schulz, K.F.; Montori, V.; Gøtzsche, P.C.; Devereaux, P.J.; Elbourne, D.; Egger, M.; Altman, D.G. CONSORT 2010 explanation and elaboration: Updated guidelines for reporting parallel group randomised trials. *Int. J. Surg.* **2012**, *10*, 28–55. [CrossRef] [PubMed]
33. Cleary, M.; Trefz, F.; Muntau, A.C.; Feillet, F.; van Spronsen, F.J.; Burlina, A.; Bélanger-Quintana, A.; Gizewska, M.; Gasteyger, C.; Bettiol, E.; et al. Fluctuations in phenylalanine concentrations in phenylketonuria: A review of possible relationships with outcomes. *Mol. Genet. MeTable* **2013**, *110*, 418–423. [CrossRef] [PubMed]
34. Yi, S.H.; Singh, R.H. Protein substitute for children and adults with phenylketonuria. *Cochrane Database Syst. Rev.* **2015**, *2015*. [CrossRef] [PubMed]
35. Singh, R.H.; Rohr, F.; Frazier, D.; Cunningham, A.; Mofidi, S.; Ogata, B.; Splett, P.L.; Moseley, K.; Huntington, K.; Acosta, P.B.; et al. Recommendations for the nutrition management of phenylalanine hydroxylase deficiency. *Genet. Med.* **2014**, *16*, 121–131. [CrossRef] [PubMed]
36. Arihan, O.; Wernly, B.; Lichtenauer, M.; Franz, M.; Kabisch, B.; Muessig, J.; Masyuk, M.; Lauten, A.; Schulze, P.C.; Hoppe, U.C.; et al. Blood Urea Nitrogen (BUN) is independently associated with mortality in critically ill patients admitted to ICU. *PLoS ONE* **2018**, *13*, e0191697. [CrossRef] [PubMed]
37. Pena, M.J.; Rocha, J.C.; Borges, N. Amino acids, glucose metabolism and clinical relevance for phenylketonuria management. *Ann. Nutr. Disord. Ther.* **2015**, *2*, 1026.
38. Proserpio, C.; Pagliarini, E.; Zuvadelli, J.; Paci, S.; Re Dionigi, A.; Banderali, G.; Cattaneo, C.; Verduci, E. Exploring drivers of liking of low-phenylalanine products in subjects with phenyilketonuria using check-all-that-apply method. *Nutrients* **2018**, *10*. [CrossRef] [PubMed]
39. Barton, S. Which clinical studies provide the best evidence? The best RCT still trumps the best observational study. *BMJ* **2000**, *321*, 255–256. [CrossRef] [PubMed]

MDPI
St. Alban-Anlage 66
4052 Basel
Switzerland
Tel. +41 61 683 77 34
Fax +41 61 302 89 18
www.mdpi.com

Nutrients Editorial Office
E-mail: nutrients@mdpi.com
www.mdpi.com/journal/nutrients

www.ingramcontent.com/pod-product-compliance
Lightning Source LLC
LaVergne TN
LVHW071945080526
838202LV00064B/6679